Tactual perception

Tactual perception: a sourcebook

Edited by

WILLIAM SCHIFF and EMERSON FOULKE

New York
University

University of
Louisville

CAMBRIDGE UNIVERSITY PRESS

Cambridge
London   New York   New Rochelle
Melbourne   Sydney

Published by the Press Syndicate of the University of Cambridge
The Pitt Building, Trumpington Street, Cambridge CB2 1RP
32 East 57th Street, New York, NY 10022, USA
296 Beaconsfield Parade, Middle Park, Melbourne 3206, Australia

First published 1982

Library of Congress Cataloging in Publication Data
Main entry under title:
Tactual perception.
Includes bibliographies and index.
1. Touch.   2. Visually handicapped – Education.   I. Schiff, William.
II. Foulke, Emerson, 1929–
BF275.T32   152.1'82   81–10172
ISBN 0 521 24095 6   CR2

Figures 12.1 through 12.7 on pages 393, 394, 395, 396, 397, 398, 400,
and 401 are reprinted from R. L. Welsh and B. B. Blasch, *Foundations of
orientation and mobility*, with the permission of the publisher,
the American Foundation for the Blind.

Transferred to digital printing 2004

This book is dedicated to two pioneers of tactual perception who conceived of the hands as a functional perceptual system for obtaining useful information from the world:

DAVID KATZ and JAMES J. GIBSON

Contents

Contributors

Nancy S. Amick
Recording for the Blind, Inc.
Princeton Unit
76 Leabrook Lane
Princeton, NJ 08540

Billie L. Bentzen
Department of Peripatology
Boston College
Chestnut Hill, MA 02167

Edward P. Berlá
Department of Special Education
University of Louisville
Louisville, KY 40292

James C. Craig
Department of Psychology
Indiana University
Bloomington, IN 47401

Emerson Foulke
Department of Psychology
Perceptual Alternatives Laboratory
University of Louisville
Louisville, KY 40292

John M. Gill
Warwick Research Unit for the
Blind
University of Warwick
Coventry CV4 7AL, UK

Grahame A. James
National Mobility Centre
22 Melville Road
Birmingham B16 9JT, UK

John M. Kennedy
Department of Psychology
Scarborough College
University of Toronto
West Hill, Ont. M1C 1A4, Canada

Jacob H. Kirman
Department of Psychology
Queens College
City University of New York
Queens, NY 11367

Lester E. Krueger
Department of Psychology
Ohio State University
Columbus, OH 43210

Susan J. Lederman
Department of Psychology
Queens University
Kingston, Ont. K7L 3K6, Canada

Jasha M. Levi
In Touch Networks, Inc.
322 West 48th Street
New York, NY 10036

Contributors

WILLIAM SCHIFF
Department of Educational
Psychology
New York University
New York, NY 10003

CARL E. SHERRICK
Department of Psychology
Princeton University
Princeton, NJ 08540

STEPHEN THAYER
Department of Psychology
The City College
City University of New York
Convent Avenue and 138th Street
New York, NY 10031

DAVID H. WARREN
Department of Psychology
University of California
Riverside, CA 92507

Editorial preface

The first purpose of this volume is to clarify the phenomena of tactual perception and bring together much of what is known about them. To the extent that we know how tactual perception operates, we should be able to help design displays for conveying information to people via touch. A second purpose of this volume, then, is to consider what is known about communication via the skin and tactual system and the utility of tangible displays developed for communicative purposes. But before we begin, perhaps we should attempt to clarify an admittedly tangled terminology.

Touch is a general term, including the study of passive and sometimes punctate cutaneous sensitivities. But it may also include the *active* exploratory and manipulative use of the skin, and hence stimulation of receptor systems in the muscles, tendons, and joints – the kinesthetic system. The term *haptic* is often used to indicate exploratory and manipulative touch, in contrast to the tactile "sensations" resulting from stimulation of passive skin receptors (Gibson, 1966; Kennedy, 1978). Whether haptic or active touch is substantively different from passive tactile sensitivity or simply refers to the means of deploying sensory surfaces remains a controversial issue. In this volume, the term *tactile* is used primarily in referring to passive touch (being touched); the terms *tactual* and *haptic* are used primarily in referring to active exploratory and manipulative touch. Whether the two differ only superficially or in some more palpable way is an issue discussed in this volume but not resolved.

The area of tactile/tactual perception has immediate relevance to students of perception, as well as to educators. Agencies in the business of producing materials for visually handicapped people should also find a summary of the field valuable. In spite of a number of fine volumes dealing with the skin senses (tactile perception or sensation) and their physiology (Kenshalo, 1978; Zotterman, 1976), no handbooks and perhaps one symposium volume attempt the leap to applications of tactile/tactual perception. Gordon's recent volume on active touch is a rare exception (Gordon, 1978). Several perceptual textbooks include mention of such showcase items as the Optacon or TVSS devices.[1] But again, the integration of research on skin sensitivities and haptics with a broad range of applications is difficult to find. Research reports and final reports are scattered widely over American and European literatures in particular, but many of them are not easy to find. As a result, agencies responsible for producing tangible graphics and mobility training devices for visually impaired people are often poorly informed about the state of the art in the science and technology of tactile/tactual perception. Similarly, graduate students of perception are often unacquainted with more than the standard psychophysical and physiological treatments of skin sensitivities and a few striking feats concerning tactile/tactual perception. The same is true of students in special education, who may focus on visual handicaps.

This book is a compilation of papers designed to be useful to advanced students, researchers, professional educators, and engineers interested in tactual perception and the production of tactile/tactual displays. The goal of the volume is to bring together up-to-date reviews of what is known and conjectured about tactile/tactual perception. The book includes reviews of basic psychophysical material without neglecting the theory of functional touching, its historical and developmental contexts, and the technology relevant to tactual perception. Although the book is an outcome of a symposium, it is more than a record of a particular meeting. We hope that for many years it will be a theoretical and practical report of the state of the art and science of tactile/tactual perception and its applications.

Each chapter begins with an overview. The author's concerns and point of view are presented, with a brief summary of the material covered in the chapter. Where appropriate, cross references are provided to other chapters that deal with related issues.

The volume includes a historical examination of tactual perception and the issues embedded in this history. Other chapters concern the tactile and tactual perception of speech, the haptic perception of pictures, educational graphics, mobility maps, and the making of tangible graphics for visually impaired people. Even the social functions of touch are explored. The book is not simply concerned with the skin senses or with practical applications or prosthetic devices. The central idea in compiling the book was to provide information pertaining to both and to other areas not explored in other volumes. The book covers the perception of objects, events, surfaces, people, the coded information of speech and of written language, and the information found in diagrams and pictures.

Yet in this case, all such information is obtained via the skin and hands. In order for the reader to understand the directions of early and recent research and theories of tactual perception, historical and developmental chapters were included. Following the late J. J. Gibson's distinction, tactual perception is considered as a set of problems concerned not only with *energy* detection and discrimination but also with how we obtain useful information about the world (Gibson, 1963, 1966).

The chapters were written by a distinguished group of sensory–perceptual psychologists, educators of visually impaired people, and producers of tactual graphics. They do not share a theory of tactile/tactual perception or a particular approach to the questions in this field. What they do share is a keen interest in discovering more about how we obtain information via touch and how this information may be better displayed to make it more readily perceptible by people deprived of one or more major perceptual contact with the world. Many of the chapters were presented and refined at a workshop and symposium on haptic perception sponsored by the National Science Foundation[2] and hosted by the University of Louisville in March 1979. Others were written expressly for this volume. The authors and editors are grateful to the National Science Foundation for supporting this project. We are also grateful to Cambridge University Press, and particularly to Susan Milmoe, for their efforts in making this material available to a broad readership. The editors are especially grateful to the other authors for their patience in rewriting their chapters to reflect the helpful criticisms of reviewers and to accommodate space limitations. In the latter case, the psychological reality of ego and the outer-world reality of economics invariably meet head-on.

Notes

1 Optacon is an acronym for *op*tical to *ta*ctile *con*version; TVSS stands for *t*actile *v*ision *s*ubstitution *s*ystem.
2 Grant No. SP178-03756.

References

Gibson, J. J. The useful dimensions of sensitivity. *American Psychologist.* 1963, *18*, 1–15.
  The senses considered as perceptual systems. Boston: Houghton Mifflin, 1966.
Gordon, G. (Ed.). *Active touch. The mechanisms of recognition of objects by manipulation: a multidisciplinary approach.* Oxford: Pergamon Press, 1978.
Kennedy, J. M. Haptics. In E. C. Carterette & M. P. Friedman (Eds.). *Handbook of perception,* Vol. 8. New York: Academic Press, 1978, pp. 289–318.
Kenshalo, D. R. (Ed.). *Sensory functions of the skin of humans.* New York: Plenum Press, 1979.
Zotterman, Y. (Ed.). *Sensory functions of the skin in primates, with special reference to man.* Oxford: Pergamon Press, 1976.

xiii

1. Tactual perception in historical perspective: David Katz's world of touch

LESTER E. KRUEGER

In Chapter 1, Lester Krueger provides a historical examination of touch based largely on David Katz's pioneer work. He discusses in some detail Katz's emphasis on activity in touch, on the importance of the role of vision in guiding touch and in interpreting tactual behavior and experience. A wealth of Katz's (and others') phenomenological material is marshalled regarding the sorts of objects, surfaces, substances, and events that are perceptible by touch and the sorts of information that mediate the particular percepts. Krueger explores in detail both the philosophical and psychological aspects of touch and other modalities. He examines the possibility of the multiple or polar nature of touch – localization functions versus identification functions, subjective versus objective poles of experience, preattentive versus focal aspects of attention, and so on. He discusses topics of touch blends, surface texture, film and volume touch, movement and vibration in both historical and contemporary contexts. In comparing Katz's and J. J. Gibson's observations on touch, Krueger intertwines phenomenology, contemporary theorizing, and recent experimental evidence concerning these intriguing topics. Such an approach makes this chapter an intellectual odyssey through the history of touch.   WILLIAM SCHIFF

Introduction

David Katz's (1925) classic monograph, *Der Aufbau der Tastwelt* (*The world of touch*), provides the main basis for the present chapter on tactual perception. Not yet available in English, this landmark volume ought to be made more widely known. Theories of tactual perception certainly must take Katz's *Tastwelt* into account. Unless otherwise specified, all references to Katz here will be to his *Tastwelt*. English summaries or synopses of this work have also been provided by Katz (1930), Krueger (1970), and Zigler (1926). Quotations presented here in English from *Tastwelt* were translated by this author.

Katz's other classic, the *Farbwelt* (*The world of colour*), first appeared in German in 1911 and then in English translation in 1935 (Katz, 1935). Robert D. MacLeod, who translated the *Farbwelt* into English, said:

1

Katz considered the *Tastwelt* [The world of touch] more important than the *Farbwelt* [The world of colour]. To some extent he was probably correct. Both are great pioneering works, but the *Tastwelt* explores a field that has never been properly cultivated and that each year gains in significance. The current interest in the body percept, for instance, would be enlightened by a reading of the *Tastwelt*. Katz had a genius for seeing problems in everyday phenomena. (pers. comm., April 1970)

James J. Gibson (pers. comm., May 1968) said of the *Tastwelt:* "The book has been neglected. I owe more to it than I have recognized recently. I had forgotten that he challenged Johannes Müller, for example . . . That was a bold stroke." Gibson himself objected to Müller's law of the specific conscious quality for each excited nerve as being too simple (Gibson, 1962, p. 484; 1966). Boring (1942) was more tentative about Katz's contribution: "The importance of such phenomenology only the future can decide. It was many years before Purkinje's comparable descriptions of visual phenomena became the basis of important chapters in the psychology of vision" (p. 512).

Katz's message

Born in 1884, Katz lived until 1954. His career roughly spanned that of the Gestalt movement, and indeed in his sympathies Katz "stood closest to the Gestalt theorists" (MacLeod, 1954, p. 3). He even wrote a textbook on Gestalt psychology (Katz, 1950). Katz was never a true Gestalt psychologist, however. Texture and ground concerned him more than did form and figure. Whereas the Gestaltists focused on the simplicity of the internal response, Katz, like Gibson, focused on its veridicality – that is, its correspondence with the external stimulus. Like Gibson, too, he was "more concerned with perceptual *contents* than with the functions through which we apprehend them" (Katz, 1935, p. 187).

Katz and Gibson. Gibson's (1966) book, *The senses considered as perceptual systems,* echoed several of Katz's main points. Both emphasized the importance of higher-order invariants in object perception and the holistic quality of perception in time as well as space. Katz deplored the typical atomism, with respect to both time and space, in the sensory psychology of touch, an atomism that bespoke a "tachistoscopic" mentality. Katz acknowledged the yeoman service of the physiologists in delineating the peripheral receptors for touch, warmth, and cold but said that psychologists ought to be studying an entirely different realm of complex phenomena. He felt that the early, intimate association between psychologists and physiologists in the tactile sensory area had stunted the independent development of the psychological side. It should be noted, though, that several physiological psychologists recently participated in a symposium on active touch (Gordon, 1978) and that Katz applauded the holistic concerns of such physiologists as Weber and Sherrington.

Both Katz and Gibson emphasized movement. Both pointed out how the hand can be wielded in active touch, so that stimulation is obtained rather than imposed. For Katz, movement of the touch organ relative to the object touched was crucial because it provided input for the sense of vibration, which Katz regarded as an important and sensitive modality and as one that is independent of the sense of pressure. For Gibson, the fact that wielding an object in different ways (tossing, shaking, etc.) usually produces a unitary impression indicates that "the merely proprio-specific information . . . [is] filtered out, as it were, leaving pure information about the object" (1966, p. 127). The permanent properties of the object, the invariants obtained over time, are isolated from the sensory input, and the perceiver "ordinarily pays no attention whatever to the flux of changing sensations" (1966, p. 3). "It's the *information* that counts, the invariants over time, and the sensations are irrelevant "(Gibson, pers. comm., May 1968).

Katz's phenomenology. Unlike Gibson, Katz did not want to rid perceptual behavior of its phenomenological aspect. True, Katz sometimes emphasized the informational aspect, as when he focused on the aid that vibrations provide in identifying various materials, rather than on the phenomenal impressions they produce. Overall, though, Katz was "one of this century's outstanding exponents of psychological phenomenology" (MacLeod, 1954, p. 1; see also Arnheim, 1953); "phenomenology for him was essentially an attitude of 'disciplined naivete'" (MacLeod, 1954, p. 3). Katz focused on the phenomenal aspect, for example, when he considered whether a perceived object was projected out in space. Like the Gestaltists, Katz was more mindful than Gibson of the perceiver's contribution to the final percept.

In reading Katz's *Tastwelt*, one is struck first by the great wealth of phenomenological details. As Kennedy (1978) noted, "Haptics was born in phenomenology" (p. 313). Phenomenological description may be a prescientific or preparadigmatic activity (Boring, 1952), but given the relatively modest progress achieved in touch perception since Katz, much more such activity may yet be needed. As Taylor, Lederman, and Gibson (1973) noted, "It is remarkable how little is known about perception by touch after more than a century of experimental sensory psychology" (p. 260).

Plan of the chapter

The present chapter treats, in turn, the external and internal determinants of tactual perception. The section entitled "The nature of the stimulus" deals with the information available in the tactual stimulus and how it is initially registered on the body surface. The section headed "The nature of the response" deals with the use made of the external input and with both phenomenological and informational aspects of tactual perception. Let us preview the two sections.

Stimulus section. The next section compares touch with other modalities and discusses the role of hand movement in obtaining tactual information, which Katz emphasized, as well as recent evidence that supports Katz's contention that the vibration sense is distinct from the pressure sense. The stimulus section deals not only with the physical stimulus – that is, with what qualitative, temporal, and spatial properties of the proximal stimulus are readily available to the observer (Gibson, 1960) – but also with the initial sensory response, which presumably is impervious to the effects of learning and conscious attention and thus ought to mirror the physical input.

Response section. The last section has separate subsections on the two main questions that may be asked about an object: Where is it? and What is it? (Shaw & Pittenger, 1978; Trevarthen, 1978; White, 1974). Katz, along with others, distinguished between the objective side or pole ("I feel a pointed object out in space") and the subjective side or pole ("I feel a prickling sensation"). The first subsection considers the conditions under which a person projects the percept out in space, that is, beyond the sensory surface. Inputs such as pain favor the subjective side, but whether they totally exclude the objective side is open to question. The second subsection considers whether touch is better equipped to detect an object's texture than its contours and to acquire information in a natural, direct fashion than in a mediated, pictorial mode.

The nature of the stimulus

Touch versus other modalities

Katz wanted to eliminate the invidious division of the senses into higher (e.g., vision, audition) and lower (e.g., touch) groups. By showing how wondrous are the abilities of touch and how rich the tactual stimulus can be, Katz hoped to regain for touch its former prominence, if not its predominance. The fingers, as wielded by the hand, he noted, obtain information on the innards of objects, whereas the eyes, remaining fixed at the outer surface of objects, play a lesser role in developing the belief in the reality of the external world. He noted, too, that the importance of touch might be better appreciated if as many people lacked the sense of touch (numbness) as lacked the sense of sight (blindness) or the sense of hearing (deafness).

Early prominence of touch. Historically, touch was considered to be a very important sense (Berkeley, 1709). Sensations of extension and resistance obtained via touch were regarded as critical in developing the concept of external objects (Brown, 1838). "If priority of sensation alone were to be regarded, the sense of *touch* might deserve to be considered in the first place; as it must have been exercised long before birth, and is probably the very feeling with which sentient life begins" (Brown, 1838, p. 212). Aristotle and the Stoic philosophers held that touch mediates every type of sense perception, even vision (Siegel, 1970); invisible particles bombard various surfaces of the body to convey smell, taste, and sound. The historical prominence of touch is evident, too, in the way touch-related words have been extended to other modalities, as in "sharp tastes," "dull sounds," and "soft colors." Rarely does the reverse occur; we never speak of "loud or fragrant touches" (Williams, 1976).

Visual capture. More recently, touch has not fared so well relative to vision and audition. It has been found that when vision and touch conflict, as when a person wears distorting goggles, vision dominates touch. When the conflict is prolonged, touch or the position sense, not vision, adapts so as to eliminate the conflict (Rock & Harris, 1967). Visual control of manual tracking movements has been found to depend on the interaction of visual and somatosensory inputs to Area 7 of the somatosensory cortex (Sakata & Iwamura, 1978; Stein, 1978). Katz was not privy to such findings, but he did cite Weber to the effect that the standard or scale used in judging an extent is that provided by the eyes, and that what is sensed by touch is reduced to the scale provided by vision. Katz also described an illusion that represents yet another instance of "visual capture" of touch (Gibson, 1933; Hay, Pick, & Ikeda, 1965; Rock & Harris, 1967). "When one cuts into some soft wood with a knife under a strong magnifying glass, the resulting visual enlargement gives rise to the impression that one is cutting deeply into a soft mass, such as cork" (Katz, 1925, pp. 240–241).

Vision and audition may dominate touch because they provide information in greater quantity and precision to the perceiver. Though the fingertips might be likened to the fovea of the retina because of their heightened acuity in discriminating tactual information, even they do not do as well as the eye. Text presented to the fingertips via braille or the Optacon typically is read quite slowly, even by well-practiced blind persons (Chapter 5; Schiffman, 1976). Katz found that materials such as kid leather, cloth, rubber, and paper are readily confused when felt by a blindfolded person, indicating that vision, not touch, makes them "feel" different in everyday life. Katz also found that recognition through touch could be considerably aided by allowing subjects a fleeting glimpse beforehand of the objects presented.

Révész (1950), similarly, said that "when we touch some common object, the tactile impression is always permeated with visual experiences" (p. 156). Vision is more highly developed and possesses properties, such as color, that haptics does not, which "explains why one speaks of 'haptic seeing,' not, however, of 'visual touching'" (p. 155). Seeing is indispensable to the sculptor, "for only vision is capable of raising the sensory impression into the sphere of aesthetic contemplation" (p. 328). All of the blind sculptors Révész discovered were late blind; "this fact and its converse – the fact that those blind from birth have never produced any plastic work of aesthetic value – leaves no doubt whatever as to the importance of visual impressions as the basis of tactile experience" (p. 234). Similar geometrical illusions have been found in haptics as in vision, but only very simple figures have been tested thus far. "The more complicated is the tactile object, the more difficult is the haptic apprehension of proportions and the more marked becomes the superiority of the visual . . . sense" (p. 141). Vision surpasses haptics, according to Révész, mainly because it examines objects simultaneously rather than in a successive or piecemeal fashion.

Information available to touch

The long-term prospects for haptics may be less gloomy than Révész thought. Vision may dominate touch, but then we should consider the other senses, such as audition, which, like touch, is limited to successive input. This subsection considers three factors affecting the quality and contents of the proximal stimulus for touch. First, must the stimulus object or source of stimulation be at the sensory surface, or may it be more distant? Second, does the stimulus object emit or reflect the energy pattern that reaches the sensory surface? Third, how does movement of the stimulus object relative to the body affect the generation and reception of the energy pattern?

Far versus near stimulation. Galen said that the skin responds to tactile stimuli only if brought into direct contact with the stimulus object, whereas the contact is mediated by moisture on the tongue in the case of taste and by the air in the case of smell and sound (Siegel, 1970). Katz, with his broader concept of the adequate stimulus in touch, would dispute the notion that the contact with the object in touch is always direct. Pressure is a near sense, Katz conceded, but vibration has many of the capabilities of a far sense. Vibration of the earth, for example, may signal the imminent approach of a train or a herd of wild buffalo. Our world, Katz contended, is not so much one of sound as one of vibration. Similarly, as Gibson (1966) pointed out, touching may be done with nails, claws, hooves, and horns, in which case the stimulus is "not a direct impression on the skin by an object, as we tend to assume" (p. 100).

Emitted versus reflected stimulation. In touch, as in vision, the stimulus energy typically originates not with the ostensive source of stimulation (i.e., the object perceived) but with another source (i.e., the press of the observer's hand on the object). The observer receives energy that the object reflects – and that typically specifies a particular surface touch. Here, the object itself plays a passive or reflective role. On the other hand, with sound, warmth, cold, passive touch, film touch, illuminant color, taste, and smell, the primary energy received is that emitted directly from the stimulus object itself; with these modalities, reflected energy may sometimes be present and may even pose serious problems, as in the acoustics of concert halls (von Békésy, 1967), but generally it is not as important as the emitted energy. Thus, one may say that a red, warm object emits warmth, but not that it emits redness (Broad, 1965). Sounds and other qualities are emitted from objects, but sights are not (Hamlyn, 1961). We say that a person can see a light and can see a chair, but not that one can hear a sound and can hear a chair (Rundle, 1972), even though chairs reflect both sound and light.

The heightened auditory attention in some blind persons, however, allows them to discriminate even textural differences in external obstacles, based on echoes from self-produced sounds (Kellogg, 1962; Schiffman, 1976), and perhaps it would be proper to say that these persons can hear a chair. In one test, blind subjects could discriminate hard surfaces (e.g., glass) from soft surfaces (e.g., denim), and even denim from velvet, with a high level of accuracy (Kellogg, 1962). With temperature too, the energy received may sometimes be reflected rather than emitted. When an object is touched, it may either absorb the skin heat or reflect it back to the person. Katz stressed the importance of the heat conductance or absorption of an object as a revealing, invariant property comparable to the light reflectance of the object in vision.

Reflected energy generally provides more information about objects than does emitted energy. This gives touch and vision an important advantage over other modalities. Emitted energy generally answers the question, Where is it? (Katz observed, for instance, that turning one's head in front of a hot oven leads to localization of the source of the emitted heat.) However, reflected energy answers both the questions Where is it? and What is it? because it provides greater information about an object's surface (texture, contours, etc.). Active touch not only depends on reflected energy but has the further advantage of giving the perceiver direct knowledge of the energy source (i.e., the hand scanning the object) and can move or redirect it in special ways so as to acquire more information about the object. With emitted energy, not even the question Where is it? may be answered in some cases, and the observer may perceive a diffuse event rather than a compact object. "The qualities which characterize smells and sounds are not located on surfaces, as colour is. They seem rather to permeate a volume, in the way that heat and cold do" (Prince, 1965, p. 417).

Movement versus stationary stimulation. Merely resting the hand on a material may evoke the impression of a surface. But to discern its surface qualities (hardness, graininess, etc.) and to recognize its specific material, movement is necessary, according to Katz. For Katz, movement obtains its power largely by producing the vital sensations of vibration. The pressure sense determines the presence of the surface, whereas the vibration sense determines the properties of the surface. Rohracher (1951) said that the vibrations produced by rubbing a surface are supplemented and perhaps aided by an ever-present, slight tremor that occurs on all parts of the body.

The role of movement differs considerably for vision and touch. In vision, movement may impede perception of surface qualities, but in touch, it is *lack* of movement that is most damaging. "The full richness of the palpable world is opened up to the touch organ only through movement" (Katz, 1925, p. 71). The touch organ, when kept motionless relative to the object, is beset with a partial anesthesia. Movement is as indispensable to touch as light is to vision. Titchener "considered movement to be necessary even for the perception of oiliness" (Katz, 1925, p. 58). Ironically, as Katz noted, apparent movement may influence the findings even of atomistically inclined sensory psychologists, as when the two-point limen is reduced by stimulating two points successively rather than simultaneously.

Katz found that adaptation occurs quickly for the motionless touch organ, but not when movement is present. With minor exceptions, "the sense of touch can be regarded as virtually indefatigable for moving stimuli" (1925, p. 62). The rapid adaptation that occurs in the absence of movement makes us largely unaware of the clothes we wear, whereas "a cloth band on a rotating disk can be moved over a fingertip with moderate speed and pressure for minutes on end – indeed, for hours, if one has the requisite patience – without one being able to establish with certainty any essential change in the touch impression" (1925, p. 61). In sum, the vibratory sense, like the auditory sense, is almost tireless (Katz, 1930). Other evidence indicates, however, that considerable adaptation occurs even with the vibration sense (Geldard, 1940a,c; Hahn, 1974).

The general direction of movement is important. Hardness–softness, as well as elasticity, is revealed by up–down movement vertical to the material, whereas roughness–smoothness is revealed by lateral movement across the material. The specific direction of lateral movement also seems to matter. Katz measured how fast three subjects moved their hands back and forth, toward and away from the body, while trying to identify flat-lying material. One subject moved his hand inward and outward at the same speed, but the other two subjects made a slow outward and a rapid inward motion. All three subjects said that the thrust toward the body was more important for their judgments. The outward movement generated less friction, was observed to a much lesser degree, and may have served merely as a necessary precondition for the inward movement, according to Katz. (Try the two motions yourself, though, and you may notice that the fingertips produce different types of shearing forces on the inward and outward thrusts [see Lederman, 1978, and Chapter 4]; when pushed outward, more resistance is encountered and the fingers move in a jerkier fashion, because they tend to dig into the surface.) Katz similarly found that the hardness of a pencil was more readily recognized by writing downstrokes than upstrokes. The preferred direction of movement reverses, though, in judging the thickness of a sheet felt between the fingers and thumb. The thumb is usually moved faster, and with heavier pressure, *away* from the wrist than toward it.

9

Touch receptor systems

Types of touch. Considerable information may reach the touch organ, especially when movement is allowed. But how much of this information is picked up by the sensory system, and in what form? The adequate stimuli for vision and audition are well known and well defined. In touch, by contrast, little is known about the operation of the mechanoreceptors and thermal receptors, let alone the effects of the intervening layer of skin, body temperature, cardiac rhythm, and so on (Petit & Galifret, 1978; Quilliam, 1978).

The most direct way to determine the adequate stimuli for touch is simply to study the peripheral receptors and their central projections. But what entities should be included in touch? For Katz, *touch* meant the four basic cutaneous qualities or specific nerve energies proposed by von Frey (pressure, pain, warmth, cold; Boring, 1942), plus a fifth (vibration) that he himself added. Considering that the receptors for these various qualities had not been identified in his day (or, except for vibration, even today; Quilliam, 1978; Vallbo & Johansson, 1978), and that Katz had more holistic concerns, such as studying the hand as a unitary touch organ, it is natural that he should sometimes have stepped beyond the bounds of touch proper. When he depicted the observer as palpating an object through a blanket or cutting through a piece of cork, he also implicated the kinesthetic or muscle sense. He thought elasticity was sensed by means of kinesthesis. The distinction between touch and other aspects of somesthesis has been blurred even further by others (with some justification; in the somesthetic cortex, for example, inputs from the joints and skin converge at some neurons in Area 5: Sakata & Iwamura, 1978). Boring (1942) noted that Révész's phenomenology on the *Tastsinnes* included all of somesthesis. The active touch used by the subjects of Gibson (1962) and Rock and Harris (1967) probably involved more kinesthetic than cutaneous sensitivity. Haptics is generally conceived to involve active touch rather than passive touch (Kennedy, 1978), and Gibson (1966) combined kinesthetic and cutaneous sensitivity in the "haptic–somatic" system. For Katz, active touch generally referred to moving the hand over a flat surface to be identified, rather than over a solid object, and thus involved mainly cutaneous sensitivity.

Touch blends. The existence of separate receptor systems may be partly concealed by interactions among their effects. If pressure and coldness are applied simultaneously to adjacent spots, for example, wetness is

10

experienced. "All perceptions of liquidity have in common one condition, namely, a fusion of pressure and temperature" (Sullivan, 1923, p. 540). When fused or blended with warmth, the pressure feels snug, and one experiences oiliness. Given Helmholtz's definition of a modality as a class of sensations connected by qualitative continua (Boring, 1942), then perhaps, given this fusion, we should not even talk about separate pressure and temperature senses at all.

Titchener and others were engaged in considerable work on touch blends or complexes at the time, which Katz reviewed to some extent. Boring (1942) gave a more complete account of this work, which stressed the contribution of the pressure sense and perhaps provoked Katz to conduct his own tests that pitted the vibration sense against the pressure sense.

In touch blends, according to Titchener, one perceives spatio–temporal patterns of pressure and temperature qualities. Pressure and cold produce felt wetness; pressure and warmth produce felt oiliness. Temperature looms larger at the liquid extreme and pressure at the solid extreme of the series of touch blends: vaporous, wet, oily, gelatinous, slimy, greasy, syrupy, muddy, mushy, soggy, doughy, gummy, spongy, and dry (Sullivan, 1923). *Touch blend* may be a misnomer in the perception of solidity, as Sullivan noted, because usually only a pattern of pressure is felt. There may be a quality of movement as well in the impression of oiliness.

In the absence of information about the receptors, it is not clear which qualities are pure and which are mixed blends, and many questions persist. Is vibration a separate modality or merely one variety of pressure sensitivity? For some persons, heat feels more like pressure and pain than like warmth and cold (Boring, 1942). Coldness, in turn, may considerably increase the sensation of pressure; Weber (1846) reported that a very cold coin laid on the forehead feels just as heavy as two warmed coins laid there. Kennedy (1978) noted that touch provides information on viscosity, slipperiness, softness, texture, and elasticity, and he said that "the possible variations in resistance are so myriad, so complex that they defy any standard physics of location and pressure, any ordinary-language categorizing schemes" (p. 294). Gibson (1966) listed such inputs as stroking, caressing, twisting, pulling, sucking, prodding, and "the crawling insect, the scratching thorn, the brushing leaf, and the shaking branch that need to be distinguished" (p. 117). He reported that blindfolded subjects can discriminate, without error, among stroking devices that rub, scrape, brush, or roll on the skin.

The vibration sense

Katz treated vibratory sensitivity as separate and superior to pressure sensitivity. He paired the vibration sense with hearing as two dynamic senses, because of the waxing and waning evident in both vibrations and tones, and the pressure sense with vision as two static senses. The affinity between vibration and hearing may run even deeper. Vibration may represent a way station on the evolutionary path leading from touch to hearing. In animals, sensitivity to oscillating stimuli preceded sensitivity to sound. Weber, too, commented on the connection between vibration and sound; for more recent research on similarities between ear and skin, see von Békésy (1967). It is conceivable that vibration sensitivity preceded pressure sensitivity as well, and that from it one branch split off and developed into the pressure sense and another into the sense of hearing (Katz, 1937a).

Skin structures seem as well constituted as those of the ear to transmit information from oscillation. The skin's sensitivity to vibration may be limited mainly by the masking effect of blood pulsation (Katz, 1937a). Katz was criticized for postulating a separate vibration sense on the skin, whereas no one would think of postulating a separate flicker sense for the eye (Geldard, 1940a). However, Katz noted that vibrations on the skin are perceived in the 50- to 500-Hz range, which makes the skin much more like the ear, which is sensitive to 20 to 20,000 Hz. For the eye, there is a single boundary value above which fusion occurs for all flicker frequencies. Katz may have overstated the difference between the skin and the eye, however. Skin vibrations in the 50- to 500-Hz range are too rapid to allow the successive indentations to be felt as separate shocks, but not so rapid that they are completely fused and felt only as pressure. In the eye, too, there might be a frequency range, say at 15 to 30 Hz, in which the successive impulses are neither totally distinguished nor totally fused.

Is there a touch analog to the distinction between pure acoustic tones and noise? Rough vibrations that Katz produced with a special apparatus led to less fine, less orderly, and less pleasing sensations than did vibrations produced by a tuning fork. Further, the latency of arousal was much longer for the tuning-fork vibrations.

Vibrations and the deaf. For Katz, the ability of deaf persons to "listen" to music through skin vibrations further attested to the close connection between skin and ear. Katz's evidence is suspect, however, because some sense of hearing might have been involved in these cases. In a person suffering from conduction or transmission deafness rather than nerve deafness, the intense vibrations produced in concert halls might well reach an intact inner ear through bone conduction (von Békésy, 1967). In any case, Katz mentioned Helen Keller's enjoyment of music, and he related a fascinating tale of Herr Sutermeister, a prominent deaf–mute, who discovered late in life that he could enjoy music. Sutermeister could appreciate different qualities of music, such as bright and somber, and seeing the conductor and the musicians enhanced his perception. The orchestra had to be situated on a podium, though, because if it was not, the oscillations would be transmitted along the floor to his feet and produce a disagreeable feeling. Transmission through the hand was also ineffective and unpleasant. The main reception point for pleasant music was the thorax or chest.

That deaf persons are very sensitive to vibrations is evident, too, in the aid they receive, in learning to speak, from putting their fingers on their own or someone else's throat or larynx (see Chapter 7). Such sensitivity indicates again that the vibration sense in the fingers is not much inferior to that in the ear. One deaf girl could understand what a normal girl was saying in a dark room if she laid her hand on the breast of the speaking girl. Another deaf person could "listen" to and understand vibrations transmitted from the speaker by means of a billiard cue stick or a bowed piece of paper. Again, however, bone conduction to an intact inner ear might explain such sensitivity.

Separate sense organs for vibration? Vibration may be a separate modality, but it need not have its own sense organs. Katz mentioned "von Frey's view that the vibration sensations are tied to the organs of the pressure sense, a view to which I, too, am inclined" (1925, p. 205). For Katz, though, "these organs can take up two states of excitation absolutely simultaneously and thus . . . their readiness to transmit vibration sensations is independent of the state of excitation resulting from a . . . pressure stimulus" (1925, p. 205). The pressure sense does *not* provide the components to form a Gestalt-like whole with a vibration; no pressure parts are recognizable as such in the vibration whole, so such parts exist for neither the skin nor the ear. Vibration, then, is no mere offshoot or variant of the pressure sensation, but something qualitatively different. Katz thus denied the validity of Müller's principle of specific nerve energy, according to which each nerve produces a specific, conscious quality when excited. Although Katz tended to agree with von Frey that vibration and pressure share a common set of peripheral receptors on the skin, he withheld making a final judgment. He noted that "the great profusion of nervous elements in the skin almost requires that even more senses be distinguished than before" and that some "structures in the skin, . . . by their size and other characteristics, seem hardly less suitable for transmitting oscillations than the elements of the basilar membrane" (1925, p. 219).

Katz presented several examples to demonstrate that felt vibration and pressure differ. Turning the hand palm up, so that the fingernail rather than the fingertip touched the material, still affords good recognition. Use of the fingernail presumably excluded the pressure sensation. When an iron nail is pulled across a rough surface, vibrations are felt in the lower arm as well as in the hand, indicating the resonance capacity of the lower arm and, again, excluding the possibility of a pressure sensation. Similarly, when the elbow is placed against a tuning fork, vibrations but no pressure sensations are felt in the hand. The pressure sense can also be excluded by holding a stick between the teeth and moving it across some material; this produces vibrations and quite accurate judgments as to the material "touched."

Katz (1925, 1936) made much of the fact that the tongue is very sensitive to pressure but very insensitive to vibration; he attributed the latter fact to the weak resonance of the tongue. Geldard (1940c), though, was puzzled as to "how the myth of lingual vibratory insensitivity ever got started" (p. 294), because several studies, including one by Müller a century ago, have shown that the tongue is highly sensitive to vibration. If the tongue's vibratory sensitivity lags somewhat behind its tactual sensitivity, "the answer lies in its lowered capacity to conduct forced vibrations"(p. 294).

A vibration sensation does not arise if a tuning fork is touched very briefly, say, for half a second. This indicates that there is a longer latency for vibration than for pressure sensations. A thousandfold variation in the physical pressure of the tuning fork on the skin has no clear effect on the vibration sensation, according to Katz. Energetically rubbing a finger with a band of pearls may raise the threshold for pressure considerably, yet it hardly affects the threshold for vibration.

Vibration sense versus pressure sense. Katz became engaged in a long, spirited debate with von Frey as to whether vibration ought to be considered a separate sense from pressure. Von Frey credited the pressure sense with our impressions of contact, pressure, vibration, and tickle. Geldard (1940a, c) reviewed both sides of this and related controversies. Based on his own data and those of others, Geldard (1940b, c) concluded that there is no separate vibratory sense.

Major evidence for separate senses had been the seemingly independent loss and retention of sensitivity for pressure and vibration on particular areas of the skin; deep receptors and bone receptors were presumed by some to be responsible for vibration sensitivity and skin receptors for contact and pressure sensitivity. Geldard pointed out, however, that the spread effects of vibration, given the mechanics of the skin and the bone (which is an excellent sound conductor), make the evidence rather dubious. "The skin transmits forced vibrations extraordinary distances with low mechanical impedance" (1940c, p. 295). The fact that the vibratory threshold may be lower than the pressure threshold, he further noted, may be due to the operation of summation of impulses to repetitive stimulation.

Geldard (1940b) confirmed von Frey's finding that the skin spots most sensitive to pressure are the ones most sensitive to vibration as well. Geldard (1940a) noted Katz's disdain for experiments involving punctiform stimulation and said that in the *Tastwelt*, Katz, "through some strange perversity, neglected to mention those proofs [of von Frey] that constitute the whole basis for the identification of pressure and vibratory sensitivities" (p. 256). But Katz readily conceded that pressure and vibration may share the same peripheral receptors. Katz's main point – which Geldard, through some strange perversity, neglected to mention – was that Müller's doctrine of specific nerve energy ought to be repudiated.

Even if vibration lacks its own receptors, it need not share the same receptors as the pressure sense. Other modalities are also available. Von Békésy (1967) reported that vibrations can be sensed by deep receptors in the joints as well as by receptors in the skin. When Katz had subjects move a body part (arm, head, etc.), for example, joint and kinesthetic sensations may have been received, and these sensations might account for the vibration impressions that were localized at the skin or out in space, but that cannot be attributed to pressure sensitivity. Thus, even if vibration can be dissociated from pressure, it need not be a separate sense but may merely be a variant of kinesthesis.

Pacinian corpuscle. Recent evidence, though, favors Katz's view that vibration is indeed a separate sense. The Pacinian corpuscle has been identified as the sensory structure responsible for the detection of vibration (Quilliam, 1978; Vallbo & Johansson, 1978). Ironically, the receptor for the less controversial pressure sense has not yet been identified. "With one notable exception (i.e., the Pacinian corpuscle), it is not yet known for certain to what kinds of physical stimuli cutaneous receptors will respond *in vitro*" (Quilliam, 1978, p. 11). The Pacinian is a large, ovoid corpuscle having onion skin coverings; it projects to the spinal cord, and possibly the brain, via a single, direct fiber. Vallbo and Johansson said that the PC units connected to Pacinian corpuscles serve large receptive fields, rapidly adapt to continued input, give an off response when the input terminates, and are sensitive to high-frequency vibration. Spatial resolution, on the other hand, seems to be handled by units having small, well-defined receptive fields (RA, SA I units); the density gradient of these units on the hand is similar to the gradient of the two-point threshold. Some of the latter units are fast adapting (RA), whereas others are slow adapting (SA I).

Gnostic units

Not only may vibration and pressure be separate senses, but various subvarieties within each sense and perhaps additional types of sensitivity may be found as well. Furthermore, sensory input may also be distinguished qualitatively by its extent and location on the body. Weber divided touch into the location sense (*Ortsinn*), the pressure sense (*Drucksinn*), and the temperature sense (*Temperatursinn*) (Boring, 1942). Perhaps we ought to replace the notion of senses with that of gnostic units, as propounded by Konorski (1967), based on the findings of Hubel and Wiesel. Gnostic units are single-cell, higher-order decision units that are responsive to particular types and patterns of input.

Konorski extended the notion of *adequate stimulus*, which refers to the type of energy to which a particular receptor is most sensitive, to the gnostic unit and lower-level detectors as well. Gnostic units, however, are defined by information sensitivity rather than energy sensitivity. "The higher the level of the given afferent system, the more complex and refined the adequate stimuli to which the units of this level react" (Konorski, 1967, p. 71). Whereas the adequate stimulus for vision is simple light energy, the adequate stimulus for a particular complex cell, say, may be light forming an edge with a particular orientation. Recent work on touch has revealed various examples of gnostic units. For example, Sakata and Iwamura (1978) described cutaneous units whose receptive fields corresponded to the skin surface areas that come into contact with objects or other parts of the body during particular stances or activities. They also reported that some neurons in a monkey fired when it grasped a cylindrical bottle or an apple, but not when it grasped a rectangular block, whereas other neurons showed the reverse pattern. Katz's stress on spatial and temporal holism can be viewed as a similar attempt to broaden the concept of adequate stimulus in touch. The vibration sense represents temporal holism. The hand as a unitary sense organ (with its own set of gnostic units?) represents spatial holism.

The hand as touch organ

Katz perhaps anticipated the notion of a gnostic unit when he suggested that the hand itself, rather than the minute receptors that the physiologists dig out of it, be regarded as the organ of touch. Katz might have gone still further and regarded the entire skin surface as the organ of touch. However, this would not have fit the general conception of a sense organ, which is compact and unitary – for example, the eye, ear, nose, mouth (Gibson, 1966). Katz's bold stroke was to propose an organ, the hand, that is as unitary as the organs of the other senses.

Versatility of the hand. Katz was not alone in his appreciation of the powers of the hand. Galen remarked on the hand's versatility as an organ equipped both for the perception of tactual qualities (warm, cold, hard, soft, etc.) and for the manipulation of objects (Siegel, 1970). Kennedy (1978) noted that the touch organ "is, in everyday use, often simultaneously or successively expressive, executive, and perceptual" (p. 293). "The hand can grope, palpate, prod, press, rub, or heft" (Gibson, 1966, p. 123).

According to Katz, Kant called the hand the human outer brain. Révész (1950) similarly said that "it may frequently be observed that the hand is more intelligent and endowed with greater creative energy than the head" (p. 58). For Révész, the hand represents the symbol and model of all our important tools. Katz (1936) noted that "the human hand makes about twelve different kinds of grasping movements" (p. 146) and that "among animals there appears to be some correlation between mental ability and manual dexterity" (p. 146). Révész (1950) also depicted a reciprocal relationship between the hand and the development of the intellect. To Révész, though, "the working hand is *the tool of the eye*" (p. 235). Untrained sighted children, working blindfolded, model in clay better than trained blind children. Furthermore, the great versatility of the hand may prove to be a mixed blessing; the performatory functions of the hand may sometimes overshadow and distract one's attention from the perceptual functions (Abravanel, 1972; Gibson, 1962; Kennedy, 1978). Movement of the hand may produce benefits as well, however, as in the case of active touch or tactile scanning.

Bridging gaps. Bridging of the gaps between the fingers provided for Katz perhaps the most persuasive demonstration that the hand is a touch organ. Close your eyes, spread your fingers somewhat apart, then draw them over a surface (preferably one that is very smooth and hard, such as metal or glass), and you will experience the surface as full and as extending into the area between the paths of the fingers. This is also an excellent example of projecting an object out in space, beyond the sensory surface. Katz had subjects move their fingers over smoked paper; when later shown the record thus obtained, they were surprised by how fragmentary the strokes were that evoked the impression of the surface. Regarding the hand as a touch organ is not so radical a notion. In the eye, as Katz pointed out, the individual receptors are spaced apart and even absent altogether in the blind spot, so there must be considerable filling in of empty spaces to produce a continuous visual field.

In various tests, Katz consistently found that a person could recognize a material more rapidly and accurately by using five fingers rather than one. Performance was as good when both hands participated in a simultaneous comparison as when a single hand made a successive comparison. However, Pick (1965) found differences in what subjects learned on simultaneous and successive tactual comparisons.

Katz said that in some cases, especially with the blind, the touch organ is not a single hand, but the two hands together. Gibson (1962) similarly noted that only a single object is perceived even when 10 different digital pressures are received from the two hands at the same time. Gibson (1962) observed that "as regards the unity of separated impressions from the two hands, there is a visual analogy in the unity of separated impressions from the two retinas" (p. 489). One obstacle to achieving reduced vision is that a person cannot dissociate and see as separate entities the two retinal fields that are fused in binocular vision (Boring, 1952). Thus, "we pass from double vision to the single object . . . when the two eyes cease to function each on its own account and are used as a single organ by a single gaze" (Merleau-Ponty, 1962, p. 232).

Memory touch. Further proof of the hand's preeminent, holistic status comes from the way in which an object retains its form and qualities when moved from the hand to less sensitive areas that, if they had received the object first, would not have yielded the same impression and recognition. Katz regarded such persistence as analogous to memory color in vision. The fingers, being very sensitive to the richness of the tactual domain, provide a memory image for other areas of the body; that is, they provide the "official" version of how some material ought to be imagined to feel. So potent is the memory image created by the fingers that the imagined touch on less sensitive areas of the body gives a clearer impression than the actual touch.

A somewhat related phenomenon Katz cited is the *tactual afterimage.* Move your hand over a material and then suddenly stop. The impression of the material may persist while the hand is at rest, even though the impression would never have arisen if the hand had been stationary in the first place and had never moved. In moving the hand and arm over an object, not only does the impression persist as the object moves to less sensitive areas of the arm, but the object maintains its identity qua object as successive sets of individual receptors are triggered, and it is felt to maintain a fixed position in space as the arm glides by it.

Active touch. Katz emphasized the role of the active, moving hand. His concern with active touch has been pursued further, most notably by Gibson (1962), who cited Katz and Révész as "the only investigators who have given much thought to . . . active touch" (p. 478). (Gordon, 1978, however, said that physiologists were well aware of the active element, and that in 1900 Sherrington explicitly contrasted *active touch* to *passive touch.*) Gibson (1962) coined the apt term *tactile scanning* for the manual activities involved in active touch or the *haptic–somatic system* (Gibson, 1966). For Gibson (1962), as for Katz, active movement favors the objective side or pole, which he termed *object-form* as opposed to *skin-form.* Thus, pressing a finger into something reveals its qualities, whereas impressing it upon a passive touch organ produces labile sensations referred to the skin. An active grasp might be needed, for instance, to convert a sensation of pressure into an impression of hardness. Similarly, William James (1890) noted that two contacts are felt if something is placed between two fingers, but a single object is experienced if the fingers are squeezed together.

A question persists, though, as to whether active touch is better because it gives the perceiver direct control of movement or because it simply increases the cutaneous information received (Gordon, 1978). Moving the hand yourself may even be a hindrance if controlling the movement diverts attention from the touch impressions. Better recognition of complex forms is sometimes obtained if the movement is made for the person after he or she has chosen what it should be (Kennedy, 1978). It should not be overlooked, though, that self-movement can provide additional information (via the efferent copy) regarding reafference and the true position out in space of the object felt. Further, motor activity may inhibit aftersensations, and this, too, should aid tactual perceptions, because it would let the perceiver concentrate more fully on the current tactual input (Heller, 1980).

Katz said that if felt roughness depended only on the friction produced by movement, and not at all on the impression of effort from having to move the hand, "then it should not matter whether the touch organ moves over a stationary tactual surface, or, conversely, the tactual surface moves at the same speed over a stationary touch organ" (1925, p. 87). Katz found somewhat better performance in judging the roughness of paper when the hand moved than when it was stationary. He did not regard his results as conclusive, however, because when the hand moved, his subjects could keep it in contact longer with the surface, could vary the speed and rhythm of movement, and could use a more sensitive portion of the fingers. He thought that the small advantage obtained for the moving hand could be accounted for entirely by these factors, and that the impression of effort in moving the hand played no role in judging roughness.

The nature of the response

The tactual input is quite varied and may involve a multitude of senses and gnostic units, as the preceding section indicated. What the perceiver does with the input, however, may be reduced to two main categories of response: localization (Where is it?) and classification and identification (What is it?) (Shaw & Pittenger, 1978; Trevarthen, 1978; White, 1974). Presumably, the location on the skin and the localization out in space are determined first (gross tuning of the percept), followed by the classification and identification of the objects localized (fine tuning of the percept). Accordingly, the subsection on localization will be presented first. The two response systems may not be fully independent of each other, though, and they may overlap in the information they use. Performance on the two functions would be negatively correlated if they operated concurrently and competed for the same limited processing capacity or attention, but they would be positively correlated if an improvement in localization, say, led in turn to better identification, or vice versa. Both systems may depend on information in the spatial domain (Paillard, Brouchon-Viton, & Jordan, 1978), although the vibration sense, as described by Katz, offers a way to specify texture in the temporal domain instead.

Many investigators have postulated two response operations or systems. Quilliam (1978) posited a gentle, soft touch followed by a more deliberate touch. Neisser (1967) proposed a general two-stage model of human information processing. In this system the initial preattentive processing, which segregates shapes and thereby determines their existence and general location, is followed by focal attention, which determines their essence and detailed properties. Trevarthen (1978) distinguished two modes of seeing, which may hold for touch as well: ambient vision (orienting in space) and focal vision (exploration of local structure for identity determination). The larger-scale patterns of orientation and coordination might be organized in the right hemisphere, with the foci of intention defined in the left hemisphere.

Von Békésy (1967) said that "the development of sensory magnitude is a slow process as compared with the process of localization" (p. 107). Localization is completed in a few milliseconds, whereas 1.2 sec are needed for the full development of the vibration sensation. Localization depends on the initial bursts of nerve discharge at stimulus onset, and it is significantly impaired when the stimulus is faded in slowly. Craig (1978) reported that with vibrotactile stimuli, detection depends on a different process than recognition. Detection is disrupted more by forward masking than by backward masking, whereas recognition is disrupted more by backward masking.

Paillard et al. (1978) obtained evidence for a double somesthetic system involving location and identification, respectively. Location is determined based on a space-coordinated system relative to the body postural reference; Paillard et al. (1978) and McCloskey and Gandevia (1978) reported evidence that cutaneous receptors participate in the position sense. Identification is based on an analysis of the relative position of the points stimulated, that is, on the acuity of the receptive surface (two-point threshold). "Thus, the mapping of the tactual space may proceed differently in each system" (Paillard et al., 1978, p. 195).

Millar (1978), conversely, proposed that tactual patterns are coded not in spatial but in textural terms, because she found that raised-dot patterns were more easily discriminated in terms of dot density than dot location. Millar observed that tactual tasks requiring reference to external spatial coordinates (horizontal–vertical, up–down, etc.) are difficult. Learning to discriminate braille patterns is difficult "because invariant spatial reference is lacking in initial explorations" (p. 224). Révész (1950) similarly reported that horizontal and vertical axes mean little to blind sculptors who are pure haptics. "The blind who live in the haptic space have but little feeling for deviations from the vertical and horizontal direction . . . The two cardinal directions owe their phenomenological character to Optics" (pp. 41–42). Likewise, Attneave and Benson (1969) found that blindfolding a person reduced the tendency to code a vibratory input in terms of physical (distal) location rather than finger (proximal) location; "this result suggests that spatial location is represented primarily in visual terms" (p. 216). Révész said that "the very fact that space as perceived by the blind completely lacks perspective, tenders any approximation to our spatial concept most problematic" (p. 160) and that "the difficulty of uniting the haptically perceived objects into a homogeneous spatial structure is further increased by the lack of a background" (p. 160). However, the fact that blind observers duck their heads when the vibratory pattern representing an external object suddenly increases in size (White, Saunders, Scadden, Bach-y-Rita, & Collins, 1970) indicates that the blind, too, may be sensitive to perspective and to "looming" (Schiff, 1965).

The localization function: where is it?

The tactual input specifies the body locations contacted (Weber's *Ortsinn*), the time and duration of contact, and the modality qualities (e.g., pressure, temperature) evoked by the contact. The localization function, which is associated with Katz's objective pole or side, enables the observer to transcend these particular specifications of space, time, and modality quality so as to place the object, as a pure, abstract entity, in its proper temporal–spatial context in the external world. In so doing, the observer maintains the identity of an object across changes or transformations in space, time, and modality quality. Suppose, for example, that two briefly presented visual dots differ somewhat in space, time, and modality quality: A red dot is followed after a brief delay by a blue dot in an adjacent location. Here the observer may perceive not the successive presentation of two independent dots but the motion of a single dot, and sometimes merely the motion itself (Wertheimer's pure phi). Insofar as similarity or identity of modality quality (color in this example) is not crucial to perceived identity, the question of existence (Where is it?) is independent of and separate from that of essence (What is it?) (Shaw & Pittenger, 1978).

To transcend the particular accidents of space, time, and modality quality means to render these dimensions transparent to the "pure information" available in the external input. Such transparency is most readily apparent in the case of space; Katz provides several illustrations of spatial transparency in touch (see below). Like space, time is a hidden or implicit dimension; objects or events occur *in* time but do not consist *of* time (Merleau-Ponty, 1962). Modality quality likewise can be conceived in this manner, as when Gibson (1966) asserted that "the evolution of sensitivity was governed by the need for the information *in* en-

ergy, not for energy as such" (p. 105). The object must be seen to stand
out as figure against the sensory flux; in phenomenological terminology,
"the relationship between matter and form is . . . [one] of *Fundierung*:
the symbolic function rests on the visual as on a ground" (Merleau-
Ponty, 1962, p. 127). To dissociate the object qua object from the modality quality, perhaps the perceiver must discern that the energy is reflected from, rather than emitted by, the stimulus object.

Let us examine separately the three defining criteria or characteristics
of the localization function: (1) spatial projection, (2) temporal projection,
and (3) absence of modality qualities.

Criterion 1: spatial projection. The projection of the object outside the
body provided Katz with the main basis for distinguishing the objective
pole or side (e.g., "I feel a pointed object out there") from the subjective
pole or side (e.g., "I feel a prickling sensation"). The objective side
predominates in the case of vision, whereas the subjective side predominates in the case of pain. The objective side has provided the prototype
or ideal for perception in general.

Thomas Reid (1878, 1970) was the first philosopher to insist on a strict
distinction between sensation and perception (Boring, 1942; Hamlyn,
1961). Perception depends on sensation but goes beyond it to provide a
conception of the object perceived and an irresistible conviction of the
object's present existence. With sensation, there is no object distinct
from the act itself; there is no difference between the sensation and the
feeling of it. Reid indicated what are generally regarded as the most
important characteristics of sensation: (1) sensation occurs prior to perception and provides the information upon which perception is based,
and (2) the object is projected beyond the receptive surface in perception
but not in sensation.

It is now generally accepted, however, that we do not have direct access
to our sensations, if such should exist, but rather must tease out our
subjective impressions via perception (Boring, 1952; Gibson, 1963). For
Gibson (1952), as for Katz and others, the subjective side (visual field) was
an *alternative* experience, not simply the basis for the other experience.
Many psychologists have been sensitive to the bimodal nature of perception (e.g., Brunswik, 1956; Mack, 1978; Rock, 1977). The perceiver may
attend either to the distal stimulus (distal or constancy mode) or to the
proximal stimulus (proximal mode) (Mack, 1978; Rock, 1977). The two
modes may sometimes alternate in rapid succession, as for example, when
railroad tracks are seen almost simultaneously as parallel and as converging (Mack, 1978). In vision, where the objective aspect normally predomi-

nates, the perceiver must take a special attitude, or the stimulus input must be reduced (e.g., by presenting a homogeneous, blurred visual field or by excluding most of the visual field with a reduction screen), in order to obtain the "basic" subjective impressions. In other cases, though, little or no effort may be needed (e.g., pains, afterimages).

Philosophers have long been interested in the subjective side, and some have recently spoken of sensationlike, immediate, and incorrigible impressions, which they have termed *sensa* or *sense data*. These are the "objects" perceived in the case of a delusion or an illusion (Swartz, 1965). A sense datum is an object of experience, not the experience (sensation) itself; we are not merely aware, but aware of. We may be aware of either a tomatoish red color patch (sense datum) or a red tomato (normal percept). Other philosophers have asserted that sense data are not objects distinguishable from the awareness of them; they do not exist apart from the sensing of them any more than does a pain or sensation (Hirst, 1967). Thus, we must distinguish between *seeing*, which refers to an activity or state, and *seeing as*, which refers to an achievement (Rundle, 1972). According to the "adverbial analysis" of these philosophers, "I sense a red color patch" merely tells *how* I sense, and sense data are only sense contents, which cannot exist unsensed. These philosophers have generalized to all sensory domains what most clearly seems to apply to pain: Reid (1970) said that the distinction between act and object in "I feel pain" is not real but grammatical. The feeling is not distinct from the pain itself, and one might equally well say, "I am being pained." Pain, it might be noted, was for Reid "the model of *all* sensation" (T. Duggan in Reid, 1970, p. XVII), and it remains today the favorite example of the subjective side.

Adopting a subjective attitude is not the same as trying to attend to punctate proximal stimuli. Sense data are not necessarily punctate; they can be entire patches of color and may be striped or variegated (Hirst, 1967). It should also be noted that realists such as Gibson (1966) and Pitcher (1971) have not regarded very favorably such nonphysical entities as sense data.

Criterion 2: temporal projection. For realists, an object out in space continues to exist even after they have stopped looking or touching. For phenomenalists, such as Berkeley and Mill, however, objects represent merely the permanent possibilities of sensation. What matters for them are the sense data, which occur and disappear as the perceiver alternately observes and ceases to observe. "It does not make sense to say that a sense-datum has existed unperceived" (Paul, 1965, p. 282).

The criteria for the objective pole, reflecting the realists' position, thus might be extended to require both temporal and spatial projection. The evidence on this point seems promising. Temporal projection is evident in vision, the sense that comes closest to the objective pole. "An object is called into being by illumination, without ceasing to exist when the illumination is removed" (Katz, 1935, p. 292).

Phenomenal permanence tends to hold in vision, but not in other modalities (Knops, 1947). Michotte (1950) reported that an object brought into contact with the skin produces two different impressions at the same time: (1) the impression of an object that had preexisted the contact, and (2) the impression of a contact that was suddenly created. This observation fits Katz's view that the objective and subjective poles are both available in touch. If the subjective pole has nearly total sway, as in the case of pain, then, according to the present criterion, no pain should persist following the termination of the painful stimulus, assuming it left no tissue damage.

Katz undoubtedly would have approved giving equal weight to the temporal and spatial domains. He attacked atomism in either time or space. His concern with active touch, movement, and vibration attests to his own commitment to temporal holism. Katz (1950) noted that the Gestalt psychologists, although professing to oppose time atomism (e.g., in movement, melody), turned readily to the tachistoscope to obtain evidence on form-creating processes. He himself overlooked time when he defined the objective pole, however. Perhaps time is so easy to overlook because of its greater transparency; insofar as it is easier to gaze mentally through a series of intervening temporal events than through a series of intervening spatial events, a person would be less aware of the presence of time.

Criterion 3: absence of modality qualities. According to Reid (1878), unless sensations are quite pleasant or quite unpleasant, it is difficult to attend to them. Because most sensations fall into the indifferent category, "they carry the thought to the external object, and immediately disappear and are forgot. Nature intended them only as signs; and when they have served that purpose, they vanish" (p. 156). Sensation and perception are always joined, but because one's attention normally is directed to the external object, "it is not easy to persuade the vulgar, that, in seeing a colored body, when the light is not too strong, nor the eye inflamed, they have any sensation or feeling at all" (p. 160).

The objective side, then, is concerned with an object's existence, whereas the subjective side is concerned with the object's essence – that is, the attributes represented in the sensa or sense data. Thus, what may most clearly characterize the subjective side is the fact that a trace of the input modality remains in the percept (Natsoulas, 1978). Whether such a trace can ever be fully removed, however, is problematic. "For Gibson, the information we acquire perceptually is . . . amodal" (Natsoulas, 1978, p. 280), but "resonating in any concrete perceptual instance is *of a modality*" (p., 281). Probably no one would confuse a sight with a sound, even if both modalities conveyed virtually identical objective information.

The subjective side is more evident in other senses, such as touch, which thus pose even larger problems for the realist. Révész (1950) said that separating form from content is more difficult in haptics than in vision. In vision, "form has an existence of its own, independent of material and object" (p. 68); a clock has the character of a circular form apart from its clock character. "It is as though the form compelled us to consider it as an independent object which we have to observe" (p. 70). In haptics, on the other hand, "the object as apprehended is so intimately associated with its form that the differentiation can only be performed by a special mental operation" (p. 69).

Katz noted that an impression of movement may always accompany that of elasticity or oiliness. For Katz, something elastic could not be imagined without also imagining a movement being carried out on an elastic object. Also, Katz could never produce in himself an imagined touch from which the touch organ was fully separated. Other persons, when asked to imagine touching various materials, invariably imagined concurrently a touch organ, which almost always was the fingertips.

By and large, though, Katz shared Gibson's emphasis on pure information and the objective pole. Movement need not be a conscious feature of the impression of stickiness, he said. Even so simple a quality as roughness bears no trace of movement in its contents. In the impression of the ordinary object, according to Katz, movement, time, and space leave no trace of themselves; the object is precipitated as an independent entity, largely uncontaminated by its journey through tactual time and space. When one's hand glides over a fixed object, say the corner of a chair, "different and constantly changing parts of the hand come into contact with the corner," yet it "persists just as unaltered in its position in tactual space as do visual objects in their position in visual space when the eye is moved" (1925, p. 69), due presumably to compensation based on central movement impulses. "It is as if the cinematic form of the stimulus is converted to the static properties of an object" (1925, p. 62).

Other qualities besides movement may also be discarded from the percept. "The structural elements [in the texture] can determine our judgment concerning the material without actually becoming conscious for us in themselves" (1925, p. 37). It is easy to underrate the role of microstructural elements in vision and in touch; "they help us the most in recognizing materials, but in a way they completely consume themselves in the process" (1925, p. 38). For Sir William Hamilton (see notes to Reid, 1878), the objective side predominates on primary qualities (extension, divisibility, figure, motion, solidity, hardness, softness, and fluidity), whereas the subjective side predominates on secondary qualities (sound, color, taste, smell, heat, and cold).

Some modalities seem more suppressed than others, and perhaps with these we could indeed speak of amodal perception, with no trace of the input modality. Vestibular sensitivity is commonly supposed to leave no trace in consciousness, serving instead to elicit directly certain postural reflexes. Similarly, "kinesthetic stimulation does not result in a distinct perceptual experience such as hearing a sound (perhaps not even to the point of immediate awareness except when the need arises)" (Schiffman, 1976, p. 94). However, it is not clear whether we can speak of perception at all when the information serves solely to trigger certain motor reflexes.

Subjective versus objective modalities. Clarification might result if we could discover why the relative preponderance of subjective and objective impressions varies across modalities. The most objective modality is vision. Hearing is not as overwhelmingly objective as seeing, Rundle (1972) said, whereas touch and temperature and perhaps taste and smell can favor either pole depending on circumstances, and pain and perhaps kinesthesis favor the subjective pole, as do the interoceptive senses (hunger, thirst, etc.). Hirst (1967) noted that, whereas sounds and colors are external and public, "tastes are a borderline case – private and in the mouth, yet in a sense external to the skin and membranes – while feelings of pressure or warmth are partly sensations proper and partly seem to be awarenesses of heavy or warm objects" (p. 408). Russell (1921) said that "public senses give us knowledge of the outer world, while the private senses only give us knowledge as to our own bodies" (p. 118). The private versus public distinction is one of degree, not of kind, though, because "no two people . . . ever have exactly similar sensations related to the same physical object at the same moment" (p. 119). According to Russell, "sight and hearing are the most public of the senses; smell only a trifle less so; touch, again, a trifle less, since two people can only touch the same spot successively . . . Taste has a sort of semi-publicity, since people seem to experience similar taste-sensations when they eat similar foods; but [they] . . . cannot eat actually the same piece of food" (p. 118).

27

Although both types of impressions, subjective and objective, are always present in touch, one pole or side may predominate in a particular instance, according to Katz. The subjective side is stronger, for example, on the parts of the body that are seldom used to obtain touch information, such as the inside of the nose or ear. The subjective side is present almost exclusively in pain sensations and can also be seen in psychopathological touch hallucinations, as well as in the phantom limb sensations of amputees.

Movement is an important factor. When the hand is moved to touch another part of the body, an objective impression occurs in the moving hand but a subjective impression occurs in the stationary area being touched. Katz cited Weber: "A peculiar dissociation arises when a warm hand touches a cold forehead; the warmth of the hand is sensed first by the cold forehead, but the forehead is felt as an object [by the hand]" (Katz, 1925, p. 20). Rieser and Pick (1976), similarly, found that the objective pole was more strongly evoked by haptic stimuli (bars that subjects grasped) than by tactual stimuli (bars pressed on the forehead); when the posture changed (90-degree change in body tilt), the spontaneous identification of a bar's direction was in terms of an objective or gravity reference system for haptic stimuli, but not for tactual stimuli.

Before concluding that the hand produces a more objective representation because it can grasp objects, whereas the forehead cannot, however, three other possible explanations should be considered. First, the hand would acquire a more precise and detailed tactual representation, given its greater tactual acuity, and this may explain why it tends to produce a more objective representation. Second, differences in arrival times of neural impulses from different parts of the body may explain why the forehead is felt as an object by the hand, and not vice versa. Coren, Porac, and Ward (1979) presented an interesting demonstration in this regard. When asked to touch the lower lip briefly and repeatedly with a fingertip and "to say where the sensation is, most people report that they feel it mostly on the lip and little or not at all on the fingertip, even though both are of about equal sensitivity" (p. 234). If the little toe or ankle is touched instead, however, then the sensation seems to be located mostly in the finger. The sensation is localized at the body area whose impulses reach the brain first, provided they arrive at least 1 msec earlier than the impulses from the other body area. Third, the hand may feel larger (and therefore less figural and objective) to the forehead than vice versa, because of a peculiar asymmetry in perceived tactual space. There seems to be a general expansion of objects located near the head; if you roll a cylinder between the finger and thumb, it feels larger near the head than when moved away with an outstretched arm (Bartley, 1953; Kennedy, 1978). Similarly, objects placed in the mouth feel larger than those placed in the hand. William James (1890) observed that when you put your finger into your mouth, the finger feels unexpectedly large to the mouth, whereas the mouth feels unexpectedly tiny to the finger. "The interior of one's mouth-cavity feels larger when explored by the tongue than when looked at. The crater of a newly-extracted tooth, and the movements of a loose tooth in its socket, feel quite monstrous" (p. 139).

A temperature sensation generally favors the subjective side, according to Katz, and warmth and cold may be experienced as pure bodily states. The temperature impression normally is not alone, but is closely bound up with an impression of touch, especially on the fingers and inner hand and when the temperature is not too high or low. When the temperature sensation is separated from the embrace of the touch or tactile sensation, the subjective side emerges strongly. The subjective side is also favored if the fingers are warmed or cooled by being dipped in water rather than by touching a solid object. Temperature can be quite objective in some cases, however. Turning the head in front of a hot oven, for example, leads to localization of the heat source out in space, which may take on a Gestalt quality similar to voluminousness. The greater skill of blind persons at localizing objects through the temperature sense (e.g., they feel the approach of a warm cylinder at three times the distance that a normal person does) suggested to Katz that such a heightened sensitivity is probably part of the so-called sixth sense of the blind.

The subjective inclination of temperature may be overridden by movement, as shown in the case of the cold foot. Keep a very cold foot absolutely motionless in bed, observed Katz, and a painfully intense impression of cold arises – one that lacks form and is not localized on any part of the body. The impression has a free-floating and purely subjective character. The least movement of the foot, though, produces localization of the cold, and the person then possesses a "cold foot." Some years later, though, Katz put some limits on a subjective impression: "There is no such thing as pure sensation, floating freely in the air, without perceptual conditions" (1950, p. 13).

It is very significant that the most prominent modality, vision, should be so heavily dominated by the objective pole. This fact may help to explain why some philosophers (e.g., Pitcher, 1971) and psychologists (e.g., Gibson, 1966) have placed a nearly total emphasis on the objective aspect. It is easy to overlook the subjective aspect if vision alone is considered, although Gibson (1950) did distinguish between the visual field and the visual world. Reid (1878) said that painters are especially adept at attending to sensations. However, if painters come closer than most persons to achieving a subjective attitude, their skill may be acquired as much by trial and error as by conscious analysis (Gombrich, 1974). Katz (1935) recommended that painters try to see colors as filmy. In general, the ability to achieve a subjective attitude in vision is limited. Observers have difficulty in judging the extent of a visual image on the retina; judgments deviate in the direction expected if the size of the distal stimulus rather than the proximal stimulus were being judged (Rock, 1977).

Is pain purely subjective? At the opposite extreme from vision, pain seems universally regarded as subjective; even Gibson (1963) acknowledged that one may say that a stomach ache is sensory rather than perceptual. Closer examination reveals, however, that the situation is not quite so simple.

Why pain is generally regarded as purely subjective seems clear. Pain seems to be an internal, private experience that corresponds directly to the sensory input acquired by the pain modality. For philosophers, it is an ideal instance of a sense datum, an experience about which the observer cannot be mistaken (see Swartz, 1965). Thus, Rundle (1972) distinguished between "feeling pains and hearing sounds, or, more generally, between 'mere' sensations and perception" (p. 201). Whereas "sounds and smells are there to be sensed by all, the pain I feel exists only insofar as I feel it" (p. 202). Furthermore, he claimed that no organ can be wielded in order to detect pain.

Rundle's points are debatable, however. The hand can certainly be wielded to verify that the pot on the stove is painfully hot, and it may be untrue that a pain cannot be a pain of anything. As Gibson (1966) noted, cutaneous pain, unlike internal pain, may carry useful information about the world. There may be just as much reason to regard certain types of pain as public as to regard sound as public. D. Owen noted that "in the same sense that we say, 'look from where I'm standing and you can see it,' we say, 'feel how much it hurts when you lie on this bed of nails like I am;' in both cases, perception is public" (pers. comm., June 1976).

To prove that pain is more than just a diffuse subjective experience, we must first determine to what object the perceiver attends. This may be difficult because with pain the "object" attended to may be an event rather than a physical object; it may be the energy source – that is, what emits the energy, rather than what reflects it. In visual perception, too, one may sometimes attend to the energy source, as when a person perceives the level of illumination in a room (emitted energy) based on the pattern of light reaching the eye, or when additional spotlighting puts a visual object into the fluorescent or illuminant mode (Beck, 1972; Katz, 1935).

Pain, too, may tend to evoke the fluorescent or illuminant mode, rather than the surface or reflectant mode, because the source of stimulation may be largely not the painful stimulus itself but the tissue damage it causes. Thus, the sensory response may strongly persist when the external stimulus is terminated. When the hand is pulled away from contact with a hot stove, it may continue to ache; the hand has become "self-luminous" with respect to pain. On other modalities, too, stimulation may be largely independent of the external stimulus. Galen noted that when the source of stimulation is removed, the changes in the eye and the ear cease, but those involving heat or cold remain (Siegel, 1970).

When the hand is self-luminous, so that a strongly persisting sensory quality moves when the hand moves, it seems quite natural that the object or event perceived should be localized at the hand, rather than at the original causal agent (e.g., hot stove). This may explain why pain, warmth, and cold seemingly favor the subjective pole. These modalities may really be just as objective as vision; it is just that their objects happen to lie at the sensory surface rather than out in space. Insofar as the pain and temperature modalities primarily monitor the state of the sensory surface, rather than provide information about external stimuli, they should perhaps be considered to be interoceptive rather than exteroceptive senses.

Whether pain is more than just a diffuse subjective experience has important practical implications. If we consider only the most subjective aspect of pain, and measure how well a person can discriminate one level of pain sensation from another, then it seems clear, for example, that acupuncture has no effect (Clark & Yang, 1974). However, although acupuncture does not affect discriminability (d'), it does prompt subjects to raise their pain criterion (β) in response to the expectation that it works. That is, acupuncture produces a placebo effect; the pain sensations apparently are the same, but they are interpreted differently when acupuncture is used than when it is not. If only sensory aspects are considered, then acupuncture appears to be worthless. If higher-level, more objective aspects are considered, however, then acupuncture is not worthless.

Much evidence indicates that the significant aspect of pain, that which makes it aversive, is *not* the pain sensation itself but what the sensation represents. The perceived intensity of pain may be influenced by the subject's own evaluation of the seriousness of the tissue damage sustained, and analgesics may affect primarily the anxiety produced by the situation rather than the pain sensation itself (Kenshalo, 1971). Lesions induced in the frontal lobes may alleviate intractable pain, with no actual sensory loss, or with even a lowering of the threshold for the sensation of pain produced by external stimuli (Association for Research in Nervous and Mental Disease, 1948; Gray, 1971). Patients with such lesions report that they still feel the pain, but that it no longer bothers them. Only if asked directly about the pain do they indicate any awareness of its presence.

Thus, before we discard acupuncture and other so-called placebos, which may include the physician's bedside manner itself, we ought to ask ourselves exactly what we are trying to alleviate. As the surgeon's scalpel penetrates the skin, the patient may attend either to the subjective pole ("I feel a sharp, tingling pressure") or to the objective pole ("I feel a sharp object out there; I perceive the presence of someone who is intent on producing some tissue damage in me"). Thus, pain, like other modalities of touch, may always have both subjective and objective aspects.

Attention. Whether the subjective or objective pole predominates may depend upon the function, rather than the structure, of a modality, and on how the tactual input is processed and to what end. Within a given modality, the two poles are generally presumed to compete with each other. Sir William Hamilton spoke of an inverse relationship between sensation and perception: The more intense the sensation the more indistinct the perception, and vice versa (Hamlyn, 1961; notes in Reid, 1878). The two poles or modes may not only compete for the same limited processing capacity but may also conflict with each other in how they set the person to perceive and act. The two poles might be complementary or functionally disjoint, so that being prepared for one would necessarily entail being unprepared for the other (Pick & Saltzman, 1978; Shaw & Pittenger, 1978). Thus, the rivalry between the two poles or modes (i.e., distal mode versus proximal mode) may be one of selective attention. Pick and Saltzman (1978) said that "mode appears to be one of that category of concepts concerned with direction of perception: set, Aufgabe, Einstellung, selective attention, and so on" (p. 9).

Switching one's attention from the subjective to the objective side, from inner to outer, may be likened to switching from one figural organization to another when presented with an ambiguous figure–ground stimulus. In both cases, an internal, stimulus-independent change in selective attention may have far-reaching consequences on the quality of the percept (cf. Hochberg, 1970). Depending upon the perceiver's attitude, an object pressed into the hand might evoke as figure either the outline of the impress from the vantage point of the hand (subjective pole) or that of the external object (objective pole). Depending on which is figural at a given moment, the body surface or the outer world, the boundary between them will serve as a unidirectional contour to cohere either an internal, subjective entity or an external, objective one.

Unlike the figure–ground case, however, the reversal of perspective on the subjective–objective dimension apparently need not be all-or-none. Attention need not be directed exclusively toward either the subjective or the objective side. For Katz, each pole or side was an imaginary or ideal type, which might never be experienced in pure form to the exclusion of the other. Katz had in mind not just two poles or extremes but an entire continuum or gradation of intermediate impressions containing both subjective and objective elements. He referred to film touch, which belongs to the objective pole, as being more subjective than surface touch, and said the same about film color vis-à-vis surface color (Katz, 1935). Gibson likewise implied that there was a continuum, rather than two opposing aspects alone, when he depicted the visual field as lying between the subjective and objective poles rather than at the subjective pole itself.

There may be a continuum rather than two ideal types, but limitations of attention seemingly demand that only one of the possible gradations be figural at a given moment or that the figural property rapidly alternate between the two extremes (Mack, 1978). "When I press my two hands together, it is not a matter of two sensations felt together as one perceives two objects placed side by side, but of an ambiguous set-up in which both hands can alternate the rôles of 'touching' and being 'touched'" (Merleau-Ponty, 1962, p. 93). Merleau-Ponty allowed for no such ambiguity, however, when an external object contacted the body; the bodily space provides "the background against which the object as the goal of our action may stand out or the void in front of which it may *come to light*" (p. 102).

The ground provided by the bodily space is easy to overlook but sometimes becomes quite evident to the perceiver. When the bristles of a stiff brush are moved over the skin, Katz noted, a person feels only those points of the brush that touch the skin, yet in another sense he or she also "feels" the spaces in between the bristle points. The person experiences not a tactile nothingness between the points but merely touch space that is empty and not covered with material. The phenomenon can be likened to the visual figure–ground relationship, Katz said, with the bristle points as figure and the empty spaces as ground. Katz reported that he was never able to reverse the tactile figure–ground relationship, though, so as to change the momentary figure of the bristle points into the ground.

A well-developed body image or percept favors the subjective pole, whereas a well-formed external object favors the objective pole, sometimes with dire results for the body percept: "If I stand in front of my desk and lean on it with both hands, only my hands are stressed and the whole of my body trails behind them like the tail of a comet" (Merleau-Ponty, 1962, p. 100). Katz (1950) said that in a standing position, in which the body image is salient and the subjective side predominates, a person may be quite insensitive to considerable changes in pressure on the soles of the feet from various exercises and shifts in posture. In a reclining position, on the other hand, pressure is sensed as coming from without and is objectified, and changes in pressure are more readily detected.

The subjective–objective dichotomy not only may be explainable in terms of attention but might in turn help to enlighten our notion of attention. According to the Yerkes–Dodson law, people perform best at an intermediate level of activation. Performance suffers when arousal is very low or very high; perhaps this is because attention in those cases is directed more toward internal events or the subjective side. With very low arousal, the person may be nearly asleep and may attend much more to internal imagery or daydreams than to objects or events out in space. With very high arousal, the person may be in a state of panic and again may attend much more to internal events, such as fear or anger, than to external objects or events. There may be several levels of internal projection, however, just as there are several levels of projection out in space (see below), and the turning inward associated with daydreaming might be at a deeper level than that normally associated with the subjective pole in touch. The subjectivity of perception is never absolute, Merleau-Ponty (1962) said, because it in turn provides an object to an ulterior *I*: "Each time I experience a sensation, I feel that it concerns not my own being, the one for which I am responsible and for which I make decisions, but another self which has already sided with the world, which is already open to certain of its aspects and synchronized with them" (p. 216).

Learning and development. Learning and prior experience might play a role in shifting the balance between the subjective and objective sides, but Katz made little mention of the modifiability of the various modalities in this regard, and he seemed to regard the modality differences as fixed and immutable. Like Gibson, he gave little attention to mechanisms of learning and, along with the Gestalt psychologists, he could be classified as a nativist. People learn to identify by touch various sorts of materials, such as paper, cloth, and metal. What seems to change with experience for Katz, however, is not the quality of a vibration or temperature impression but the ease with which it can be named. People are innately equipped to project objects out in space. As children grow older, what may develop in vision, for instance, is not the ability to cohere stimulus patterns into objects but rather the ability to adopt a subjective attitude (Katz, 1935).

For von Békésy (1967), on the other hand, the external projection in vision and audition is learned early in life. Similarly, according to Berkeley, "a man born blind, being made to see, would at first have no idea of distance by sight; the sun and stars, the remotest objects as well as the nearer, would all seem to be in his eye, or rather in his mind . . . each . . . as near to him as the perceptions of pain or pleasure, or the most inward passions of his soul" (1910, p. 187). For Katz and others, on the other hand, all visual impressions are automatically projected out in space, even when one views an afterimage with the eyes shut or experiences spots produced by pressure on the eyeball.

Modes of touch: film, surface, volume. Katz provided important details on how objects might be cohered on the objective side when he described three specific modes of touch that are analogous to the film, surface, and volume color modes of vision (Katz, 1935). The objective pole predominates to varying degrees in all of these modes, because objects, materials, and space are projected out in space. Conceiving of a touch analog to surface color is not difficult, because surface touch is readily experienced when one touches an object made of some solid substance (e.g., metal, glass, wood) and having a continuous, unbroken surface. In surface touch, one experiences a definite surface at a definite distance and orientation.

But what touch impression would correspond to film color, whose misty, spongy appearance, produced by homogeneous illumination, contrasts sharply to the hard, impenetrable, and definitely localizable appearance of surface color? A strong (and sufficiently rapid) stream of air or liquid, Katz said, produces a space-filling film touch or immersed touch (*raumfüllendes Tastquale*). The stream feels indeterminate in form, and though there may be a suggestion of a certain thickness, the form lacks a rear boundary and is always perceived as lying in the frontoparallel plane. Katz (1936) said that film touch also arises in drawing the hand through water or a thick liquid. Kennedy (1978) provided yet another example: Think of brushing cobwebs aside. Film touch or immersed touch does not represent the qualities of a body; it characterizes a substance, not an object. In film touch, the resistance that the material offers the hand is experienced as elastic rather than stiff or rigid. According to Katz, moving the fingers through loose sand or flour produces neither a surface touch nor a film touch, but I would submit that the impression comes closer to that of a film touch.

Volume touch occurs when a solid object is felt through a soft material, and the soft material seems to fill the intervening space between the hand and the object, producing a spacelike touch (*raumhafte Tastphänomene*). To try this yourself, just lay a blanket over a matchbox or book. (The solid object must have sharp contours; putting the blanket on a flat surface, such as the floor, does not produce volume touch.) The ability to feel two layers at the same time allows the physician to feel organs through the skin by means of palpation and percussion. The physician directs attention to the organ itself, of course, and ignores the voluminous feel of the intervening tissue. Katz (1930, 1936, 1937a) devised a "percussion phantom" to help train medical students in the art of percussion. The device consists of a cardboard square placed over an opening in a box. Subjects tap the cardboard with their fingers or a percussion hammer in order to determine the shape of a lead plate that is attached underneath the cardboard and absorbs the vibrations produced by tapping. "In general, the thicker the plate, the easier the task" (Katz, 1930, p. 84). The subject draws the outline of the shape perceived on a piece of paper clamped on top of the cardboard. The paper can then be placed directly on top of the lead plate to determine the accuracy of the drawing. Katz (1930) said that percussion has also been used to test Swiss cheese: "In a first-class cheese the holes must be of the right size and number, and this can be determined by the percussion method" (p. 86).

A person wearing gloves feels a surface lying beyond a thin covering layer. With close-fitting, very thin rubber gloves, the impression of a veiling layer may give way to the impression of "deafness" in the fingers. Katz (1935) said that there is nothing in touch that is comparable to the impression of illumination in vision, but perhaps this diminution could be likened to a dimming of illumination. It should be noted, too, that the existence of volume touch disproves the ancient notion that the skin is special because it responds only to direct contact with objects (Siegel, 1970).

Transparency may persist even when the intervening material is quite rigid. Katz's subjects felt the hardness and softness of a pencil at the writing point rather than in the hand holding the pencil. Katz also noted Lotze's observation that touching an object with a stick gives the feeling of being in immediate contact with the object, just as though one's hand were actually touching it. Lotze also observed that "while sewing, our perception seems to be immediately present in the point of the needle" (Katz, 1925, p. 116). By the same principle of external or eccentric projection, Katz noted, an automobile driver feels the goodness of the road and an airplane pilot feels the elastic qualities of the air rather than merely the local jiggling of a steering wheel or rudder against the hand. Merleau-Ponty (1962) observed that "the stick is no longer an object perceived by the blind man, but an instrument *with* which he perceives" (p. 152). The blind man is aware of the length of the stick "through the position of objects [rather] than of the position of objects through it" (p. 143). In general, according to Merleau-Ponty, "to get used to a hat, a car or a stick is to be transplanted into them, or conversely, to incorporate them into the bulk of our own body" (p. 143).

Von Békésy (1967) noted that "every well-trained machinist projects his sensations of pressure to the tip of a screwdriver, and it is this projection that enables him to work rapidly and correctly" (p. 225). In one test, von Békésy attached microphones to two vibrators on the chest and alternated the presentation of a click between two loudspeakers. The vibration was felt more strongly at one vibrator or the other, depending on which microphone was closer to the loudspeaker currently being sounded. At first the person experienced the vibratory sensation jump from one side to the other, but with practice the sensation moved continuously in accordance with the lateral position of the sound source. (When he successively pulsed vibrators on the two knees, the sensation moved continuously from one knee to the other in the free space between them; Katz, 1930, 1937a, reported a similar phenomenon.) The sensation was felt to move on the surface of the chest, but some persons, by following with the eye the alternate sounding of the two loudspeakers, "became able for no obvious reason to locate the vibratory sensation close to the loudspeaker when its distance from the chest was no greater than 2 or 3 feet" (p. 225). "After several months of training it became possible to localize the vibratory sensation, even with eyes closed, at a position outside the body, though usually this position was closer to the body than to the loudspeaker" (p. 225).

When a bank of 400 vibrators forming a tactile vision substitution system (TVSS) is placed on the back of a blind person and connected to a television camera so that the light received from a particular point out in space can turn on one vibrator, the person not only discerns the shape and orientation of objects scanned by the camera but also projects them out in front of the self (White, 1974; White et al., 1970). When the tactile image was made to "loom" by suddenly being magnified with a turn of the zoom lever on the camera, blind observers ducked startled. Certain occlusion effects found in vision are not found in touch, however (White, 1974).

Katz (1937a) reviewed research by himself and his associates (Kietzmann, Klemm, Noldt, Petzoldt, Thiel) on the ability to localize vibratory sources beyond the body's surface. Normal and deaf subjects who touched a dinner plate with their hands could accurately report where on the plate a vibrator was applied. Further tests involved placing the subject's fingers or hands at various distances along a bar and having the subject report the side (left, right) on which a vibrator was applied. Even with a single hand or with the two hands crossed (i.e., the left hand on the right side), the vibration could be properly localized. A slightly earlier and slightly stronger stimulation on one side of the hand prompted the subject to localize the source toward that side. Given the fact that vibrations travel through wood at a rate of 5,000 meters per second, the time difference could not have exceeded a fraction of a millisecond. Using separate vibrators for the two hands confirmed that localization could be based on either a time or an intensity difference. More recently, Gescheider (1974) reported on further tests in which a time difference was traded off against an intensity difference in determining the apparent localization (see also von Békésy, 1967).

Projecting an object farther out in space, past an intervening medium, might be conceived as going beyond the processes evident in the subjective and objective poles. The punctate stimuli are not only organized into coherent entities or patches but are filled out so as to encompass regions not in immediate contact with the sensory surface. The perceiver may project not only objects out in space but also empty space (Katz, 1935) or a three-dimensional, visual world (Gibson, 1950). According to Katz, the projection is not a cold-blooded, nonspatial inference, such as might be based on past experience and well-learned association; the notion of external objects seems to be innate (Katz, 1935).

What does it mean, though, to say that the percept of an object is projected out in space? Is the objective side so dominant in vision that persons really perceive themselves as standing in space when they look into the mirror in the morning? "Significantly, those who speak of the 'projection of sensations' do not attempt to define the notion. An acceptable definition is extremely difficult to obtain at best, and impossible at worst" (Savage, 1970, p. 42). Are all impressions (as opposed to real objects) locatable? When someone projects a visual afterimage onto a wall, Savage asked, does he or she genuinely believe it *is* on the wall? "In the phantom-limb phenomenon the subject 'projects' sensations to the place previously occupied by the limb, although he knows full well that no limb is there"(1970, p. 44). Does projection merely provide suggestions via our imagination?

The notion of projection out in space may be vague and ill-defined in part because there may be several possible levels or even a hierarchy of projection. A person may project in space an object that is pricking the skin or may project beyond this point to perceive the causal agent or energy source that is making the object press against the skin. If the person taps with the object, he or she may either feel it externally or, more likely, project beyond it to perceive the surface it is tapping. The percept might even go beyond this surface and capture a glimpse of the Kantian thing in itself. Katz (1950) noted that the visible expression perceived on a face is displaced inward and located within the person at whom we are looking. In particular, "most persons think of the eyes as revealing the minds of others" (Katz, 1950, p. 83).

The classification and identification function: what is it?

Two types of answers might be obtained for the question, what is it? (White, 1974): (1) an immediate, natural identification, as when the outline of a familiar object is discerned; (2) a mediated, coded identification involving a more arbitrary social meaning, as when a word is read. The second type, the mainstay of work on information processing, is typically studied with reductive procedures (i.e., using brief, static, two-dimensional, black-and-white arrays). As such, it ought to be more closely associated with the subjective side than with the objective side. A person reading a book must attend less to the book out in space than to the internal identification responses made while reading. A person studying a painting likewise must attend not simply to the literal shapes on the canvas but to what they represent.

Katz gave scant attention to symbolic or coded identification, however. His concern was with surface qualities (*Modifikationen*), which lead to the classification of a material on such dimensions as hard–soft and rough–smooth, and with the identifying characteristics (*Spezifikationen*) which tell us whether the material is paper, leather, metal, or something else. Like Gibson, Katz was interested primarily in natural, physical objects, not in coded or social objects. (Katz perhaps best revealed his preference for texture over shape when he equated texture or microstructure with the natural form or grain of a material and shape or macrostructure with the artificial form impressed upon the material.) Katz's findings concerning the role of vibration, temperature, pressure, and elasticity in the classification and identification process will be considered below.

Symbolic or coded identification. Katz did not uncover any phenomena involving symbolic or coded identification. The reason may be that the skin is relatively unsuited for that type of communication. The 50- to 60-word-per-minute reading rate attainable with braille or the Optacon (Chapter 5; Schiffman, 1976) is not that impressive. Widening the window past which text moves to include more than one letter aids reading if the material is presented to vision, but not if it is presented to touch (White, 1974). Perhaps people too readily adopt the objective pole in touch, thus causing the natural identification of the pattern out in space to overshadow the coded identification of the words received. Perhaps braille readers tend to fill in the region between the fingers and merge the letters received on different fingers into a single Gestalt. Révész (1950) noted, similarly, that form and content are more difficult to separate in haptics than in vision. Perhaps a reductive or analytical procedure – for example, using electrical or thermal stimulation instead of mechanical stimulation – would heighten the subjective side and thus aid reading via touch.

The basic identification problem with the skin may lie not with attention, however, but with the general poorness of tactual acuity or spatial resolution. After all, the eye fares no worse at natural identification because of its considerable powers in symbolic identification. Even the fingertips with their extensive cortical innervation, do not possess the same acuity as the fovea: "The skin cannot rival the eye in purely spatial perception" (Kirman, 1973, p. 66). As Katz noted, there is nothing comparable to a magnifying glass or microscope to improve one's touch. In the haptic world of the blind, as a result, objects may lose their individualizing or distinctive features; different forks may all be apprehended simply as "fork" (Révész, 1950). The common view is that young children are especially prone to deal with objects manually, yet Abravanel (1972) found that young children compared visual shapes more accurately than haptic shapes and even preferred to rely on visual information when comparing test shapes with a haptic standard.

The lack of spatial acuity in touch ought to be less of a drawback in discerning texture or hardness than in discerning shape or contour, because no particular detail on a surface is critical for defining its texture or hardness. Thus, "texture perception, unlike shape perception, is performed frequently and easily by *both* vision and touch" (Chapter 4). In touch, texture might be encoded in a temporal or spatiotemporal manner, rather than in a spatial manner, by the vibration sense.

Révész (1950) emphasized the temporal factor, too, when he said that haptics suffers because, unlike vision, it receives its input in a piece-meal, successive manner. A blind person's "tactile movements are too many and too much divided into separate acts to enable him to arrive at a . . . total impression" (p. 83) of a form. Révész thus raised "a strong challenge to the pretended *universality* of the so-called Gestalt laws of perception" (p. 130), which had been developed in vision, with its si-multaneous mode. In haptics, "in which the comparatively independent parts tend to retain their independence, one can hardly speak of an integrative function" (p. 202); the sculptures of the early blind "lack the totality of form which we encounter in those who have lost their sight at a later period of life" (p. 233).

Kirman (1973) has said that whereas the eye excels in coding spatial patterns and the ear in coding temporal patterns, the skin is best suited for coding spatiotemporal patterns. Braille has been relatively successful because it provides spatiotemporal, rather than spatial information to the reader, but it might be much improved, according to Kirman, if the successive stimuli could be related to each other in a more coherent manner allowing an extended spatiotemporal pattern to emerge from their sequential presentation.

Texture. Katz dealt with a wealth of tactual information, but above all, he was concerned with texture or microstructure. As Gibson (1962) pointed out, Katz was more interested in the fine structure of the surface, the substance of the object, rather than its shape. Katz considered the micro-structure to be independent of the macrostructure; no matter how a piece of wood is carved, for example, it keeps the same grain or texture. It is interesting to speculate on whether Katz's intense involvement with vi-bration preceded and thus led to that with texture, or vice versa.

In his classic volume on vision, Katz (1935) showed perhaps an even greater concern for microstructure. A similar emphasis is evident, too, in Gibson's (1950) analysis of visual texture gradients. Gibson (1966) said that the visual "texture of a surface is probably even more important to animals than its pigment color in identifying it" (p. 126). Similarly, Katz said that "color can deceive, but texture cannot do so as easily" (1925, p. 33). Thus, Katz and Gibson both saw great potential in texture, even though it is very irregular at the lowest level: "We might even say that regularity within irregularity of elements is the law of material structure" (1925, p. 36; 1935, p. 88). Katz's concern with microstructure (ground) goes somewhat against the grain of Gestalt psychology, in which macro-structure (form and its contours – figure) seems largely to preempt other concerns. Nuances, textures, and meanings may attach to events that involve holistic perception but do not properly fall under the rubric of form. "All forms are wholes, but . . . not all wholes are forms" (1950, p. 39). Admittedly, shape typically provides better information for identifying objects than does texture, especially if solid, three-dimensional objects are presented, and older children seem to prefer to match on the basis of shape rather than texture (see Chapter 4). However, Katz was more interested in substance identification (e.g., whether an object is made of cloth or paper–*Spezifikationen*) than in object identification (e.g., whether an object is a hammer or a hoe).

In achieving the objective pole, reflected energy may be crucial because of the information it provides on texture or microstructure, both in vision and in touch. Among exteroceptive systems, then, vision and touch may most fully favor the objective pole, because these two senses are best suited to conveying considerable information about the fine-grain structure of materials and objects. It may be no accident, then, that Katz devoted his main attention to touch (Katz, 1925) and vision (Katz, 1935), and that Gibson likewise devoted his attention to touch (Gibson, 1962, 1966) as well as to vision (Gibson, 1950, 1979).

In vision, according to Katz (1935), the presence of a heterogeneous microstructure enables the observer to perceive surface (vs. film) colors and thereby to dissociate the illuminated objects or surface (reflectance or albedo) from the illumination (emitters). The film mode is more subjective, but the illuminant mode is seemingly the most subjective of all, because in that mode the only external entity perceived is the emitter itself. In touch, the presence of surface texture enables the observer to use felt vibration to identify various materials.

Texture differs from edges in terms of the spatial frequency information available. If the edges are not abrupt and the regions bounded are large, then the changes present will be solely of low spatial frequency. On the other hand, texture involves closely spaced discontinuities, so its changes will be mainly of high spatial frequency. High spatial frequency information is also present in the fine details and features of the letters and words we read, though low spatial frequency information may help us to segment and segregate the words. It will be interesting to see whether the spatial frequency work in vision can be generalized to the tactual domain; the fundamental spatial frequency of a grating seems not to affect its felt roughness, however (see Chapter 4).

Vibration. What may initially have turned Katz from the pressure sense to the vibration sense was the great sensitivity of his subjects to differences

42

in the smoothness of paper and other flat materials, a sensitivity evident in the lips and toes as well as the fingers. (Toe sensitivity he took to indicate that the particular prior experience of a touch organ does not affect the surface quality perceived. As to lip sensitivity, he detected differences in odor among the papers he used, but he thought, perhaps incorrectly, that these cues did not contribute to the performance with lips.) His subjects readily discriminated whether two sheets of paper had the same surface texture, even when the papers did not differ enough to have produced different pressure sensations. Performance was surprisingly good when blindfolded subjects made absolute judgments of what they were touching and what material it was (e.g., wood, glass, metal, cloth). Differences in heat transfer and the temperature impression of the materials also aided identification (see below). When surface irregularities or bumps were large enough to be felt by the pressure sense, as with raised braille characters, subjects moved the hand in slow sweeps, in contrast to the fast passes made in judging roughness.

That vibrations did occur when the fingers swept over the materials is attested to by the need for Katz to stop up the subjects' ears to keep out telltale noises. Recognition and discrimination were almost as good when the subjects ran a pencil, rather than their fingertips, over the material. Performance was greatly disrupted, though, when the pencil was swaddled in felt or cloth to damp the transmitted vibrations. When later questioned, subjects said that the vibrations felt in the fingers and hand provided the basis for their judgments. Recognition declined very little, much less than would be expected if pressure sensations played a major role, when Katz coated subjects' fingers with a 0.1-mm layer of collodion or a 0.2-mm layer of adhesive tape. The collodion fills in irregularities on the skin surface, thus perhaps excluding the pressure sense, yet only slightly dampens the vibrations, producing slightly "deaf" fingers. The collodion layer transforms the felt impression, so that when each hand touches a different surface, the surfaces are discriminated better if both hands are coated, or both are uncoated, than if one is coated and the other is not. Katz likened the effect of the coating to the veiling effect of an episcotister. Katz could have gone further and likened the veiling to the perception of the illumination level in vision, as noted above.

Subjects could even discriminate fairly well among such materials as wood, porcelain, metal, and paper by hitting them with a hammer. Even when the hammer made contact with an iron plate for barely 3 to 5 msec, the blow and the resulting vibrations nevertheless produced confident recognition of the material.

Katz found that the felt roughness increased when materials were moved across the stationary fingers with increased force. Lederman (1974, 1978; Chapter 4) similarly found that felt roughness increased when the fingertip force exerted on a grooved plate or piece of sandpaper increased. Katz said that increasing the force may increase the felt roughness either (1) by increasing the resistance of the hand to the movement or (2) by producing stronger vibrations on the skin. Katz demonstrated that the perception of roughness and the recognition of a material could not be based on the frictional resistance. He glued two sheets of different texture back to back, then ran one hand down the composite sheet with the thumb on one side and the index and middle fingers on the other. He clearly perceived two different impressions at the same time. That the resistance felt in the hand is irrelevant to the judgment of roughness has been demonstrated, too, by Taylor and Lederman (1975). They lubricated a grooved aluminum plate with liquid detergent to reduce the coefficient of friction, and thus the resistance felt in the hand, but found no change in felt roughness when subjects moved their fingers across the soaped plate rather than a dry one.

Katz found that applying sticky glue to the fingers increased the resistance felt, yet made all papers feel very smooth, because no vibrations were produced. The absence of vibrations was confirmed by the lack of noise heard when the ear was brought close to the touched surface. (An increase in lateral or shearing force, rather than a decrease in vibrations, might account for the increased smoothness in this case, however; see Chapter 4.)

Cooling "deafened" the fingers and rendered Katz's subjects incapable of discriminating between some papers and recognizing some materials. Such a loss shows once again that the roughness felt does not depend exclusively on how much force is expended in moving the touch organ. Finally, touching a paper with five fingers, instead of one finger, increases the resistance but not the roughness felt.

Medium hand speed gave the best performance, but Katz's subjects by no means maintained a constant speed. Moving the hand faster produces a "higher-pitched" vibration, so to maintain an invariant impression of a material, the subject must take both pitch and hand speed into account. Katz wrapped a long strand of wire around a pencil, thus forming a series of ridges, and had subjects move their fingers, at different speeds, over the ridges. Judgments on roughness remained essentially the same over a 10-fold range in speed (1 to 10 cm per second). Lederman (1974) likewise found little change in felt roughness over a 25-fold range in speed (1 to 25 cm per second). Like Katz, she found that a material feels slightly smoother at a higher rate of hand movement.

Pressure. Katz conceded that in some cases, such as when there are high bumps on a surface, pressure sensations may greatly influence judgments of roughness. He also noted, from his own experience, that vibration sensations contribute little to the impressions produced by broken-up materials, such as sand, sugar, and meal. And the pressure sense may contribute to the fair discrimination obtained when the fingers are moved above and then down onto a material. Increasing the pressure changes the impression qualitatively; Katz cited Titchener, who said that as the pressure grows, the sensation first is bright, then becomes heavier and more fixed, and finally takes on a grainlike feel.

Katz said that the ability to recognize slight differences in level on a surface may be greatly developed with practice. He cited the case of a deaf–blind girl who could read large headlines in newspapers and the numbers on paper money simply by feeling the slight indentations. "Indeed, the refinement of the sense of touch, brought to a peak by practice, should be able to explain many performances by mediums who claim to have a telepathic power"(1925, pp. 109–110).

Pressure sensitivity may be involved in other complex phenomena as well. When Katz's subjects tried to discriminate papers that differed in thickness, the difference thresholds he found were very small for his thinnest sheets and very large for the thicker sheets. More interestingly, he found three distinct stages in the judgmental process as thicker and thicker sheets were compared. With the thinnest sheets, the fingers could feel each other, and the sheet served as a thin veil; a difference in the thickness of such a veil could be easily detected. With intermediate thickness, the major clue was flexibility and how the sheet bent. The thickest sheets, which bent little, finally forced subjects to differentiate sheets by how far apart the fingers felt, a rather imprecise piece of information.

Elasticity. The pressure sense is not necessary for the impression of elasticity, because the elasticity of a rubber band may be felt by crunching it between the teeth. Katz regarded the articular or muscle sense as the chief participant in the feeling of elasticity. Katz and Stephenson (1938) found that a weight on a spring felt equally as heavy as a free weight weighing only 60 percent as much. Thus, an elastic pull of 4 kg felt only as heavy as a 2.5-kg dead weight. I would posit that a fixed weight feels heavier because it tends to be objectified and apprehended as something more distinct from the person. This factor, along with the elastic properties of the muscles themselves, might account for a related effect. Katz and MacLeod (1949) asked subjects to lift a weight and then squeeze a dynamometer with the same amount of effort. Subjects produced 10 times as large a pull on the dynamometer as justified by the weight lifted.

There may be a simpler explanation for these results, however. The elastic pull or grasp may have triggered sensory inputs, such as vibrations, that provided feedback to facilitate the motor commands and thus reduced the heaviness experienced. Functional cooperation between index finger and thumb provides the highly evolved human precision grip, and McCloskey and Gandevia (1978) reported that electrical stimulation of the index finger makes a weight lifted by the thumb feel lighter. They also found that a weight lifted at the wrist feels lighter if a piece of rubber tubing is grasped by the hand rather than just rests on the hand. When the hand grasps a vibrating object, there may be a "magnet reaction," with the fingers adhering to the object and forming a grip that is difficult to loosen (Torebjörk, Hagbarth, & Eklund, 1978).

Yet another explanation is also possible. An object on an elastic band may feel lighter because the bounce or movement it gets makes it feel larger or more voluminous out in space. An object on a fixed-length string, by contrast, ought to feel denser or more concentrated, because it can be more definitely localized at a single point in haptic space. Thus, Katz may have uncovered a touch analog to the size–weight illusion in vision, in which a pound of feathers feels much lighter than a pound of lead. In both vision and touch, perceived heaviness may depend in part on perceived density.

Katz (1937b) investigated what bakers meant when they used terms such as *good body, good spring, lively, good elasticity,* and *claylike* to describe flour. He found that good body means that a dough has a minimum of stickiness. The "general feeling of unpleasantness towards sticky things is very likely to be an important factor in the tendency of the baker to make his dough as little sticky as possible" (p. 389). Katz did not report, though, whether using sticky dough produces bread that is any less appetizing after it is baked. He found that increasing the water added by 1 to 2 percent was sufficient to produce a discriminable difference in stickiness. He observed, too, that "in the impression of stickiness we have coolness as an important component" (p. 388). Sullivan (1923) similarly reported that a temperature component was needed in order for liquidity or semiliquidity to be felt instead of solidity.

Katz thought that the difference between lively and claylike or dead was based upon the coordination of antagonistic muscles. After the fingers move together and touch, there is a short opposite movement or bounce. An elastic dough will help this reflex movement, but not a dough of poor elasticity. One feels full of life, the other feels dead.

In one test, bakers judged the dough very well just from watching Katz handle it. Thus, in one case at least, "the sense of vision is very likely to be educated by the sense of touch" (p. 388). Similarly, Kennedy (1978) noted that complex visible events often reveal the underlying nonvisual features; we can tell which of two objects is harder, for example, when we see them collide. "In the jerk of the twig from which a bird has just flown, we read its flexibility or elasticity" (Merleau-Ponty, 1962, p. 230).

Temperature. Katz considered the temperature sense, not the pressure sense, to be the second most important source of tactual information after vibration. This reveals again that Katz was more concerned with an object's substance or material than with its shape or contour. A material's ability to conduct heat represents the same kind of invariant property as its ability to reflect light (reflectance or albedo). Metals feel positively cold. And wools feel positively warm, even though wool must rise to body temperature if it is initially cooler. In one task, blindfolded subjects were able to order materials that had about the same specific heat in a series according to heat conductance. Recognition of materials such as glass and metal was markedly disrupted by shortening the presentation interval or by artificially heating the materials. The temperature Gestalt of a material also depends on its capacity to absorb heat; if the material takes an unusual form (e.g., tin foil), or if the perceiver is in a very warm environment, I might add, then an anomalous temperature Gestalt may arise.

Temperature sensitivity aids more in identifying characteristically cold materials, perhaps because such materials are relatively rare. Katz might have considered other explanations as well. Cold materials might be more salient because they deviate more from the neutral point than do warm materials, due to the great ability of the metals to conduct heat away from the skin surface, or because there are nearly 10 times as many cold spots as warm spots on the skin (von Frey, 1904). In any case, shortening the duration of contact impedes recognition more for cold than for warm materials. Also, Katz's subjects made larger movements over the cold materials, perhaps to prevent any local buildup of heat on the surface of the materials and thus to sharpen the sensation of cold.

A buffer medium between the skin and an object may let vibrations through but seriously disrupt temperature sensitivity, thereby destroying the liveliness of the touch impression. The resulting stiff, dead feeling may explain why amputees often prefer to touch things directly with the bare stump rather than by means of an artificial device, Katz noted. However, the temperature sense is in part a distance sense, because a person may form a temperature impression of a material that is felt through a thin layer of another substance.

Touching through a cloth. The procedure that craftsmen such as carpenters (Kennedy, 1978) and automobile body inspectors (Lederman, 1978; Chapter 4) use to examine the finish on surfaces – wiping the surface with a paper or rag, or while wearing a cotton glove – has recently been studied (Gordon & Cooper, 1975; Lederman, 1978). Gordon and Cooper found that the orientation of a surface undulation is better detected when one runs a thin, intermediate paper across a surface rather than the bare fingers. An intervening paper or cloth might also help in reading braille. Katz described one blind person who "could read Braille text well with cloth or suede gloves, and very well through kid leather gloves" (1925, p. 150). According to a teacher at a home for the blind, some blind girls who have to memorize material "try to make this task easier for themselves by placing the Braille text under an apron and then reading it through the apron" (1925, p. 150).

There is an interesting visual analog to touching through a cloth. Contrast effects between adjacent regions are greater with textureless, filmy stimuli, and color contrast is enhanced if a thin tissue paper blurs the surface texture. "Viewing a gray paper on a colored background through a thin tissue paper enhances contrast. The phenomena of tissue contrast has been known for a hundred years, but the basis for it is still unknown" (Beck, 1972, p. 41). This visual effect differs from the one involving touch, however, in that the intervening paper does not move as the eye scans over it; if the hand likewise were to scan over a stationary intervening paper, performance would be hurt, not improved by inserting the paper (S. J. Lederman, pers. comm., November 1979).

The thin intermediate paper or cloth may improve performance by turning off the light–pressure system that produces felt roughness and that might normally mask the deeper receptors (Gordon & Cooper, 1975). The paper might also help by eliminating potentially distracting temperature sensations. What Katz might have said, too, is that by veiling the vibrations that normally reveal the surface texture, the paper would allow one to attend more fully to the surface contours via the pressure sense. Vibrations might be felt to occur on the intervening paper, but the object's contours would be localized farther out in space.

With the bare fingers, the impression of surface bumps might tend to be merged with other properties perceived at the same location. Information on roughness and hardness may be salient when least wanted. Thus, "touching movements which endeavor in vain to discern the sequence of Braille letters, nevertheless provide us spontaneously with information on the roughness of the paper upon which they are pressing" (Katz, 1925, pp. 111–112). A reductive procedure, such as using an intervening paper or apron, might aid touch by enabling the person to attend to the bumps rather than to the surface. Katz cited a case in which the surface impression changed radically, depending on whether an intervening medium was used. "A glass plate was set into vibration. When I move my bare finger over it, then I feel a vibrating surface of smooth glass. If I touch the glass with a little rod, however, then the illusion of a rough surface comes through quite clearly" (1925, p. 236).

Contrary to Gordon and Cooper, however, the thin intermediate paper may not work in a reductive fashion. Lederman (1978; Chapter 4) found that the paper increased rather than decreased the felt roughness. This might be due to a reduction in shear force, but it is also possible, Lederman said, that the intermediate paper is an amplifier, not an attenuator, because its edges catch on surface irregularities. The intervening paper might have been an effective amplifier because the skin itself is too smooth to catch on small surface irregularities. If so, then a rough paper ought to work better than a smooth paper. Lederman (pers. comm., November 1979) confirmed this prediction; the rougher (nonglossy) side of the intermediate paper works better, and she always uses this side in her tests.

If the paper amplified the roughness present in the sandpaper Lederman (1978) used, then its effect ought to become more evident as the coarseness of the sandpaper increases (i.e., grit number decreases). However, Lederman's data indicate little or no tendency for the roughness added by the intervening paper to grow as coarseness increases. The contribution of the intervening paper to perceived roughness remained constant in absolute magnitude, and even decreased in relative magnitude, as grit number decreased and the sandpaper felt rougher. This indicates that the paper's effect is largely independent of, or additive to, the effect of the underlying sandpaper. Perhaps slight tremors or micro-motions, which must have occurred between paper and hand as the paper was wiped across the sandpaper, generated the separate roughness component added by the paper. If the paper had been glued to the fingers, it might have added less to the felt roughness.

The problem with the bare fingers may be that they have evolved so as to enhance the performatory function of the hand rather than its perceptual function. Katz mentioned that workmen moisten their hands in order to get a better grip on an ax or spade, and that for the same reason the hand may be well endowed with sweat glands and not covered with hair. Even the slight normal moisture on the fingers ought to make them somewhat sticky. As mentioned above, when Katz applied sticky glue to the fingers, all papers felt very smooth. An intervening paper thus might increase felt roughness, as well as sensitivity to details, merely by eliminating the stickiness due to perspiration. Perhaps an antiperspirant applied to the fingers would work just as well as an intervening paper in improving one's touch.

Acknowledgments

The author is grateful to Denis J. D'Avello, Richard D. Gilson, Seth N. Greenberg, John M. Kennedy, Susan J. Lederman, Michael Luthman, Dean H. Owen, Ronald G. Shapiro, and William Schiff for helpful comments on earlier versions of this chapter.

References

Abravanel, E. How children combine vision and touch when perceiving the shape of objects. *Perception & Psychophysics*, 1972, *12*, 171–175.

Arnheim, R. David Katz, 1884–1953. *American Journal of Psychology*, 1953, *66*, 638–642.

Association for Research in Nervous and Mental Disease. *The frontal lobes*. Baltimore: Williams & Wilkins, 1948.

Attneave, F., & Benson, B. Spatial coding of tactual stimulation. *Journal of Experimental Psychology*, 1969, *81*, 216–222.

Bartley, S. H. The perception of size or distance based on tactile and kinaesthetic data. *Journal of Psychology*, 1953, *36*, 401–408.

Beck, J. *Surface color perception*. Ithaca, N.Y.: Cornell University Press, 1972.

Békésy, G. von. *Sensory inhibition*. Princeton, N.J.: Princeton University Press, 1967.

Berkeley, G. Essays toward a new theory of vision, 1709. In A. C. Fraser (Ed.), *Selections from Berkeley* (ed. 6). Oxford: Clarendon Press, 1910.

Boring, E. G. *Sensation and perception in the history of experimental psychology*. New York: Appleton-Century-Crofts, 1942.

Visual perception as invariance. *Psychological Review*, 1952, *59*, 141–148.

Broad, C. D. Some elementary reflexions on sense-perception. In R. J. Swartz (Ed.), *Perceiving, sensing, and knowing*. Garden City, N.Y.: Doubleday, 1965, pp. 29–48.

Brown, T. *Lectures on the philosophy of the human mind*, vol. 1. Hallowell: Glazier, Masters and Smith, 1838.

Brunswik, E. *Perception and representative design of psychological experiments*. Berkeley: University of California Press, 1956.

Clark, W. C., & Yang, J. C. Acupunctural analgesia? Evaluation by signal detection theory. *Science*, 1974, *184*, 1096–1098.

Coren, S., Porac, C., & Ward, L. M. *Sensation and perception*. New York: Academic Press, 1979.

Craig, J. C. Vibrotactile pattern recognition and masking. In G. Gordon (Ed.), *Active touch. The mechanism of recognition of objects by manipulation: a multidisciplinary approach*. Oxford: Pergamon Press, 1978, pp. 229–242.

Frey, M. von. *Vorlesungen über Physiologie*. Berlin: Springer, 1904. Excerpt reprinted in R. J. Herrnstein & E. G. Boring (Eds.), *A source book in the history of psychology*. Cambridge, Mass.: Harvard University Press, 1965, pp. 49–58.

Geldard, F. A. The perception of mechanical vibration: I. History of a controversy. *Journal of General Psychology*, 1940, 22, 243–269. (a)

The perception of mechanical vibration: II. The response of pressure receptors. *Journal of General Psychology*, 1940, 22, 271–280. (b)

The perception of mechanical vibration: IV. Is there a separate "vibratory sense"? *Journal of General Psychology*, 1940, 22, 291–308. (c)

Gescheider, G. A. Temporal relations in cutaneous stimulation. In F. A. Geldard (Ed.), *Conference on cutaneous communication systems and devices*. Austin, Tex.: Psychonomic Society, 1974, pp. 33–37.

Gibson, J. J. Adaptation, aftereffect, and contrast in the perception of curved lines. *Journal of Experimental Psychology*, 1933, 16, 1–31.

The perception of the visual world. Boston: Houghton Mifflin, 1950.

The visual field and the visual world: a reply to Professor Boring. *Psychological Review*, 1952, 59, 149–151.

The concept of the stimulus in psychology. *American Psychologist*, 1960, 16, 694–703.

Observations on active touch. *Psychological Review*, 1962, 69, 477–491.

The useful dimensions of sensitivity. *American Psychologist*, 1963, 18, 1–15.

The senses considered as perceptual systems. Boston: Houghton Mifflin, 1966.

The ecological approach to visual perception. Boston: Houghton Mifflin, 1979.

Gombrich, E. H. The sky is the limit: the vault of heaven and pictorial vision. In R. B. MacLeod & H. L. Pick, Jr. (Eds.), *Perception: essays in honor of James J. Gibson*. Ithaca, N.Y.: Cornell University Press, 1974.

Gordon, G. (Ed.) *Active touch. The mechanism of recognition of objects by manipulation: a multidisciplinary approach*. Oxford: Pergamon Press, 1978.

Gordon, I. E., & Cooper, C. Improving one's touch. *Nature*, 1975, 256, 203–204.

Gray, J. *The psychology of fear and stress*. New York: McGraw-Hill, 1971.

Hahn, J. F. Vibratory adaptation. In F. A. Geldard (Ed.), *Conference on cutaneous communication systems and devices*. Austin, Tex.: Psychonomic Society, 1974, pp. 6–8.

Hamlyn, D. W. *Sensation and perception: a history of the philosophy of perception*. New York: Humanities Press, 1961.

Hay, J. C., Pick, H. L., Jr., & Ikeda, K. Visual capture produced by prism spectacles. *Psychonomic Science*, 1965, 2, 215–216.

Heller, M. A. Tactile retention: reading with the skin. *Perception & Psychophysics*, 1980, 27, 125–130.

Hirst, R. J. Sensa. In P. Edwards (Ed.), *The encyclopedia of philosophy*, vol. 7. New York: Macmillan, 1967, pp. 407–415.

Hochberg, J. Attention, organization, and consciousness. In D. I. Mostofsky (Ed.), *Attention: contemporary theory and analysis*. New York: Appleton-Century-Crofts, 1970, pp. 99–124.

James, W. *The principles of psychology*, vol. 2. New York: Holt, 1890.

Katz, D. Der Aufbau der Tastwelt. *Zeitschrift für Psychologie*, 1925, Ergänzungsband 11. (The monograph was originally published by Johann Ambrosius Barth in Leipzig and was reissued in German in 1969 by Wissenschaftliche Buchgesellschaft in Darmstadt.)

The vibratory sense and other lectures. University of Maine Studies, Second Series, No. 14. *The Maine Bulletin*, 1930, 32, 1–163.

The world of colour. (Translated by R. B. MacLeod & C. W. Fox.) London: Kegan, Paul, Trench, Trubner, 1935. (Reissued by Johnson Reprint, a subsidiary of Academic Press.)

A sense of touch: the technique of percussion, palpation and massage. *British Journal of Physical Medicine*, 1936, 11 (Old Series), 146–148.

Methoden zur Untersuchung des Vibrationssinnes. In E. Abderhalden (Ed.), *Handbuch der biologischen Arbeitsmethoden*. Section 5, Part 7, II. Berlin: Urban & Schwarzenberg, 1937, pp. 879–918. (a)

Studies on test baking. III. The human factor in test baking. A psychological study. *Cereal Chemistry*, 1937, *14*, 382–396. (b)

Gestalt psychology: its nature and significance. (Translated by R. Tyson.) New York: Ronald Press, 1950.

Katz, D., & MacLeod, R. B. The mandible principle in muscular action. *Acta Psychologica*, 1949, *6*, 33–39.

Katz, D., & Stephenson, W. Experiments on elasticity. *British Journal of Psychology*, 1938, *28*, 190–194.

Kellogg, W. N. Sonar system of the blind. *Science*, 1962, *137*, 399–404.

Kennedy, J. M. Haptics. In E. C. Carterette & M. P. Friedman (Eds.), *Handbook of perception*, vol. 8. New York: Academic Press, 1978, pp. 289–318.

Kenshalo, D. R. The cutaneous senses. In J. W. Kling & L. A. Riggs (Eds.), *Woodworth & Schlosberg's experimental psychology* (ed. 3). New York: Holt, Rinehart & Winston, 1971, pp. 117–168.

Kirman, J. H. Tactile communication of speech: a review and an analysis. *Psychological Bulletin*, 1973, *80*, 54–74.

Knops, L. Contribution à l'étude de la "naissance" et de la "permanence" phénoménales dans le champ visuel. In A. Michotte et al. (Eds.), *Miscellanea Psychologica Albert Michotte*. Louvain: Publications Université de Louvain, 1947, pp. 562–610. (Reprinted in A. Michotte et al. (Eds.), *Causalité, permanence et réalité phénoménales*. Louvain: Publications Université de Louvain, 1962, pp. 299–346.)

Konorski, J. *Integrative activity of the brain: an interdisciplinary approach*. Chicago: University of Chicago Press, 1967.

Krueger, L. E. David Katz's Der Aufbau der Tastwelt (The world of touch): a synopsis. *Perception & Psychophysics*, 1970, *7*, 337–341.

Lederman, S. J. Tactile roughness of grooved surfaces: the touching process and effects of macro- and microsurface structure. *Perception & Psychophysics*, 1974, *16*, 385–395.

"Improving one's touch" . . . and more. *Perception & Psychophysics*, 1978, *24*, 154–160.

Mack, A. Three modes of visual perception. In H. L. Pick, Jr., & E. Saltzman (Eds.), *Modes of perceiving and processing information*. Hillsdale, N.J.: Erlbaum, 1978, pp. 171–186.

MacLeod, R. B. David Katz, 1884–1953. *Psychological Review*, 1954, *61*, 1–4.

McCloskey, D. I., & Gandevia, S. C. Roles of inputs from skin, joints and muscles and of corollary discharges, in human discriminatory tasks. In G. Gordon (Ed.), *Active touch. The mechanism of recognition of objects by manipulation: a multidisciplinary approach*. Oxford: Pergamon Press, 1978, pp. 177–187.

Merleau-Ponty, M. *Phenomenology of perception*. (Translated by C. Smith.) London: Routledge & Kegan Paul, 1962.

Michotte, A. A propos de la permanence phénoménale faits et théories. *Acta Psychologica*, 1950, *7*, 298–322. (Reprinted in A. Michotte et al. (Eds.), *Causalité, permanence et réalité phénoménales*. Louvain: Publications Université de Louvain, 1962, pp. 347–371.)

Millar, S. Aspects of memory for information from touch and movement. In G. Gordon (Ed.), *Active touch. The mechanism of recognition of objects by manipulation: a multidisciplinary approach*. Oxford: Pergamon Press, 1978, pp. 215–227.

Natsoulas, T. Residual subjectivity. *American Psychologist*, 1978, *33*, 269–283.

Neisser, U. *Cognitive psychology*. New York: Appleton-Century-Crofts, 1967.

Paillard, J., Brouchon-Viton, M., & Jordan, P. Differential encoding of location cues by active and passive touch. In G. Gordon (Ed.), *Active touch. The mechanism of recognition of objects by manipulation: a multidisciplinary approach*. Oxford: Pergamon Press, 1978, pp. 189–196.

Paul, G. A. Is there a problem about sense-data? In R. J. Swartz (Ed.), *Perceiving, sensing, and knowing*. Garden City, N.Y.: Doubleday, 1965, pp. 271–287.

Petit, J., & Galifret, Y. Sensory coupling function and the mechanical properties of the skin. In G. Gordon (Ed.), *Active touch. The mechanism of recognition of objects by manipulation: a multidisciplinary approach*. Oxford: Pergamon Press, 1978, pp. 19–27.

Pick, A. D. Improvement of visual and tactual form discrimination. *Journal of Experimental Psychology*, 1965, *69*, 331–339.

Pick, H. L., Jr., & Saltzman, E. (Eds.). *Modes of perceiving and processing information*. Hillsdale, N.J.: Erlbaum, 1978.

Pitcher, G. *A theory of perception*. Princeton, N.J.: Princeton University Press, 1971.

Prince, H. H. The causal theory. In R. J. Swartz (Ed.), *Perceiving, sensing, and knowing*. Garden City, N.Y.: Doubleday, 1965, pp. 394–437.

Quilliam, T. A. The structure of finger print skin. In G. Gordon (Ed.), *Active touch. The mechanism of recognition of objects by manipulation: a multidisciplinary approach*. Oxford: Pergamon Press, 1978, pp. 1–18.

Reid, T. *An inquiry into the human mind*. Originally published in 1764. T. Duggan (Ed.). Chicago: University of Chicago Press, 1970.

Essays on the intellectual powers of man. Originally published in 1785. Abridged edition with notes from Sir William Hamilton and others. J. Walker (Ed.). Philadelphia: J. H. Butler, 1878.

Révész, G. *Psychology and art of the blind*. (Translated by H. A. Wolff.) London: Longmans, Green, 1950.

Rieser, J. J., & Pick, H. L., Jr. Reference systems and the perception of tactual and haptic orientation. *Perception & Psychophysics*, 1976, *19*, 117–121.

Rock, I. In defense of unconscious inference. In W. Epstein (Ed.), *Stability and constancy in visual perception: mechanisms and processes*. New York: Wiley, 1977, pp. 321–373.

Rock, I., & Harris, C. S. Vision and touch. *Scientific American*, 1967, *216*, 96–104.

Rohracher, H. Tastvorgang, Vibrationssinn und Körperschwingung. In *Essays in psychology dedicated to David Katz*. Uppsala: Almqvist & Wiksell, 1951, pp. 235–239.

Rundle, B. *Perception, sensation, and verification*. London: Oxford University Press, 1972.

Russell, B. *The analysis of mind*. New York: Macmillan, 1921.

Sakata, H., & Iwamura, Y. Cortical processing of tactile information in the first somatosensory and parietal association areas in monkeys. In G. Gordon (Ed.), *Active touch. The mechanism of recognition of objects by manipulation: a multidisciplinary approach*. Oxford: Pergamon Press, 1978, pp. 55–72.

Savage, C. W. *The measurement of sensation: a critique of perceptual psychophysics*. Berkeley: University of California Press, 1970.

Schiff, W. Perception of impending collision: a study of visually directed avoidant behavior. *Psychological Monographs*, 1965, *79*, whole no. 604.

Schiffman, H. R. *Sensation and perception: an integrated approach*. New York: Wiley, 1976.

Shaw, R., & Pittenger, J. Perceiving change. In H. L. Pick, Jr., & E. Saltzman

(Eds.), *Modes of perceiving and processing information*. Hillsdale, N.J.: Erlbaum, 1978, pp. 187–204.

Siegel, R. E. *Galen on sense perception*. New York: S. Karger, 1970.

Stein, J. Effects of parietal lobe cooling on manipulative behaviour in the conscious monkey. In G. Gordon (Ed.), *Active touch. The mechanism of recognition of objects by manipulation: a multidisciplinary approach*. Oxford: Pergamon Press, 1978, pp. 79–90.

Sullivan, A. H. The perceptions of liquidity, semi-liquidity and solidity. *American Journal of Psychology*, 1923, *34*, 531–541.

Swartz, R. J. (Ed.). *Perceiving, sensing, and knowing*. Garden City, N.Y.: Doubleday, 1965.

Taylor, M. M., & Lederman, S. J. Tactile roughness of grooved surfaces: a model and the effect of friction. *Perception & Psychophysics*, 1975, *17*, 23–36.

Taylor, M. M., Lederman, S. J., & Gibson, R. H. Tactual perception of texture. In E. C. Carterette & M. P. Friedman (Eds.), *Handbook of perception*, vol. 3. New York: Academic Press, 1973, pp. 251–272.

Torebjörk, H. E., Hagbarth, K. E., & Eklund, G. Tonic finger flexion reflex induced by vibratory activation of digital mechanoreceptors. In G. Gordon (Ed.), *Active touch. The mechanism of recognition of objects by manipulation: a multidisciplinary approach*. Oxford: Pergamon Press, 1978, pp. 197–203.

Trevarthen, C. Modes of perceiving and modes of acting. In H. L. Pick, Jr., & E. Saltzman (Eds.), *Modes of perceiving and processing information*. Hillsdale, N.J.: Erlbaum, 1978, pp. 99–136.

Vallbo, A. B., & Johansson, R. S. The tactile sensory innervation of the glabrous skin of the human hand. In G. Gordon (Ed.), *Active touch. The mechanism of recognition of objects by manipulation: a multidisciplinary approach*. Oxford: Pergamon Press, 1978, pp. 29–54.

Weber, E. H. Der Tastsinn und das Gemeingefühl. In R. Wagner (Ed.), *Handwörterbuch der Physiologie*, vol. 3, 1846, pp. 481–588. Excerpt reprinted in R. J. Herrnstein & E. G. Boring (Eds.), *A source book in the history of psychology*. Cambridge, Mass.: Harvard University Press, 1965, pp. 34–39.

White, B. W. What other senses can tell us about cutaneous communication. In F. A. Geldard (Ed.), *Conference on cutaneous communication systems and devices*. Austin, Tex.: Psychonomic Society, 1974, pp. 15–19.

White, B. W., Saunders, F. A., Scadden, L., Bach-y-Rita, P., & Collins, C. C. Seeing with the skin. *Perception & Psychophysics*, 1970, *7*, 23–27.

Williams, J. M. Synaesthetic adjectives: a possible law of semantic change. *Language*, 1976, *52*, 461–478.

Zigler, M. J. A review of David Katz's Der Aufbau der Tastwelt. *Psychological Bulletin*, 1926, *23*, 326–336.

2. The psychophysics of touch

CARL E. SHERRICK & JAMES C. CRAIG

In Chapter 2, Carl Sherrick and James Craig examine problems of measuring tactile capabilities in the context of structural and functional characteristics of receptors, physiological recording techniques, and in classical psychophysical experiments on passive touch. Theoretical issues and empirical work on active touch are then introduced, with the authors noting that the issue of what information is added by using active touch, and whether the addition appreciably improves performance, is far from settled. What seemed perfectly clear from the phenomenology of Katz, and from some early demonstrations by Gibson and co-workers, is a slippery issue as crucial experiments are attempted. The authors consider separating the exploring functions of the hand from its sensing functions. But such strategies for tactual perception might deter production of useful stimulus information via the exploratory process. If, as the authors suggest, we are in the midst of the liveliest controversy since the era of Hunter and Lashley, it is hoped that the heat generated by the questions may produce rapid advances in the field. For active touch, although recognized as important, has received far less research attention than the sensory physiology and psychophysics of the skin senses. WILLIAM SCHIFF

In preparing a chapter for a specialized handbook such as the present one, the authors are faced with at least two obligations beyond the usual ones of clear exposition and concise description. These are (1) to provide a sufficiently scholarly deposition on the fundamentals of the subject so that the reader will accept the authority of the writers when they (2) speculate on the application of those fundamentals to the topic at hand. In the best of possible worlds, the two functions of research in basic problems and the development of methods and devices for real-world application would seem to be most efficient when they are combined in a single individual. Unfortunately, this is commonly not the situation, largely because of attitudinal and motivational differences among persons in basic and applied research and partly because of the limitations of world and time.

The next best alternative to the expert in both basic and applied

55

knowledge is the dyad formed by an expert in each area, or, better yet, a triad formed by the basic researcher, the applied researcher, and the clinical or educational investigator. The latter has, one hopes, through diligent observation of cases from day to day, arrived at a system of description of problems of adaptation by patients to illness or handicaps that suggests what functions are best candidates for study in the application process, i.e., what needs there are to be met by applied research.

In searching for such triads, one finds only too rarely the appropriate environmental niche for their appearances and survival, in places such as research institutes within or across university departments or medical schools, or in industrial, government, or business organizations. In the school or associated institute, one may find the fourth member of the group – the user – who gives ultimate meaning to the efforts of the other three.

The working substitute for coherent groups of this kind is usually the scientific meeting, conference, or workshop, such as the one from which the present chapter has emerged. It may seem pessimistic to state at the outset that what is gained by the participants at these brief encounters is a fraction of the potential insight that might be achieved, a fraction whose value is proportional to the duration and intensity of the intellectual contact. The former quantity may be only the duration of the meeting itself, or it may be extended by continuing correspondence. In view of the fact that intellectual conspecifics and sympatrics tend to assemble in separate groups at conferences, the hope for cluster formations of the kind described above is justifiably faint but nonetheless eternally resilient. It is with the full awareness of the need to integrate basic research and apply it to clinical problems, as well as of the difficulty of achieving it to a significant degree, that the following exposition is presented.

The measurement of tactile capabilities

The history of attempts to use touch as a communicative sense is very long, as Geldard (1977) and Krueger (Chapter 1) have pointed out. Psychophysical measurement, involving systematic procedures for tapping relatively simple discriminative capacities of the skin, was developed toward the middle of the 19th century, mainly through the efforts of E. H. Weber (see Boring, 1942). Succeeding generations of psychologists and physiologists have often found it convenient to liken one or another capacity or quality of experience to that of one of the major senses in order to promote student understanding of the meaning of the function described. Thus, whereas for temperature sensations there are no generic terms in the major senses (quite the opposite; colors may be "warm" or "cool"), touch has made several borrowings. Pressure may be "bright," the two-point limen likened to minimum separable visual acuity, or the difference limen (DL) for vibration rate compared to the pitch difference threshold in hearing. It is well to remind ourselves at this juncture that all such analogies are supported by a few bare threads spun originally from phenomenal or physical analysis or general neuroanatomic or physiologic homologs. The danger in pursuing them for the purposes of designing communications devices is that attributes not covered by the original analogies are implied or accepted in situations in which they are wholly unsuitable. Indeed, the history of sensory substitution devices and techniques is a documentation of the evolution of thought from simplistic touch–vision or touch–hearing analogs to more sophisticated analyses that insist on testing the perceptual hypotheses with techniques developed for the tactile system (see Craig, 1976; Geldard, 1977; Kirman, 1973).

Receptor systems for touch

Structural features

There are several excellent modern sources for a description of the kinds and location of tactile receptors and their allied neural connections (see Burgess, 1974; Iggo, 1973; Quilliam, 1978). For present purposes, the receptor systems of greatest interest must be those that lie in or just proximal to the hand, especially those found in the digital skin, joints, and tendons, as well as muscles involved in hand and digit movement.

Among the receptors to be found in digital skin, there are two major groupings, free nerve endings and encapsulated nerve endings. Figure 2.1 is a semischematic depiction of endings in the human digit. Of the first group, there is inferential evidence that some of these may be embedded in intraepidermal tissue, which is the relatively thin, waterproof covering or cuticle, whereas others are more clearly visualized (in histological preparations) in the dermis as papillary nerve endings. The term *papillary* refers to the highly corrugated appearance of the skin in cross section, where the dermis alternately advances into and retreats from the epidermis. The fingerprint pattern is produced by these dermal undulations. The second group of receptors consists of Merkel disks, found in the intraepidermal tissue, Meissner corpuscles, and Pacinian corpuscles. Meissner corpuscles, like Pacinian corpuscles, are egg-shaped, but the former are found in or near the papillary tissues at the dermoepidermal

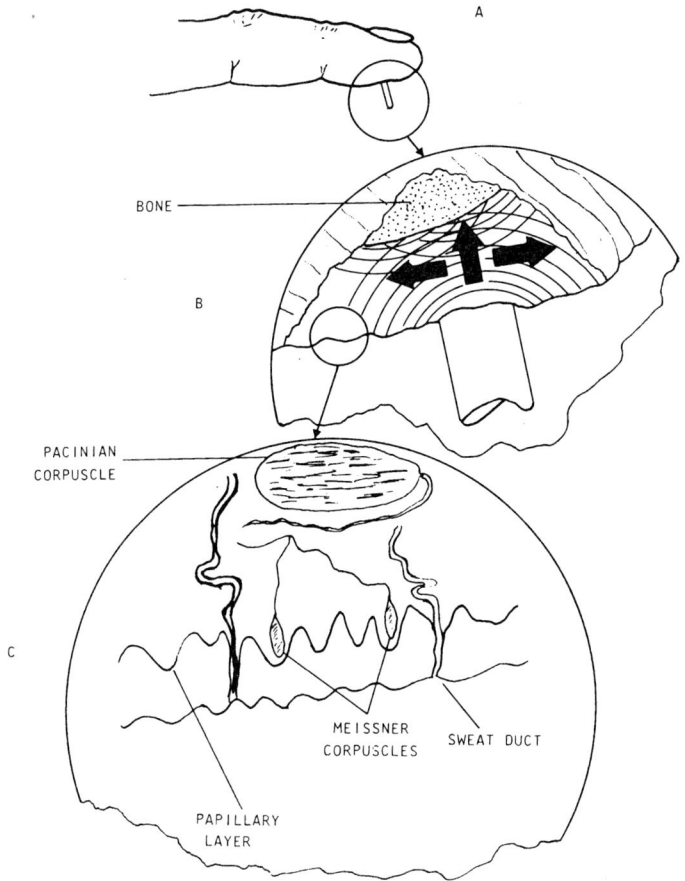

Figure 2.1 A highly schematized representation of some sensory receptors of the human finger. *A*. The index finger pressing on a small probe. *B*. A magnified cutaway view of the internal tissues, showing the physical effects of palpating. Large arrows are static forces of internal pressure; radiating lines are transient shear or compression waves propagated through the tissue and reflecting from bone. *C*. Further magnification of the subdermal area to show the disposition of receptor structures in the skin. Only two types of receptor are shown, and the congeries of other cell types are omitted for clarity.

junction and are about one-twentieth the size of the Pacinians. The latter corpuscles are probably the largest single receptor in the body, achieving a size of 1.5 by 0.5 mm, and are usually found in the subcutaneous tissues at least 2 to 3 mm below the cuticle. A third feature that differentiates the Pacinian corpuscle from the other encapsulated receptors is its frequent monopoly of a single nerve fiber, whereas the others must share their nerve fiber with several fellows. In addition, a single Meissner corpuscle may have three or more nerve fibers converging upon it. It is apparent that the structure of the peripheral cutaneous nervous system alone is a complex one, involving one-to-one receptor–nerve relations as well as many-one and one-many relations. The precise character of this schema is not yet clear, but the potential it offers for spatiotemporal coding of a great variety of mechanical impact patterns is enormous.

Functional features

Because of its large size, its characteristic appearance (oval shape, lamellated outer hull like an onion), and its dedication to a single axon, the Pacinian corpuscle is the best-understood mechanoreceptor in the somesthetic system, excluding the nonauditory labyrinth (see Loewenstein, 1971). Although there are estimated to be only about 500 to 1,000 Pacinian corpuscles in all 10 human fingers (Quilliam, 1978), the sensitivity of these bodies to mechanical impacts is such that a tissue displacement of the order of the wavelength of blue–green light (500 nm) is sufficient to trigger a nervous discharge in them. Because of their mechanical character and neurochemical properties, and those of the tissue in which they lie, these receptors show only an "on" and "off" response to the beginning and end of a static or constant displacement. For this reason, they are called *rapidly adapting receptors* and are usually spoken of as velocity-, acceleration-, or jerk-sensitive receptors (Burgess, 1974).

In a painstaking study of the distribution, receptive fields, and functional characteristics of nerves excited by sensitive tactile areas on the skin of the hand, Vallbo and Johansson (1978) described units that they characterized as Pacinian bodies, as mentioned above. These authors recorded from individual neural units in humans, mainly in the median nerve of the upper arm of alert, healthy young adults. With carefully controlled tactile stimuli and recording methods, a large number of units were examined for a variety of functional characteristics by means of this relatively new technique, called *microneurography* by some investigators. Once a typical Pacinian corpuscle response pattern is discovered by this method, its receptive field is examined by stimulating around the original "strike" with the mechanical probe and noting the nerve response. For the Pacinian body, the receptive field is usually large, with poorly defined borders and a single point of maximum sensitivity. A single Pacinian body may show a receptive field of several square centimeters. Clearly, the response of such a receptor can tell us of a minute mechanical event, as well as of its time of occurrence, but only in general where on the skin the event occurred.

In addition to finding nerve responses corresponding to the typical Pacinian corpuscle, Vallbo and Johansson found a second rapidly adapting receptor having a receptive field somewhat smaller and with more sharply defined borders, as well as several areas of peak sensitivity rather than just one. The authors have suggested that the location and behavior of this group correspond to those imputed to the Meissner corpuscle. The relatively high sensitivity of this group to transient stimuli, coupled with very good spatial "tuning," indicates its potential for registering the location as well as the timing of stimuli.

A second group of units characterized as *slowly adapting* emerged from the same experiments. Such units typically exhibit a burst of neural spikes at the onset of a static deformation, followed by a slowly diminishing firing rate over the next few seconds (Burgess, 1974). These could be subdivided, as the rapidly adapting units were, into two types with respect to receptive field size and definitiveness, and number of sensitivity peaks. The slowly adapting unit with small receptive fields showed little sensitivity to skin stretching, requiring instead an almost direct impact to excite it. The second type of slowly adapting unit, in addition to its larger, indistinct receptive field, showed sensitivity to skin stretching in particular directions. The receptor for the former unit has been tentatively identified as Merkel's disks, and for the latter as Ruffini endings, but the findings are not yet certain.

Integration of neural signals

The question that follows from the description of a set of signaling sources such as those listed above is, how are the signals coded for transmission to the brain? It is well beyond the scope of this chapter to recount in great detail the numerous investigations of nervous activity at the peripheral nerve level, in the spinal cord, and in the brainstem, thalamic nuclei, and somatosensory cortex (see Wall, 1973; Werner and Whitsel, 1973). It has been shown, for example, that the activity patterns of peripheral nerves are preserved by some fibers in the CNS, whereas other fibers respond only to the onset of activity, or its offset, or both. Yet others are quieted by the upstream (peripheral) signal, and still others respond only when correlated activities of two or more peripheral nerves occur.

At the cortex, we find a preservation of the body space across the surface of the brain, pictured in some textbooks as the *sensory homunculus* (see Geldard, 1972, p. 289). There is some preservation of temporal coding as well, and there are indications that receptor groups enjoy sepa-

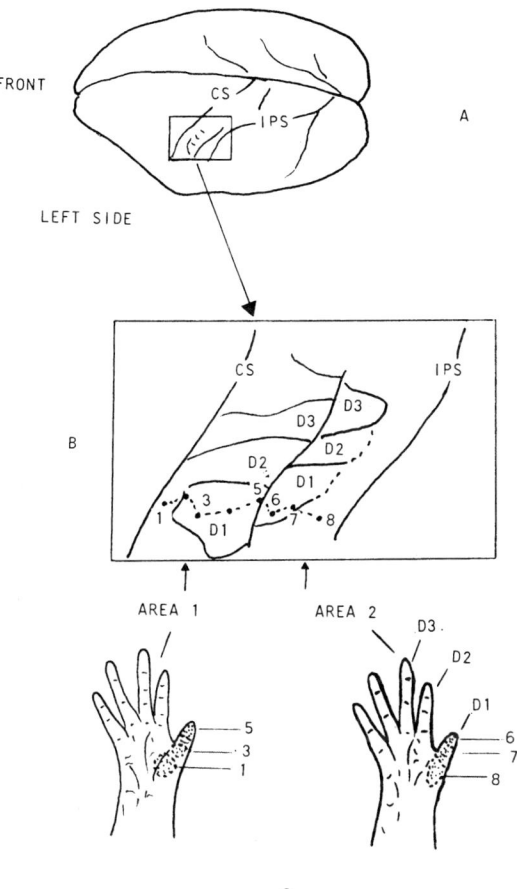

Figure 2.2. The location of fields of tactile sensitivity in the macaque (monkey) cortex, from data obtained by Kaas et al. (1979). A. The entire cortex, showing the region in which recordings were made. B. The region of recording enlarged, showing the duplex arrangement of representation (for tactile stimuli) of the digits. C. The numbered zones on the monkey's paw shown here correspond to the numbered points of recorded electrical response shown in B. The mirror-image representation is apparent from the ordering and position of the numbers. Abbreviations: CS — central sulcus; IPS — interparietal sulcus; D1, D2, D3 — digits 1 (thumb), 2 (index finger), and 3 (middle finger).

rate representation in columnar arrays in the cortical assembly (Werner and Whitsel, 1973, p. 649). Figure 2.2 depicts the location in the macaque monkey of cortical areas that respond to tactile stimuli. The diagram is derived from those of Kaas, Nelson, Sur, Lin, and Merzenich (1979), who made microelectrode recordings of potentials from the exposed cortex of

61

anesthetized monkeys while probing various sites on the body. Besides determining that there appear to be two cortical areas that completely duplicate representation of the body surface, these investigators have found evidence that a third area represents the sensitivity to heavier pressures, and that a fourth area may be present as well. The mirror-image character of two of these areas is well illustrated by Figure 2.2, which shows how recording sites (numbered on the drawing of the cortex) match the areas of stimulation on the monkey's first digit. Not all primates show evidence of redundant configurations such as those illustrated here, but it appears to be generally true that the CNS, like all bureaucratic organizations, prefers multiple copies. Even in the presence of impressive information such as this, it should be remembered that the cortex is not the proven seat of sensation but only an important link in the catenary of information processing.

It has already been stated that in attempting to determine what particular receptor systems do, the physiological technique most commonly applied is electrophysiological recording. In peripheral nerve studies, the physical stimulus of choice (say, a mechanical probe applied to a small area of intact skin) is presented to an animal (including human) preparation in which the nerve has been exposed, or in which fine, sharp electrode wires have been inserted into the tissues overlying the nerve fibers. The mechanical stimulus is moved about until the recording system shows a regular and preferably unitary neural activity in the presence of the stimulus. Once the receptive field is outlined, the investigator examines the unit's pattern of response to variations of the pattern of stimulus input. On the basis of the input–output relations thus obtained, the investigator will characterize the receptor as one of the several groups already described.

It is important to note that this method of describing receptor function, in the absence of other converging experimental operations, cannot guarantee the identification of either receptors or sensory experience, as Melzack and Wall (1962) and Wall and Dubner (1972) have pointed out for touch and Bartley (1959, p. 739) has emphasized for visual neurophysiology. It is only with the findings of psychophysical or histological parallels to neurophysiological findings that the identity of functions and structures becomes more probable. Indeed, the parallels must become more than analogies. As Mueller has noted, "Our eventual goal . . . must be to establish a correspondence between the physiological data and the behavioral data, a correspondence that must be more than generally reasonable, it must be numerically sensible" (1965, p. 101).

One may conceive of a set of receptors, A, B, C, D, in a given skin area. It is determined that receptor B responds to a sudden, brief mechanical indentation but fails to respond, after its initial activity, to a prolonged indentation. In physiological parlance, B is a rapidly-adapting tactile receptor. In the past, the term *touch receptor* has been used to describe such identifications, but this implies that when the receptor–nerve system is excited, "touch" would be the report of the subject stimulated. This is almost never the situation, of course. The subject is usually an animal that gives no behavioral evidence of experiencing touch at all; indeed, the physiologist is typically interested in receptor function, not the subject's perceptions.

In more recent years (see Hensel and Boman, 1960; Merzenich and Harrington, 1969; Talbot, Darian-Smith, Kornhuber, & Mountcastle, 1968), it has been possible to compare physiological and psychophysical performance records within or across species, sometimes within the same subject at the same time (Gybels & van Hees, 1972; Uttal, 1959) to provide the converging psychophysical–physiological operations desired for the fuller description of receptor function. Even in these cases, where the results are "numerically sensible," caution in interpretation is wanted, because one may present the stimulus, see the neural response, and hear the subject's report, yet not be certain of the total underlying process. The reason is that, whereas receptor B is on record, receptors A, C, and D are not, but their activities may well influence the final outcome as a result of the integrative processes in the CNS. That is, if one is committed to knowing the neural basis of behavior, one may not end the search when one or two functions are found to parallel the behavioral data. Receptor B's solitary activities are not the neural substrate for touch, but only an example of the contingencies that suggest the structure of the substrate. Within the substrate may be a multiplicity of neural codes that correlate with the manifold aspects of tactile perception.

Psychophysical studies of passive touch

Absolute sensitivity and its distribution over the body

In comparison with the visual and auditory systems, the sense of touch requires a large expenditure of energy for its excitation. Even so, the amount of energy required to displace a single hair on the arm enough to produce a sensation of touch was calculated by von Frey (1920) as only 0.014 erg. That would be the amount of kinetic energy in a piece of paper the size of the letter *O* on this page if dropped from a height of 1 cm. Measurements of the power delivered to the skin by a threshold vibrotactile stimulus at a frequency of 250 Hz yield values of about 0.01 μW (Sherrick, unpublished data).

A number of studies have shown that the general bodily distribution of sensitivity to tactile stimuli favors the frontal facial region and the hands of humans and other primates, with maximal sensitivities at the fingertips and lip borders (Geldard, 1972). This appears to be true not only for absolute sensitivity but for accuracy of localization and acuity for two points as well. Anatomically and physiologically, this distribution of sensitivity is supported by a high density of receptors in these regions and a large amount of available cortical space responsive to excitation of these regions.

The sensitivity of the skin to repetitive pressures or vibrotactile stimuli varies over the body, much as static pressure sensitivity does. The propagation of vibratory disturbances of long duration and the effects of temporal and spatial summation of repeated impacts combine to yield some apparent differences in distribution of sensitivity, to a degree that caused some early investigators to postulate a separate "vibratory sense" (cf. Geldard, 1940).

The response of the human observer to vibrations of different frequencies or rates is of considerable interest at present because of a series of findings by Verrillo (1963, 1968) and by Mountcastle and his colleagues (Talbot et al., 1968). The sensitivity to vibration, measured as the absolute threshold of the amplitude of skin displacement over a frequency range of 10 to 1,000 Hz, varies as a ladle-shaped curve, with the handle extending from 10 to 50 Hz and the bowl of the ladle describing a sharper-sided curve from 50 to a minimum near 250 Hz, rising quickly to a high value beyond 1,000 Hz (see Figure 2.3). It is important to note here that the function described is a highly complex one that requires carefully controlled conditions for stable replication. Moreover, modification of the contactor area, the presence of additional mechanical loads on neighboring skin surfaces, and static contactor pressure can all produce significant changes in the form of the function. In light of such effects, the complications presented by the usual paradigms in active touch are staggering.

It is the contention of Verrillo that two functions can be partialed from this complex curve by appropriate experimental means, and that they represent the response of two or more receptor systems. The physiologists agree that Pacinian corpuscles probably produce the steeper function comprising the middle frequency range, but they are uncertain about the identity of the system responsible for the low-frequency sensitivity (see, however, Merzenich & Harrington, 1969). What should be

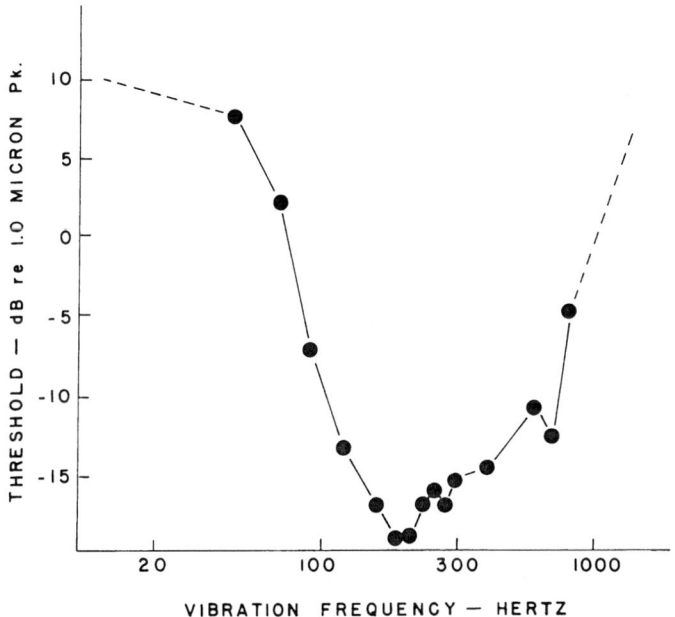

Figure 2.3. The absolute threshold for mechanical vibration of the fingertip as a function of frequency. The contactor was a 9-mm-diameter probe held to the finger with a 15-gm static force. No surround was present, and the direction of vibration was perpendicular to the skin surface. Data are the means for two observers. (From Sherrick, unpublished work)

remembered about vibrotactile sensitivity is that any transient or repetitive mechanical disturbance can be characterized as a distribution of energies across the frequency spectrum, and the frequency response of the system to sinusoidal vibrations is a reliable method for assessing the performance and sensitivity of the skin. It will not, however, disclose all the response characteristics of the system, in particular those evoked by brief, quasi-random events. Hence it cannot predict the outcome of experiments that involve complex patterns of stimulation varying both spatially and temporally.

Discrimination

What is frequently desired in a sensing system is not a high absolute sensitivity to energies but rather a high degree of selectivity, that is, a differential response to stimuli that vary in one or more aspects. In theory, there could be as many kinds of discrimination as there are aspects of a stimulus pattern, including complexes made up of simple aspects. The

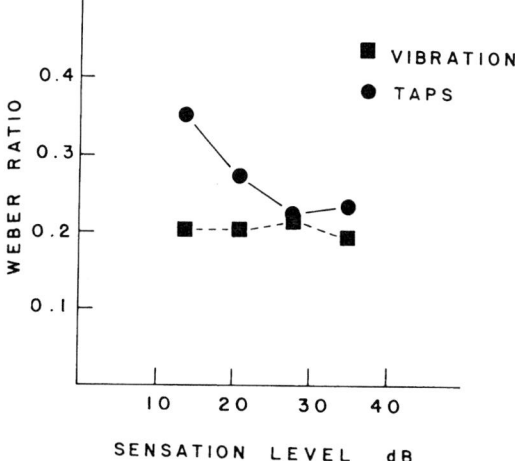

Figure 2.4. The DL for intensity of vibrotactile bursts and tactile pressure pulses, measured on the index finger with a 6-mm-diameter contactor at a static force of 20 gm and with a fixed surround present. (After Craig, 1978)

major lines of investigation have generally involved only the simple aspects, however: intensive, spatial, rate, or numerosity discriminations.

A study of the difference limen for pressure was made by E. H. Weber in the mid-nineteenth century (see Boring, 1942). The study examined what was to be called the *Weber ratio* for two different modes of applying force to the hand. The Weber ratio is defined as the increment (or decrement) of intensity required to detect a change, divided by the intensity that already exists, that is, the baseline intensity. Thus, if a person is presented with a 200-gm weight and requires on the average an additional 10 gm to note a weight increase, the Weber ratio is calculated as 10÷200 or, decimally, 0.05. The basis of classical psychophysics consists in part of the postulate that the Weber ratio is constant for all intensities. It is apparent that this assumption resembles the Perfect Gas Law of physics; it is approximately true for a large middle range of values but breaks down badly at the extremes.

The relative *difference limen (DL)*, as the Weber fraction is also called, has been determined for static pressure by a number of investigators to be about 0.14 (Boring, 1942). For impulse (tap) stimuli, Craig (1972,1974) has determined it to be about 0.2 when the signal/noise ratio is sufficiently high. For vibrations, Craig found a value of 0.2 (see Figure 2.4). It is of some interest to note that the size of the intensive DL is generally regarded as an index of acuity, that is, the smaller the DL, the more sensitive the system is. Von Békésy (1947) has noted, however, that skin

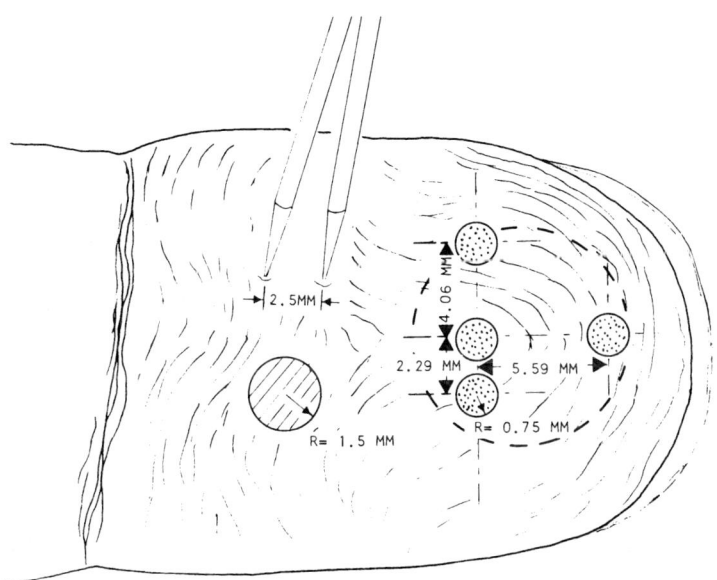

Figure 2.5. The size of the two-point limen and the error of localization on the palmar side of the index finger. Data are from Weinstein (1968). The size of the circle for the error of localization is based on the mean estimated error as described in the text. For comparison, standard braille dots are shown to scale, with the diameter of a single dot given at its base. Other dimensions shown are, in order of increasing size, the interdot, intercell, and interline distances. Values are from Nolan and Kederis (1969, p. 5). The large dashed circle around the dots represents the area covered by the vibrator used in obtaining the curve of Figure 2.3.

that has been obtunded by a topical anesthetic has a smaller DL than normal, at least near the threshold. Thus, by the criterion of absolute sensitivity, the skin is less sensitive, but by the criterion of relative sensitivity it is more sensitive.

There are many ways of measuring spatial discrimination. Of the classic methods, the two-point limen and the error of localization are the best known, and Boring (1942) has noted that there are 121 ways of determining values for the latter capacity. Weinstein (1968) has made systematic explorations of the body for these two measures and found values very similar to those of Weber, who originated the measures of spatial acuity. Figure 2.5 shows the comparative sizes of the two-point limen and the localization error on the human finger, according to Weinstein's data. The two-point limen was obtained by touching the observer's skin with the two tips of a modified draftsman's compass simultaneously and asking whether one or two points were felt. By progressive increases or decreases in the compass span over successive trials, the experimenter can determine the average separation above which the observer can always discriminate two points from a single point and below which he or she begins to fail to do so. The localization error was determined by inking a Y-shaped mark on the skin and touching the observer with a single probe at the junction point of the Y. When a second touch was presented on one of the branches of the Y, the observer was asked whether the first locus or a new locus had been touched. The farthest distance at which an incorrect response occurred was averaged over the three branches, and this mean was taken as the error of localization.

A notable anomaly found in comparing the results of the two measures has been that the error of localization is smaller than the two-point limen. One would think that it might be easier to detect the separation of two objects placed on the skin simultaneously than if the two objects were placed on the skin successively. Boring (1930) has discussed the problem at some length and has offered an explanation in terms of the methods employed, not physiology. Von Békésy (1960) has suggested that the two-point limen is evidence of what he calls *neural funneling*, a concept that involves a central core of excitation surrounded by an annular inhibitory zone. When two such funneling processes are set up in adjacent skin regions, the ratios of excitation to inhibition and their lateral spread will determine the acuity of the system. Little has been done to advance the psychophysical aspects of neural funneling theory since von Békésy's death.

Vierck and Jones (1969) tested the ability of subjects to discriminate the difference in size between two cylinders. They reported that the discrimination is surprisingly good, amounting to a value of 0.13. When compared with the value of the two-point limen for a given area, it seems to be smaller than might be predicted if the outer edges of the cylinders to be compared were viewed as point stimuli. The measurement techniques are hardly comparable, however, because the two-point limen represents a categorical judgment. One can measure the DL for greater or lesser "one-nesses" and "two-nesses," as, in fact, Friedline did (Boring, 1942, p. 482), and found them to be one-fourth of the limen.

Recently, Green (see Geldard, Sherrick, & Cholewiak, 1980) examined judgments of absolute distance between pairs of blunt probes placed on various body areas and found that there is a tendency for observers to perceive placements transverse to the body axis as shorter than longitudinal ones. Moreover, simultaneous dual stimulation will produce a definite compression or shrinkage of distance judgments in comparison to successive stimulation. These effects are not constant over all areas, nor will they persist if the spatial or temporal separation of the points exceeds certain limits. For the palm of the hand, distortions of this kind have not been so readily demonstrated as for areas such as the arm, but a complete analysis of the phenomena has not been made. It should be noted, in this connection, that small spatial and temporal separations of tactile events will generally improve the discrimination of them. The two-point limen is significantly reduced if the compass points are "rocked" over the tangent loci. We may presume that when the nervous system views events through more than one window it can detect more features, hence more potential differentia.

For the measures discussed above, time as a dimension was usually not a part of the fabric of events, except as one or more epochs in which the mechanical impacts to be compared were delivered. Thus, for example, when two disparate points were pressed on the skin in the two-point limen studies, their impacts were intended to be simultaneous in onset and offset. Similarly, studies of rate or frequency discrimination involving vibratory stimuli have usually provided controls for the simultaneous variation of spatial or intensive cues to permit assessment of "pure" rate discrimination, because it is commonly observed that frequency changes produce magnitude as well as localization shifts (Goff, 1967). A number of studies of the DL for rate of vibration have been made, of which the recent one by Rothenberg, Verrillo, Zahorian, Brachman, and Bolanowski (1977) is probably the most thorough and reliable. These authors found a relative rate DL of 0.2 at the best frequency of about 200 Hz, with a variation, over the useful frequency range of 10 to 300 Hz, of 0.5 to 0.25, for sinusoids on the forearm.

Aside from rate judgments, there are several other discriminations possible in the time domain: numerosity, successiveness, and temporal order. All of these have been examined at one time or another, with the consistent finding that the skin is inferior to the ear and superior to the eye in many of these tasks (Geldard, 1970). Lechelt (1975) has shown that the skin fails to count accurately if five pulses are presented over a 700-msec epoch, placing it between the ear and the eye in this respect. Gescheider (1974) has shown the threshold for successiveness to be about 4 msec, and Hirsh and Sherrick (1961) found the limen for perceived order to be about 20 msec, a figure matched by the ear and the eye almost exactly.

Adaptation

One of the classic studies of adaptation in the area of cutaneous sensitivity is that of Nafe and Wagoner (1941), who determined that static weights allowed to rest on the skin of the thigh were reported as yielding pressure sensations so long as the skin was moving, as determined by sensitive physical measurement. With the slowing and cessation of displacement came the report of the disappearance of sensation. In the view of these authors, adaptation of the pressure sense was synonymous with stimulus failure, that is, the disappearance or subliminal existence of the adequate stimulus of tissue movement (see Geldard, 1972, p. 300). The conclusion to be drawn is that for effective processing the skin–contactor interface must always be in motion, a lesson learned more recently (see Riggs, Ratliff, Cornsweet, & Cornsweet, 1953) for the human eye.

When the stimulating device vibrates continually, one might expect from the above conclusion that adaptation would not occur. Hahn (1966, 1968) has shown, however, that it does, in significant degrees, and takes place in at least two independent systems depending on the frequency of vibration. In a sense, the skin can be temporarily "deafened" by prolonged application of time-varying patterns, although never totally so. Von Békésy (1967, p. 11) has suggested that adaptation, far from being a failure of processing, is a built-in mechanism that serves to reduce the information load to the CNS. Thus, persisting steady-state conditions are attenuated in their level, but new transient conditions may still be effectively processed (von Békésy, 1960, p. 364; Geldard, 1972, p. 58). The mechanisms for such action are not nesessarily confined, by the way, to the periphery or to the CNS but may occur redundantly at several levels.

Masking of tactile stimuli

Like adaptation, masking generally is taken as a condition that exemplifies the failure of a sensory system to process incoming information. The usual situation for masking involves the simultaneous presence of wanted and unwanted signals, and the failure to apprehend the former or the noticeable diminution of its sensory magnitude. If the times of appearance of the two are not simultaneous, we speak of *forward* and *backward masking* effects. The first effect implies that the masker (unwanted signal) precedes the wanted signal in time, and vice versa for the second effect. In addition, the source of masking may be local, when the same general portion of the sensory surface is involved, or remote, when the masker and desired signals affect separate areas. When contralateral areas of the body are thus stimulated, the term *central masking* is sometimes used, but this application must be taken with the caveat that all processing is ultimately central, and spatial separation is only one way of partitioning blocks of input information. The famous Weber "thaler experiment" demonstrates that two putatively independent sensory systems can interact under the appropriate conditions. Weber could show that a single cold thaler (a German coin) felt heavier than two stacked warm coins. It is possible, of course, that the temperature was acting directly on the pressure receptors, and not by way of the temperature sense (cf. Stevens & Green, 1978). In connection with these observations, Sherrick (1976) has reviewed some investigations that demonstrate masking or interference effects across the major modality boundaries of touch, hearing, and vision.

The effect of masking is usually to degenerate the wanted signal, as most of us commonly note when listening to a speech in a noisy environment. In the design of tactile codes, one part of the wanted signal may mask another (see Geldard, 1962; Pickett & Pickett, 1963). Kirman (1978) has argued that there may be display designs that require mutual masking effects for the best processing (but see Chapter 6). More complex masking effects are discussed in other chapters.

Active touch

Definition of active touch

In past discussions of the distinction between active and passive touch, the hand and digits have been the primary objects for differentiation. These remarkable appendages enjoy their highest development in humans, who by virtue of their exquisite sensitivity in control, perception, and coordination with the visual system have become tool makers and users *par excellence*. As a complete closed-loop system for exploration and manipulation, the hands and fingers (in connection at times with that other sensitive area, the mouth) are second only to the visual–motor system in extracting information from space-occupying objects. For J. J. Gibson, the differentiation is straightforward: "In passive touch, the individual makes no voluntary movements" (1962, p. 489). We assume that an elaboration of this sentence would contain the qualification that those voluntary movements and their associated information input not correlated with the cutaneous stimulus patterns of interest would not be considered examples of active touch. In other words, if you are scratching your head while the experimenter places a two-point esthesiometer on your skin, the latter performance may still be regarded as passive touch, albeit a poor example of it, given the possibility of attentional perturbations and remote masking.

The point of the preceding discussion is that there is no real necessity, given present-day technology, for the touched skin to belong to the exploring hand. In the TVSS of Collins (1970), the vibrators on the back of the observer were coupled optico-electronically to the objects being "felt"; similarly, the letters being "read" by the Bliss Optacon (Bliss, Katcher, Rogers, & Shepard, 1970) are "felt" at the tactile matrix when in fact they are otherwise intangible. One of us has pointed out elsewhere that direct coupling of the sensory surfaces to the exploring member is no longer the limiting nor necessarily the preferred condition (Sherrick, 1974). The major reasons for continuing to employ the same hand for exploring and sensing are those of familiarity and convenience – by no means, let us be the first to admit, the least of considerations in any aid for the handicapped. An object that is never more than an arm's length away certainly must be both familiar and convenient, if at all usable. To return to the point of the discussion, a recent study by Schwartz, Perey, and Azulay (1975) argues against the assertion that the passive hand is less perceptive than the exploring hand. In J. J. Gibson's original experiments on passive-active perception of objects (1962, p. 486), the observers were either allowed to palpate the forms of six small cookie cutters and identify them, or they were to present the palm to the experimenter, who pressed the forms into the passive hand. For active touch, the mean percent of correct identifications was 95, whereas for the passive condition it was 49; and if in the latter condition a lever-operated (hence, more uniform) presentation was used, correct performance fell to 29 percent. In another series of trials, the forms were continually rotated after being pressed on the palm, and accuracy increased to 72 percent. Schwartz et al. compared the accuracy of identification for the same forms and some additional ones for the two conditions; in passive the restrained finger had the form moved over it in such a way that the complete contour was felt once. No difference in accuracy of performance was obtained, suggesting that, at least for contour recognition, exploratory activity is not a necessary accompaniment for accurate performance. These results do not necessarily undermine Gibson's position concerning active touch, but they suggest that the modifier "active" should not be taken to mean that motor outflow is the exclusive condition for accurate processing.

Gibson's fascinating theoretical exposition, along with his experimental orientation to the problem of active touch as an information-gathering process (1962) and his fuller elaboration of haptics in relation to other systems of perception (1966), has been advanced and extended in recent years by Taylor and Lederman (see Lederman & Taylor, 1972; Taylor and Lederman, 1975; Taylor, Lederman, & Gibson, 1973) and by Gordon (1978). The last reference is a book in which contributions from the above-mentioned authors as well as several others appear, including neuroanatomic as well as neurophysiological studies of receptor and motor functions. The different approaches taken by the contributors are evidence of the variety of disciplines that seek to comprehend how palpable information is acquired.

If we accept uncritically the position that the study of haptic processing demands the inclusion of proprioceptive-motor systems for its comprehension, we find ourselves in the middle of one of the most lively controversies since the era of Hunter and Lashley. We allude to the current dispute concerning the problem of motor control and the question of closed-loop (i.e., proprioceptive feedback) systems versus open-loop (motor program) systems (see Adams, 1977; Stelmach, 1976). If we assume that the study of Schwartz et al. (1975) can be generalized, we are free to concentrate on the perception of complex tactile patterns as separate from the performance aspect. It is only in relatively recent times that complex patterns have been examined by quantitative means (see Lederman, 1978; Millar, 1978; Nolan & Kederis, 1969). Indeed, only the past quarter-century has seen quantification of dimensions such as hardness, roughness, and viscosity, all of which, though probably not unitary phenomenal dimensions, have correlate physical scales (Harper & Stevens, 1964; Stevens & Guirao, 1964; Stevens & Harris, 1962). Similarly, only a few attempts have been made to combine dimensions of tactile experience in the interest of improving discrimination and processing of complex patterns (see Foulke & Warm, 1967; Lappin & Foulke, 1973; Schiff & Isikow, 1966; Taylor, 1977, 1978).

The alternative to divorcing the exploratory from the sensing function by fiat is to encourage what might be called *separate maintenance*. By this we refer to a statement made earlier concerning the separation of performatory from perceptual processes with electronic aids such as the TVSS and Optacon. It is also possible to employ the digital computer for this purpose (see Chapter 6; Mann, 1974).

The applied psychophysics of touch

We have outlined in brief some of the discriminative capacities of humans in situations marked by careful stimulus controls, selection and training of observers, standardized testing situations, the minimization of extraneous environmental influences, and the maintenance of unidimensional variations of the stimulus pattern. The results tell us something of the limits of processing capabilities when the input channel and the receptive organism are relatively unperturbed. What is wanted by the handicapped individual, however, is a useful grammar of touch that is applicable to the problem of braille, the Optacon, or tactile map reading. Our knowledge of the size of the DL for touch is as useless to the blind person stranded in the middle of O'Hare Airport as the chemical composition of Polaris was to the navigator of the Santa Maria.

Synthesis of signs by dimensional combinations

The problem in application for communicative purposes is one of coding, that is, in the selection and specification of readily learned values along the various dimensions of tactile experience. Further, the proper combination of these values is required to produce unique clusters that can be smoothly processed in yet larger combinations as rate and complexity grow with task demands, skill, and experience. The task is a complicated one, for it requires the generation, testing, and revision of repeated versions of codes and clusters, as the history of braille itself will testify (see Chapter 5). An attempt at an alternative "skin language" can be found in the work of Geldard and co-workers (see Geldard, 1957). The object of the research was to produce an alphabetic code for the skin that allowed the transmission of words at moderate rates, employing what was known of the best processing capabilities of the skin. Accordingly, three dimensions of tactile experience were chosen: stimulus location, intensity, and duration. Five values of location (on the chest) were selected, along with three values of intensity and three of duration. In addition, each cluster of locus, intensity, and duration was assigned a single letter of the alphabet or short word in such a way that the most frequently appearing letters in the English language were the shortest durations of vibration (see Figure 2.6). The Vibratese alphabet thus produced was taught to a subject who, over a period of weeks, acquired sufficient processing skills so that he or she could translate, at a low error rate, about 35 words per minute.

In an analysis of errors made by subjects, Howell (1956) pointed out that a common source was the confusion of letters having low intensity and long duration with those of high intensity and short duration. Basic research in vibrotactile sensitivity has shown that temporal summation

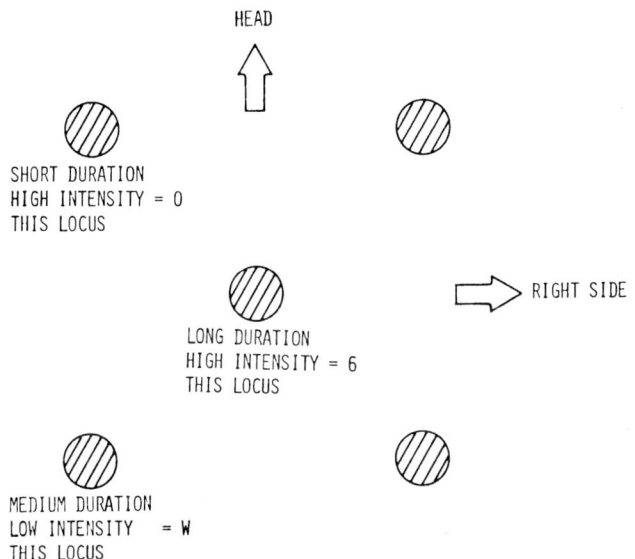

HEAD

SHORT DURATION
HIGH INTENSITY = 0
THIS LOCUS

RIGHT SIDE

LONG DURATION
HIGH INTENSITY = 6
THIS LOCUS

MEDIUM DURATION
LOW INTENSITY   = W
THIS LOCUS

Figure 2.6. The Vibratese code, after Geldard (1957). The five locations shown are on the chest. Examples of letters are shown for some positions, to illustrate the various possible combinations of locus, intensity, and duration of vibration.

effects may cause brief, intense signals to appear equal in magnitude to longer-lasting but less intense signals (see Verrillo & Smith, 1976), a fact that would have to be incorporated in any revision of the Vibratese system, but that exemplifies as well the importance of basic research findings to application.

A notable feature of the Vibratese language is its lack of redundancy (in the common usage of the term), that is, it is not possible to remove a dimension from any code cluster that stands for a letter and still identify it as that letter. What is required for redundancy of this type is to supply at least one additional dimension or feature set that lends superfluous information to the code. Thus, for Vibratese, adding frequency as a dimension in such a way that a low frequency accompanied weak levels of vibration, a medium frequency moderate levels, and a high frequency intense levels would make the clusters partially redundant. The effect of redundancy is, in part, to offset the deterioration of signals in noisy conditions. The idea is that if one dimension is interfered with by noise, the second may not be (cf. Howell, 1958).

Redundancy was the subject of Taylor's dissertation at the Princeton Cutaneous Communication Laboratory (Taylor, 1978). As his criterion for processing efficiency, Taylor chose the judgment of temporal order of tactile patterns presented in close succession. The dimensions chosen for manipulation were locus and frequency of the vibrotactile stimulus, specifically the ring, middle, and index fingertips of one hand, and frequencies of about 50, 150, and 450 Hz. Observers were required to judge which of the six possible orders of three stimuli was presented on a given trial. In one set of conditions, the judgment was to be based on locus alone, and frequency was the same for each locus; in a second set, locus was the same, and frequency was the basis of judgment. In the third set, which is the condition of interest, locus and frequency were varied redundantly, that is, the third finger was always stimulated with the lowest frequency, the middle finger with the middle frequency, and the index finger with the high frequency. This is the condition of correlated redundancy. By comparing the percentage of correct judgments for the three conditions, Taylor could estimate the effect of redundancy, because the time between the three successive stimuli was always the same.

The results were clear in yielding significantly and consistently superior performance over several blocks of trials for the two-dimensional redundant as compared to the one-dimensional conditions. Moreover, for control trials in which the locus and frequency sets were paired but not correlated, performance was no better than for the comparable one-dimensional condition. There are reasons for thinking that the basis for improvement is not simply the addition of information from two sources; nonetheless, improvement in channel capacity via the use of correlated redundancy has been clearly demonstrated by Taylor's experiments. A surprising by-product of the investigation was the demonstration that some observers processed frequency of vibration as well as or better than locus. We have already pointed out, however, that frequency changes may not induce unidimensional effects phenomenally, that is, apparent rate, location, and extensity of the pattern may all be changed with frequency. Taylor had, of course, controlled for the obvious shifts in sensory magnitude that accompany frequency changes.

Experiments such as Taylor's and others already mentioned demonstrate what may be done by combining dimensions to encode language or other complex sequences of information (e.g., tracking skills; see Hahn, 1965; Hill, 1970). Such investigations inquire whether generating more complex patterns enhances acquisition or performance of a skill by increasing or enriching the cues available in its exercise. A task that comes to mind, particularly in the present context, is that of the finger maze, a device that had a prominent place in undergraduate psychology laboratories of the 1920s and 1930s. The mazes took many shapes but were commonly of the multiple-T variety, having tactually distinctive start and goal points, but with a perfectly uniform interior character that required the subject to learn the appropriate sequence of right or left turns to find the shortest path to the goal. It would be interesting to determine whether such a maze might be resurrected and standardized to test the relative efficacy of tactual patterns for haptic displays.

One may wonder if, in a sense, the haptic explorer constructs what Tolman (1948) called a *cognitive map* when he or she palpates a space-occupying object. Early trials with unfamiliar stationary objects might resemble mazelike (strip map) behavior, with the subject moving the fingers along a surface and noting its texture while at the same time storing the angle of the fingers and the appearance of edges, corners, or rounded surfaces in a programmed sequence. For portable objects, the lack of a fixed orientation may be offset by feelings of heft or density, the symmetry of the center of mass (see Kreifeldt & Chuang, 1979), and overall size relative to the hand. As learning progresses, the function of cues may change from that of benchmarks at choice points to that of confirmations of anticipated sequences that serve to lubricate the "sticking points" or disjunctions in a perceptual-motor series, resulting in a fusion of a large number of the separate acts into a continuous, uninterrupted movement.

Synthesis by dimensional reduction

Gregory (1978) has noted that a subject whose sight was restored was often confused by the visual environment, but some of the subject's behavior suggested that the reduction of vistas to simple line drawings might have aided considerably in their recognition. It is possible that a similar treatment of complex haptic displays would expose their essential aspects, in the present situation by subtraction of features or dimensional values. For this purpose, it might be necessary to create a series of tactile patterns of systematically varying complexity, to arrive at "haptic equivalents" (see Chapter 6). The differences between the resulting patterns would then rank low on the scale of important features or dimensional values, because they are not useful differentia. From the opposite standpoint, extracting features from a display until recognizability dropped quickly should yield a set of aspects high on the scale of importance. Whether these approaches will work at all is a matter to be settled by experiment. Indeed, the question of simple scaling of important stimulus aspects is moot, because we are not certain that the integration of dimensions proceeds in a linear fashion for all individuals at all stages of skill development.

Acknowledgments

Portions of this chapter were prepared under DHEW Grant NS 04755 to Princeton University and under Grant NS 09783 to Indiana University from the National Institutes of Health.

References

Adams, J. A. Feedback theory of how joint receptors regulate the timing and positioning of a limb. *Psychological Review*, 1977, *84*, 504–523.

Bartley, S. H. Central mechanisms of vision. In H. W. Magoun (Ed.), *Handbook of Physiology*. Sect. 1, Vol. 1: *Neurophysiology*. Washington, D.C.: Physiological Society, 1959, pp. 713–740.

Békésy, G. von. A new audiometer. *Acta Otolaryngologica*, 1947, *35*, 411–422.

Experiments in hearing. New York: McGraw-Hill, 1960.

Sensory inhibition. Princeton, N.J.: Princeton University Press, 1967.

Bliss, J. C., Katcher, M. H., Rogers, C. H., & Shepard, R. P. Optical-to-tactile image conversion for the blind. *IEEE Transactions on Man–Machine Systems*, MMS-11, no. 1, 1970, 58–64.

Boring, E. G. The two-point limen and the error of localization. *American Journal of Psychology*, 1930, *42*, 446–449.

Sensation and perception in the history of experimental psychology. New York: Appleton-Century-Crofts, 1942.

Burgess, P. R. Cutaneous mechanoreceptors. In E. C. Carterette & M. P. Friedman (Eds.), *Handbook of perception*, Vol. 3: *Biology of perceptual systems*. New York: Academic Press, 1973, pp. 219–249.

Collins, C. C. Tactile television: mechanical and electrical image projection. *IEEE Transactions on Man–Machine Systems*, MMS-11, no. 1, 1970, 65–71.

Craig, J. C. Difference threshold for intensity of tactile stimuli. *Perception & Psychophysics*, 1972, *11*, 150–152.

Vibrotactile difference thresholds for intensity and the effect of a masking stimulus. *Perception & Psychophysics*, 1974, *15*, 123–127.

Vibrotactile letter recognition: the effects of a masking stimulus. *Perception & Psychophysics*, 1976, *20*, 317–326.

Foulke, E., & Warm, J. S. Effects of complexity and redundancy on the tactual recognition of metric figures. *Perceptual & Motor Skills*, 1967, *25*, 177–187.

Geldard, F. A. The perception of mechanical vibration, IV. Is there a separate "vibratory sense?" *Journal of General Psychology*, 1940, *22*, 291–308.

Adventures in tactile literacy. *American Psychologist*, 1957, *12*, 115–124.

(Ed.). *Virginia cutaneous project, 1948–1962*. Charlottesville, Va.: University of Virginia Psychological Laboratory. Ann Arbor, Mich.: University Microfilms, OP 16, 352, 1962.

Vision, audition, and beyond. In W. D. Neff (Ed.), *Contributions to sensory physiology*, vol. 4. New York: Academic Press, 1970, pp. 1–17.

The human senses, (rev. ed.). New York: Wiley, 1972.

Tactile communication. In T. A. Sebeok (Ed.), How animals communicate. Bloomington, Ind.: Indiana University Press, 1977, pp. 211–232.

Geldard, F. A., Sherrick, C. E., & Cholewiak, R. W. *Princeton cutaneous research project progress report no. 36*. Princeton, N.J.: Princeton University, 1980, pp. 30–36.

Gescheider, G. A. Temporal relations in cutaneous stimulation. In F. A. Geldard (Ed.), *Cutaneous communication systems and devices*. Austin, Tex.: Psychonomic Society, 1974, pp. 33–37.

Gibson, J. J. Observations on active touch. *Psychological Review*, 1962, *69*, 477–491.
The senses considered as perceptual systems. Boston: Houghton Mifflin, 1966.

Goff, G. D. Differential discrimination of frequency of cutaneous mechanical vibration. *Journal of Experimental Psychology*, 1967, *74*, 294–299.

Gordon, G. (Ed.). *Active touch*. Oxford: Pergamon Press, 1978.

Gregory, R. L. Remarks in discussion period of a session on "Research Horizons." Conference on Interrelations of the Communicative Senses, Asilomar, Calif., Sept. 29–Oct. 1, 1978.

Gybels, J., & van Hees, J. Unit activity from mechanoreceptors in human peripheral nerve during intensity discrimination of touch. In G. G. Somjen (Ed.), *Neurophysiology studied in man*. Amsterdam: Excerpta Medica, 1972, pp. 198–206.

Hahn, J. F. Unidimensional compensatory tracking with a vibrotactile display. *Perceptual & Motor Skills*, 1965, *21*, 699–702.
Vibrotactile adaptation and recovery measured by two methods. *Journal of Experimental Psychology*, 1966, *71*, 655–658.
Low-frequency vibrotactile adaptation. *Journal of Experimental Psychology*, 1968, *78*, 655–659.

Harper, R., & Stevens, S. S. Subjective hardness of compliant materials. *Quarterly Journal of Experimental Psychology*, 1964, *16*, 204–215.

Hensel, H., & Boman, K. Afferent impulses in cutaneous sensory nerves in human subjects. *Journal of Neurophysiology*, 1960, *23*, 564–578.

Hill, J. W. Describing function analysis of tracking performance using two tactile displays. *IEEE Transactions on Man–Machine Systems*, MMS-11, no. 1, 1970, 92–100.

Hirsh, I. J., & Sherrick, C. E. Perceived order in different sense modalities. *Journal of Experimental Psychology*, 1961, *62*, 423–432.

Howell, W. C. Training on a vibrotactile communication system. Unpublished master's thesis, University of Virginia, 1956.
Discrimination of rate of amplitude change in cutaneous vibration. Unpublished doctoral thesis, University of Virginia, 1958.

Iggo, A. (Ed.). *Handbook of sensory physiology*, Vol. 2: *Somatosensory system*. New York: Springer, 1973.

Kaas, J. H., Nelson, R. J., Sur, M., Lin, C. S., & Merzenich, M. M. Multiple representations of the body within the primary somatosensory cortex of primates. *Science*, 1979, *204*, 521–523.

Kirman, J. H. Tactile communication of speech: a review and an analysis. *Psychological Bulletin*, 1973, *80*, 54–74.
Tactile pattern perception and tactile displays. Paper presented at the Conference on Interrelations of the Communicative Senses, Asilomar, Calif., Sept. 29–Oct. 1, 1978.

Kreifeldt, J. G., & Chuang, M.C. Moment of inertia: psychophysical study of an overlooked sensation. *Science*, 1979, *206*, 588–590.

Lappin, J. S., & Foulke, E. Expanding the tactual field of view. *Perception & Psychophysics*, 1973, *14*, 237–241.

Lechelt, E. C. Temporal numerosity discrimination: intermodal comparisons revisited. *British Journal of Psychology*, 1975, *66*, 101–108.

Lederman, S. J. Heightening tactile impressions of surface texture. In G. Gordon (Ed.), *Active touch. The mechanism of recognition of objects by manipulation: a multidisciplinary approach*. Oxford: Pergamon Press, 1978, pp. 205–214.

Lederman, S. J., & Taylor, M. M. Fingertip force, surface geometry, and the perception of roughness by active touch. *Perception & Psychophysics*, 1972, *12*, 401–408.

Loewenstein, W. R. Mechano-electrical transduction in the Pacinian corpuscle: initiation of sensory impulses in mechanoreceptors. In W. R. Loewenstein (Ed.), *Handbook of sensory physiology*, Vol. 1: *Principles of receptor physiology*. New York: Springer, 1971, pp. 269–290.

Mann, R. W. Technology and human rehabilitation: prostheses for sensory rehabilitation and/or sensory substitution. In J. H. Brown & J. F. Dickson (Eds.), *Advances in biomedical engineering*, vol. 4. New York: Academic Press, 1974, pp. 209–253.

Melzack, R., & Wall, P. D. On the nature of cutaneous sensory mechanisms. *Brain*, 1962, *85*, 331–356.

Merzenich, M. M., & Harrington, T. The sense of flutter-vibration evoked by stimulation of the hairy skin of primates: comparison of human sensory capacity with the response of mechanoreceptive afferents innervating the hairy skin of monkeys. *Experimental Brain Research*, 1969, *9*, 236–260.

Millar, S. Aspects of memory for information from touch and movement. In G. Gordon (Ed.), *Active touch. The mechanism of recognition of objects by manipulation: a multidisciplinary approach*. Oxford: Pergamon Press, 1978, pp. 215–227.

Mountcastle, V. B., Talbot, W. H., Darian-Smith, I., & Kornhuber, H. H. Neural basis of the sense of flutter-vibration. *Science*, 1967, *155*, 597–600.

Mueller, C. G. *Sensory psychology*. Englewood Cliffs, N.J.: Prentice-Hall, 1965.

Nafe, J. P., & Wagoner, K. S. The nature of pressure adaptation. *Journal of General Psychology*, 1941, *25*, 323–351.

Nolan, C. Y., & Kederis, C. J. *Perceptual factors in braille word recognition*. New York: American Foundation for the Blind, Research Series No. 20, 1969.

Pickett, J. M., & Pickett, B. H. Communication of speech sounds by a tactual Vocoder. *Journal of Speech and Hearing Research*, 1963, *6*, 207–222.

Quilliam, T. A. The structure of fingerprint skin. In G. Gordon (Ed.), *Active touch. The mechanism of recognition of objects by manipulation: a multidisciplinary approach*. Oxford: Pergamon Press, 1978, pp. 1–27.

Riggs, L. A., Ratliff, F., Cornsweet, J. C., & Cornsweet, T. N. The disappearance of steadily fixated test objects. *Journal of the Optical Society of America*, 1953, *43*, 495–501.

Rothenberg, M., Verrillo, R. T., Zahorian, S. A., Brachman, M. L., & Bolanowski, S. J. Vibrotactile frequency for encoding a speech parameter. *Journal of the Acoustical Society of America*, 1977, *62*, 1003–1012.

Schiff, W., & Isikow, H. Stimulus redundancy in the tactile perception of histograms. *International Journal for the Education of the Blind*, 1966, *15*, 1–11.

Schwartz, A. S., Perey, A. J., & Azulay, A. Further analysis of active and passive touch in pattern discrimination. *Bulletin of the Psychonomic Society*, 1975, *6*, 7–9.

Sherrick, C. E. Current prospects for cutaneous communication. In F. A. Geldard (Ed.), *Cutaneous communication systems and devices*. Austin, Tex.: Psychonomic Society, 1974, pp. 106–109.

The antagonisms of hearing and touch. In S. K. Hirsh, D. H. Eldredge, I. J. Hirsh, & S. R. Silverman (Eds.), *Hearing and Davis: essays honoring Hallowell Davis*. St. Louis: Washington University Press, 1976, pp. 149–158.

Stelmach, G. E. (Ed.). *Motor control: issues and trends*. New York: Academic Press, 1976.

Stevens, J. C., & Green, B. G. Temperature–touch interaction: Weber's phenomenon revisited. *Sensory Processes*, 1978, *2*, 206–219.

Stevens, S. S., & Guirao, M. Scaling of apparent viscosity. *Science*, 1964, *144*, 1157–1158.

Stevens, S. S., & Harris, J. R. The scaling of subjective roughness and smoothness. *Journal of Experimental Psychology*, 1962, *64*, 489–494.

Talbot, W. H., Darian-Smith, I., Kornhuber, H. H., & Mountcastle, V. B. The sense of flutter-vibration: comparison of the human capacity with response patterns of mechanoreceptive afferents from the monkey hand. *Journal of Neurophysiology*, 1968, *31*, 301–335.

Taylor, B. Dimensional interactions in vibrotactile information processing. *Perception & Psychophysics*, 1977, *21*, 477–481.

Dimensional redundancy in the processing of vibrotactile temporal order. Unpublished doctoral thesis, Princeton University, 1978.

Taylor, M. M., & Lederman, S. J. Tactile roughness of grooved surfaces: a model and the effect of friction. *Perception & Psychophysics*, 1975, *17*, 23–36.

Taylor, M. M., Lederman, S. J., & Gibson, R. H. Tactual perception of texture. In E. C. Carterette & M. P. Friedman (Eds.), *Handbook of perception*, Vol. 3: *Biology of perceptual systems*. New York: Academic Press, 1973, pp. 251–272.

Tolman, E. C. Cognitive maps in rats and men. *Psychological Review*, 1948, *55*, 189–208.

Uttal, W. R. A comparison of neural and psychophysical responses in the somesthetic system. *Journal of Comparative and Physiological Psychology*, 1959, *52*, 485–490.

Vallbo, A. B., & Johansson, R. S. The tactile sensory innervation of the glabrous skin of the human hand. In G. Gordon (Ed.), *Active touch. The mechanism of recognition of objects by manipulation: a multidisciplinary approach*. Oxford: Pergamon Press, 1978, pp. 29–54.

Verrillo, R. T. Effect of contactor area on the vibrotactile threshold. *Journal of the Acoustical Society of America*, 1963, *35*, 1962–1966.

A duplex mechanism of mechanoreception. In D. R. Kenshalo (Ed.), *The skin senses*. Springfield, Ill.: Charles C. Thomas, 1968, pp. 139–159.

Verrillo, R. T., & Smith, R. L. Effect of stimulus duration on vibrotactile sensation magnitude. *Bulletin of the Psychonomic Society*, 1976, *8*, 112–114.

Vierck, C. J., Jr., & Jones, M. B. Size discrimination on the skin. *Science*, 1969, *163*, 488–489.

von Frey, M. Ueber die zur ebenmerklichen Erregung des Drucksinns erforderlichen Energiemengen. *Zeitschrift für Biologie*, 1920, *70*, 333–347.

Wall, P. D. Dorsal horn electrophysiology. In A. Iggo (Ed.), *Handbook of physiology*, Vol. 2: *Somatosensory system*. New York: Springer, 1973, pp. 253–270.

Wall, P. D., & Dubner, R. Somatosensory pathways. *Annual Review of Physiology*, 1972, *34*, 315–336.

Weinstein, S. Intensive and extensive aspects of tactile sensitivity as a function of body part, sex, and laterality. In D. R. Kenshalo (Ed.), *The skin senses*. Springfield, Ill.: Charles C. Thomas, 1968, pp. 193–218.

Werner, G., & Whitsel, B. L. Functional organization of the somatosensory cortex. In A. Iggo (Ed.), *Handbook of physiology*, Vol. 2: *Somatosensory system*. New York: Springer, 1973, pp. 621–700.

3. The development of haptic perception

DAVID H. WARREN

In Chapter 3, David Warren examines the development of haptic perception, that is, the related acts of reaching, touching, grasping, and manipulating. He also grapples with the complex issues of cross-modal relations in the course of human development – issues of how haptic activities are coordinated with vision and audition. He notes that according to Piaget and other classical theorists, visual and haptic activities begin as separately organized processes, with visual activity gaining gradual control over manual activity. This view is then contrasted to Bower's, that one system cannot calibrate the other in the course of early development, because both are undergoing substantial physical development at the same time. Bower has argued for some time that visual–motor correspondences are unlearned and unintegrated. Rather, there is an initial primitive unity of the senses, with *differentiation* progressing in the course of development. This view is, of course, based on E. J. Gibson's conceptualizations of perceptual development.

Genevan, Russian, and American literatures bearing on later childhood are examined by Warren for clues to the development of haptic perception in the postinfancy period of early childhood. Controversial views, such as the questionable facilitative role of haptic information in enhancing visually obtained information are explored. The cross-modal developmental literature is then reviewed with specific reference to exploratory strategies in directing haptic activity. This issue is critical to theories of the superiority of active touch over more passive forms of touch. In particular, the questions may boil down to whether it is a relative lack of haptic *sensitivity* or haptic *strategies* that limits the child's performance on haptic tasks. Although there is evidence of developmental improvement during early childhood, much of it seems due to shifts in haptic strategies.

Warren also explores coding and memory research relevant to haptics, noting the extreme uncertainty of conclusions in this area. The development of haptic perception involves some fascinating questions, but few clear answers are available. Warren's summary of this enormous literature provides a firm base for further work by developmental psychologists, perceptual psychologists, and educators who wish to pursue these topics.   WILLIAM SCHIFF

For the purposes of this chapter, I will limit the definition of haptic perception to perception of information gained through the active use of the hands and fingers. Thus excluded will be passive skin receptivity, as in the perception of temperature, pressure, and so on. Also excluded, aside from an occasional point of contrast, will be the passive stimulation of the hands and fingers and active exploration in which the primary activity is created by arm movements as opposed to hand and finger movements.

One has the choice, in such an analysis, of two distinct approaches. One involves deciding, a priori, what the significant issues are and organizing the available literature to bear on them. The other involves collecting *all* the available literature and allowing the organization to emerge from the major topics contained therein. The latter approach is inherently constrained by the nature of previous research and is thus an inadequate venture by itself. It is particularly inadequate for the treatment of the development of haptic perception, because, as it happens, much of the interesting information that we have is a by-product of research on other issues, such as the development of intermodality organization. The former approach is also inappropriate by itself, because it presupposes an a priori knowledge of what is important and what is not, a risky assumption at best. For better or worse, I have attempted a compromise between these two opposites.

The adult: product of development

It is often useful, in approaching developmental issues, to begin by drawing a picture of the adult, so that the reader has a notion of the final result of the developmental trends that are presented. This approach is particularly useful when the adult is fully understood, because then the end point of development serves as a fixed benchmark against which the successive developmental approximations may be evaluated.

In the case of haptic perception, this approach is of only limited value. It may be said that adults (in contrast to infants) have quick and effective haptic capabilities, can manipulate objects with facility and identify them accurately and with ease, can remember the characteristics of objects contacted haptically, can compare objects presented visually with those presented haptically, can abstract important information gained haptically, and the like. Further, they can do all of these tasks so quickly that it is not always evident, even upon close analysis, exactly how they are being done. Indeed, as is often the case, the nature of adult behavior and capabilities can be substantially elucidated by the study of development. Just as the complex cognitive capabilities of the adult can be better understood if their development is examined, so that the emerging components of adult competence can be evaluated both as elements and as contributors to overall adult competence, so too can adult haptic perception be better understood in a developmental context.

One reason adult haptic perception is a less than solid benchmark is that the adult's haptic capabilities have simply not been studied with the sophistication that has in recent years been brought to bear on haptic developmental issues. For example, only in the context of developmental research has the importance of haptic search strategies been realized. Moreover, it is in the context of nonnormal perceptual development (primarily that of visually impaired children) that even the developmental importance of haptic search strategies has been fully recognized. Small wonder, then, that the adult serves as a less than optimally effective anchor for the consideration of developmental trends. If anything, adult haptic perceptual issues will be clarified by the continuing study of the corresponding developmental issues.

Nonetheless, it may be said that the adult can make extremely fine haptic discriminations; can use the haptic sense to mediate the perception of shape, size, texture, location, temporal rate, and other properties of objects and events; can, for the most part, make effective comparisons of haptically, visually, and even auditorally perceived events; and above all, has the haptic capabilities under the effective guidance of a mature perceptual–cognitive control system. None of this can be said of the infant, and the purpose of this chapter will be to chart, to the extent possible given the existing literature, the territory that the infant traverses in becoming the adult.

Infancy

Beginning at a very tender age, the human infant moves its arms and hands, contacting objects at first sporadically and accidentally, then intentionally and regularly. This developmental progression involves, briefly, a transition from what is perhaps initially a disorganized set of physical contacts to an intentional and coordinated manner of gaining significant information about the world. The first set of questions, then, has to do with the nature of this progression, what experience the development depends on, what the significant events are along the way, and how haptic perception initially becomes coordinated with, or differentiated from (depending on one's theoretical stance) other means of perceiving the physical environment. In short, how does the human infant learn to use haptically gained information to contribute to his or her perception of the world?

The developmental integration view

As is often the case in considering developmental issues, it is instructive to look first to Piaget, who provides a valuable account of the developmental acquisition of reaching and grasping in the young infant. In *The Origin of Intelligence in the Child*, Piaget (1953) characterizes five stages in the development of prehension, stages that progress from the simple, reflexive behavior that characterizes the newborn infant to a well-integrated coordination of vision, reaching, and grasping. The details of the stages are not important for this treatment, nor are the ages. But the sequence is interesting. In the *first* stage, impulsive movements occur, with reflexive grasping (no thumb used). The grasping is reflexive in that it is nonvoluntary, but this grasp at least momentarily attracts the infant's attention. The *second* stage involves circular reactions related to hand movements. The infant grasps and holds for the sake of the repetitive activity, but there is no coordination with other schemas such as looking and sucking. The hand is not used as a tool to operate on the environment, but clearly it is delivering sensations that the infant prolongs and repeats. In the *third* stage, vision gradually becomes involved as the eyes are attracted to the hand's behavior. Vision does not yet control the hand, but it is beginning to attend to the hand. The hand is involved in its own activity, grasping for the sake of grasping but not for the purpose of bringing an object into view. (By contrast, at the same age, the hand *does* grasp an object with the goal of bringing it to the mouth to suck.) Gradually vision begins to influence the hand, as the hand tends to remain more and more within the visual field. Only in the *fourth* stage does any significant degree of visual control over the hand's behavior emerge. That is, now the hand acts in a different manner when it is in view than when it is not, and in particular it moves to grasp a viewed object. (This behavior is characteristic of the 3- to 4-month period.) The limitation of the fourth stage, which is overcome in the final stage, is that the eye–hand coordination occurs only when the hand is in the visual field with the object to be grasped. In the *fifth* stage, if the object is in the visual field and the hand is not, the hand will be brought from out of sight to grasp the object. That is, the visually perceived object serves as the stimulus for reaching wherever the hand is.

Two important points should be noted about this developmental progression. First, there are initially independent schemata, whose coordination develops. It is not that the hand does nothing until visual control is established; rather, the hand has its own behaviors, and gradually these become integrated with visual behavior. Second, the hand is, through its reaching and grasping activities, independently delivering interesting information (as in stage two) to the infant before becoming functionally integrated with vision.

Other infancy observers have, for the most part, corroborated the substance of Piaget's observations on the development of grasping and vision. For example, White (1971) presents observations on the development of visually directed reaching and grasping. White describes both the eye and the hand behavior characteristic of quiet, supine behavior, as well as the response to the presentation of a visually interesting and graspable test object. White organizes the sequence by age periods, in contrast to Piaget, who chooses to identify stages, with the implication that in each successive stage, a significant change in the nature of the behavior has occurred. Nevertheless, there is a great deal of similarity in the two accounts. Visual attention to an object precedes visual–manual coordinated activity. Visual regard of the hand occurs before visual direction of the hand's activities. The hand becomes an interesting visual stimulus. There is a gradual emergence of looking back and forth between hand and object. White emphasizes several components that Piaget does not, however, such as the increase, then decrease, in bilateral manual activity and, at around 4 months, the anticipatory opening of the hand as it approaches a test object.

The interpretations offered by White and Piaget are also similar in important respects. Both postulate the initial independence of hand and eye activities, with the gradual emergence of visual control over the hand's behavior. Thus both offer an integration theory in which initially separate activity patterns (schemas) become integrated under the direction of vision. White summarizes this point succinctly:

> A number of relatively distinct sensorimotor systems contribute to its [prehension's] growth . . . These systems seem to develop at different times, . . . and may remain in relative isolation from one another. During the development of prehension these various systems gradually become coordinated into a complex superordinate system which integrates their separate capacities. (p. 63)

Uzgiris (1967) also presents observational evidence that generally supports the initial separateness of schemas, such as touching, mouthing, and vision, which tend developmentally toward a gradual organization. Uzgiris stresses the role of cognitive factors in this development, particularly the shift from primary to secondary circular behaviors, a development that proceeds from operations on the self to operations on external objects.

Uzgiris observed infants from 1 to 23 months of age. Objects were presented to the infant for unstructured play, and the infant's spontaneous behaviors were recorded. Various modes of interaction with the objects were categorized. Of interest are the following. *Holding:* Once the very early reflex grasp ceases to occur, an object placed in the hand is dropped, because the infant does not maintain a hand position that is suitable for holding on to the object. Following the first month, some object retention begins. However, the infant does not bring the object up for visual regard and "hardly shows any reaction when the object finally drops from his hand" (p. 322). But holding provides tactual experience "and is a prerequisite to the coordination of grasping with mouthing, looking, and other reactions" (p. 322). *Mouthing:* Hand–mouth coordination occurs very early, even before the hand is successful in grasping long enough to bring an object to the mouth. *Visual inspection:* This is described as looking intently at an object that is held practically motionless. At first, looking seems to be a by-product of bringing an object to the mouth: "The infant obtains fleeting glances of the object held in his hand. He shows no distress as the object moves out of sight and makes only minimal attempts to follow with his eyes" (p. 323). Gradually coordination occurs so that sustained looking is possible. This behavior occurs before the infant is able to bring an object, placed in the hand out of sight, into view. *Examining:* Visual inspection becomes more integrated and is then called examining. The infant no longer simply views an object held stationary but "turns it around, pokes at it, feels its surface, manipulates its parts while observing the object and the effect of his manipulations on it" (p. 324). Uzgiris stresses that "the infant shifts his attention from the use of a given schema to interaction with a particular object" (p. 324): That is, initially the infant experiences subjective sensations, created by repetition of primary circular reactions, moving later to operations on objects (secondary circular reactions).

Uzgiris interprets these behaviors within the context of the infant's developing cognitive abilities: "The sequential acquisition of schemas in relation to objects is assumed to represent a developmental hierarchy growing out of the infant's numerous interactions with objects in the environment, rather than just reflecting his increasing motor capacities or haphazard learning" (p. 331). Like Piaget and White, she hypothesizes that initially separate modality experiences come to be coordinated, thereby allowing the development of interest in objects, as opposed to sensations. This is, then, an interactive view of development, but a view that leans on cognitive factors: "Attention to objects facilitates differentiation between them and may contribute to the acquisition of object permanence, interest in novelty, and numerous new schemas. Interest in novelty, in turn, may promote further exploration of objects" (p. 331).

The developmental differentiation view

Bower has a different view of development in early infancy, and he offers data and interpretation that conflict with those of Piaget, White, and Uzgiris. Bower argues that both visual and hand systems are undergoing significant physical growth during early infancy, and that neither can serve as an invariant reference system for (or teacher of) the other: "The theoretical problem of how one growing system is calibrated onto another growing system is very difficult and creates the greatest single methodological problem in the study of infancy" (1974a, p. 77).

Bower suggests that there are different types of reach, with different characteristics and intentions. Bower (1974a) found that 2-week-old infants reached for an object that was too far away to obtain; the infants showed little or no upset at their failure to grasp the object, and they gradually ceased reaching for it. Reaching for an object that was within range continued to occur. The results of another study corroborate the young infant's capability for appropriate reaching: Bower, Broughton, and Moore (1970) used Polaroid filtering to produce a virtual image of an object within reach, but of course, the object was not tangible under this condition. Reaching occurred in 2-week-old infants, and their failure to attain the virtually imaged object produced upset and continued attempts to reach for it. Bower argues that these infants were reaching appropriately, based on the visual information, and that their upset occurred because the expected concordance between visual information and tactual attainment did not occur.

Bower argues that this visual–motor concordance is unlearned, and thus he rejects the developmental integration notions of White and Piaget. Regarding the virtual image study, he states: "All the newborn infants touched and grasped real objects without any sign of being disturbed. They also grasped at empty air without upset when no visible object was present. The virtual object, however, produced a howl as soon as the infant's hand went to the location of the intangible object. Here too, then, we have evidence of a primitive unity of the senses . . . This unity is unlikely to have been learned, given the early age and the history of the infants studied" (1974a, pp. 113–114). Further, "such arguments cannot *prove* that the coordination is not learned; one-trial learning is, after all, possible. But the subsequent history of the development of visual–tactual coordination would seem to argue against a learning-theory explanation" (1974a, p. 114).

In the virtual object situation, the reported behavior pattern continued until 6 months of age. Then, the infants still became startled, but their grasping behavior showed important changes. They stopped grasping with their hands still open, looked at their hands, rubbed the hands together, and banged them on a surface, together with further attempts to grasp the virtual object. Bower suggests that "one could say that the infants were trying to verify that their hands were really working and had not suffered a loss of sensitivity" (1974a, pp. 114–115). They also showed exploratory visual behavior, swinging the head from side to side (producing motion parallax that is opposite in direction, because of the filters, to the normal motion parallax result). They stopped reaching for the virtual object. When a new object was introduced, these now skeptical 6-month-olds apparently tested their vision first and reached only if they experienced normal parallax. Thus the older infants apparently knew that something was wrong with their visual–tactual coordination, and they systematically checked the tactual and visual components. "The responses of older infants are differentiated; they seem to be aware of vision and touch as separate modalities, unlike the younger infants who apparently have a wholistic, unanalyzed awareness of the situation . . . One must conclude that they [the young infants] have not yet differentiated the visible qualities of an object from its tangible qualities" (1974a, p. 116).

Bower suggests that vision becomes dominant and controlling at 5 to 6 months of age: "An infant will drop an object that he is grasping if he can no longer see it. One only has to cover the infant's hand with a cloth for him to drop a grasped object . . . It thus seems that one consequence of the differentiation of vision from touch is that touch loses its ability to specify the presence of an object and regains this ability only after a prolonged period [i.e., after this 6-month phase] . . . Developmentally, visual tangibility precedes tactual tangibility, whereas undifferentiated visual–tactual concordance precedes both" (1974a, pp. 116–117).

Bower thus suggests that ontogenetically, infants progress through stages from an initial unity of the senses (primitive unity) to a gradual differentiation. He argues (1974b) that this ontogeny recapitulates a phylogenetic progression: "Intermodal unity is greater the lower or younger an experimental organism is" (p. 148). He suggests that the phylogenetically early system was one that probably responded to pressure variations. Then:

> The system gradually evolved eyes, ears, nose, all of which were designed to allow it to use the same internal apparatus to respond to the same information within different energy spectra. As organisms evolved, and particularly as they began to grow their parts at different rates and to different sizes, this early unity had to be

abandoned . . . The proprioceptive and visual unity we find early in infancy cannot survive the different growth patterns of the eye and of the skeleton. The information load necessary to maintain it is simply too great. Therefore, the initial primitive unity must go, leaving undifferentiated sensory systems in place of a unitary perceptual world. (1974b, p. 151)

A related issue concerns the adjustment of the reaching hand to the size of the object. White (1971) suggests that such adjustment occurs relatively late in the development of visually guided reaching behavior, in the 4- to 4.5-month phase, when the hand begins to open in anticipation of contact with the object. Only a "closed fisted swipe" is seen around 2.5 months of age. Bower, by contrast, presents evidence that appropriate preparation of the hand occurs much earlier in development, and in fact he uses such observations as further support for the hypothesis that the senses are initially undifferentiated. The subjects in Bower's (1972) experiment were between 7 and 15 days of age. Balls and cylinders, varying in diameter, were presented to the infant at shoulder height, and the nature of the hand and arm activity was observed and videotaped. The separation between thumb and forefinger, or between the two hands when both were used, was measured from the records. The separation was found to vary consistently with the diameter of the object presented, indicating that the size information gained visually was effective in directing the anticipatory movements of the hands.

With such evidence of visual direction in very young infants, why do other investigators (e.g., Piaget, White) find the development occurring only around 4 or 5 months of age? Bower suggests that in White's study, the earlier anticipatory movements occurred but did not continue because of the relative impoverishment of the institutional environment, which did not contain many objects for the infant to reach for. In an unpublished study, Bower (1973, cited in 1974a) provided reachable objects for infants continually throughout the first several months of life and found no disappearance of the early reaching. Although reaching occurred continuously, however, the nature of the grasping attempts changed. Grasping under the direction of vision declined, whereas tactually guided grasping remained. Bower suggests that the visually guided grasping was not reinforced, whereas tactually directed grasping resulted in the attainment of the grasped object and was thus reinforced. Bower also stresses the importance of developing attentional capabilities in these early months: Early in the process, the infant does not have sufficient attentive capacity to attend simultaneously to both the hand and the object being reached for, and must therefore shift limited attention back and forth. Later, increased attention allows the simultaneous visual registry of hand and object.

To summarize, then, Bower distinguishes an early type of reaching (phase I) from a later kind (phase II) that other investigators have described. In phase I, reaching and grasping are not differentiated and cannot be separately directed. Then, as a result of the development of tactually initiated grasping and the relative nonreinforcement of visually initiated grasping, grasping and reaching become separated. In phase I, the reaching–grasping unit is visually initiated, but in phase II, reaching is visually initiated and grasping is tactually initiated. A related distinction is made between visually initiated and visually controlled reaching: In phase I, reaching is visually initiated but not visually controlled (presumably because of attentional inadequacies and/or motor control), whereas in phase II it is visually initiated and visually controlled (Bower, 1977).

This distinction between visual initiation and visual guidance is an important one. Bruner and Koslowski (1972) observed the manual activity of infants from 10 to 22 weeks of age in response to the presentation of a graspable object (a small ball) as opposed to a nongraspable object (a large ball). Both objects were placed within reach, with their near surface (10-cm, or 4–5 in) in front of the infant's eyes. The key question was whether the infant would show appropriately differentiated manual activities to the two objects *before* the onset of successful reaching in which tactual feedback would occur. That is, would the visual information, developmentally prior to the receipt of tactual feedback from a successful reach, initiate manual activities that would be appropriate to the object presented? The answer was a clear yes: "Forward swiping," an activity that was assumed to be more appropriate for large, ungraspable objects, occurred more in response to the visual presentation of the large ball, whereas several manual activities that were assumed to be more suitable for grasping small objects (bringing the two hands toward the midline, midline activity by the two hands) occurred more frequently in response to the visual presentation of the small ball. The differential distribution of these two kinds of manual activity continued after successful reaching began (around 5 months), but the key finding was that the differentiation occurred *before* the onset of successful reaching. Thus, visual information served to *initiate* appropriate manual behavior before it began to guide reaching: Tactually reinforced activity is not a prerequisite to the differentiation of hand activity. Bruner and Koslowski argue, contrary to Piaget and White, that "the issue in visual–motor coordination has not to do with the integration of two separate sensory systems or modalities, but rather with the differentiation and serial ordering of the constituent acts involved in achieving an objective like object capture" (p. 13). Implicitly, their stance supports Bower's view, in that they discuss a "preadapted coordination of visual and manipulatory space in children still too young to have had any experience of feedback from visually controlled grasping" (p. 13). However, they seem to stop short of a definitive argument that there is a "primitive unity," as proposed by Bower. The interpretation presumably centers on the possible equivalence of "preadapted coordination" and "primitive unity."

McDonnell (1975) presents results that suggest a relatively early effective guiding of reach by vision. In contrast to visual *triggering* of reaching, visually *guided* reaching is attentionally much more demanding, because the infant must attend to the position of the object, the position of the hand, and the difference between them, with movement as a further complication. McDonnell observed infants reaching toward objects viewed through 30-diopter prisms. There was evidence for continuous guidance (shown by appropriate trajectory changes) for even the youngest infants, and McDonnell concluded that reaching was at least partly visually guided, although he did find an improving degree of visual control over the, 4- to 10-month range, with corrections and monitoring becoming more coordinated. McDonnell suggested that increasing attention is a factor in increasing control of the hand in the visual periphery.

Use of haptic information by infants

Regardless of differences in their arguments about whether the haptic and visual senses are initially nondifferentiated (Bower) or initially separate (White, Piaget), the theorists discussed so far are in reasonable agreement that by the middle of the first year or so, the hand's activity is largely under visual control. Two questions then arise: To what degree is the haptic system capable of mediating perceptual and cognitive events in the absence of vision? When both are available, does haptic experience add anything to visual experience?

Gratch and Landers (1971) studied 6-month-old infants on several tasks related to the development of object permanence. A visual task, in which the infant had continuous sight of a test object, produced sustained visual attention to the object. In a task in which the subject grasped the object, then had it covered by an opaque cover, the infant would, until about 7.5 months, simply hold the now-covered object while looking around for something to see. There was no evidence that haptic contact with the object mediated the infant's knowledge that the object continued to exist: "They were not able, through touch, to recognize the presence of an object" (p. 369). Older infants would bring out the object from under the cover. Thus visual information was clearly capable of mediating object awareness earlier than haptic information. An intermediate condition, involving partial covering of a previously grasped object, produced success earlier than the complete covering condition. Gratch (1972), further interested in the conditions under which haptic information might be useful, used a condition in which an already grasped object was covered with a transparent cloth, compared with an opaque cloth. As measured by the child's success in bringing the object out from under the cloth, there was considerable success with the transparent cloth but little with the opaque cloth in the group of 6-month-olds. For the subjects who failed on the opaque cloth task but succeeded on the transparent cloth task, the continued sight of the object in the latter condition was clearly the key. Thus the addition of visual information to haptic information facilitated performance.

Other evidence also supports the notion that the effective use of visual information developmentally precedes the effective use of haptic information. Bower, Broughton, and Moore (1970) were interested in this question, among others. They observed, with infants from 6 days to 6 months of age, the efficiency and nature of grasping under conditions in which an object was placed in the infant's hand out of his or her sight, or presented visually and the infant allowed to reach for it. Visual presentation of the object produced anticipatory hand shaping in all subjects, even the youngest. Thus visual information directed manual activity, a phenomenon also noted by Bruner and Koslowski (1972). However, when the object was placed in the infant's hand out of his or her sight, hand shaping was poor, involving a "stereotyped closure movement – which was not adapted to the object" (p. 52). Nor did placing an object in the hand elicit attempts to look at the object until about 3 months of age. It was concluded that early in development, visual information is more effective than tactual information in directing the course of grasping (the prehensile system). At around 5 months, though, the grasping movement began to come under the control of tactual information rather than being wholly commanded by vision. Bower et al. (1970) suggested that the emergence of tactual information salience could at least in part be accounted for by assuming a maturation of the tactual system, resulting in an increase in its rapidity and efficiency.

Results from a study by Schaffer and Parry (1970) add to this picture of the haptic system as developmentally delayed, compared with the visual system. An object was presented for inspection, either visually or visually with haptic access. Then the familiarized object was presented together with a novel object, and visual and haptic behaviors were assessed for the two objects. Three age groups were studied: 5 to 7 months, 8 to 10 months, and 11 to 13 months. At all ages, there was more visual attention to the novel object than to the familiar one. For the two older groups, there was also more hand manipulation of the novel object. For the youngest group, however, there was no differentiation of hand manipulation of the two objects. Clearly, the younger infants could discriminate the two objects, as evidenced by their differential visual activity, but this discrimination did not occur in their hand behavior, suggesting that "it is only at subsequent age levels that the regulation of manipulative behavior by the visual system with respect to the processing of familiarity was observed to occur" (p. 567).

Because visual processing apparently precedes haptic processing developmentally, perhaps we should conclude that haptic information does not play a role in perception when both modalities are available. Such a conclusion is not supported, however. Harris (1971) examined 8- and 12-month-olds in a test of this question. Two groups were used at each age level. One was allowed only visual examination of an object, which was covered by Plexiglas, whereas the other could both see and handle the object. The dependent measure was the persistence of search for the object after it was taken away. For the 8-month-olds, visual + haptic examination produced a much longer search than visual examination alone. For the older infants, the same trend occurred, but to a lesser extent. Harris concluded that haptic contact enhanced the infant's conception of the object's existence, at least for the younger children.

In a similar experiment, Harris (1972) again used 8- and 12-month-old groups. In a familiarization phase, two objects were presented, one that could only be seen and one that could be seen and handled. After this phase there was a 15-sec delay; then the objects were presented for the discrimination phase, in which the infant could both touch and see the objects. Visual inspection time for the two objects was recorded during this phase. The object presented only visually during familiarization received significantly more visual attention during discrimination, a pattern that was more marked for the older group. The availability of haptic inspection changed the pattern of visual examination during discrimination, presumably by making the visually + haptically inspected object more familiar; this relatively novel object would be expected to receive more attention. In any case, explanations aside, it is clear from the results that the availability of haptic information during inspection did contribute to the overall processing of information about the object.

A similar experiment was reported by Gottfried, Rose, and Bridger (1977) with 1-year-old infants. This experiment demonstrated not only the usefulness of haptic information but also the availability of haptically processed information for cross-modal transfer to a visual task. First, a familiarization phase occurred in which the infant examined one object. Examination occurred either visually or haptically with the hand (and in one condition, with the mouth). Then a 20-sec visual recognition memory interval occurred in which a novel object was paired with the familiar one and both were presented for visual inspection out of reach. Visual fixation was recorded during this phase. Finally, a reaching preference test was conducted by moving the two objects within the infant's reach. Regardless of the manner of initial examination (visual, oral, or manual), there was more visual fixation on the novel object in the middle phase. The subsequent reaching results also showed a significant preference for the novel object. Clearly, habituation had occurred in the oral and manual inspection conditions as well as in the visual condition. Further, though, the haptic familiarity with the inspected object transferred cross-modally, such that the differentiated experience with the two objects affected subsequent visual attention.

The experiment by Gottfried et al. (1977) should also remind us of the importance of the mouth as an organ of haptic experience. It is almost trivial to note the role of oral sensitivity in directing the mouth appropriately to the nipple in extremely young infants. Gesell, Ilg, and Bullis (1949), among many others, note the importance of "mouthing" behavior as a means of exploring the size, shape, and texture of objects. It is also worthy of note that Piaget and others have reported the tendency of young infants to bring handled objects to the mouth for exploration, as a stage developmentally prior to the examination of handled objects with the two hands in concert, and even prior to the manipulation of an object for the purpose of visual inspection.

Infancy issues

What conclusions can we draw from this literature on haptic development in infancy? There is no need here to review specific results, and in any case the findings may be interpreted in different ways. Indeed, there is a major unresolved theoretical issue, with Bower on one side and Piaget, for example, on the other. There is agreement that by the middle of the first year, vision exerts significant control over hand activity. Disagreement occurs on a developmentally earlier issue. Bower argues that the initially undifferentiated senses gradually become differentiated, with vision then taking over direction as organization occurs. Piaget, by contrast, sees the hand and eye as initially independent (and thus, by implication, initially differentiated), with vision gaining control as organization occurs.

In my view, the critical test has not been made. And it will be a difficult test to conceptualize, let alone conduct. The conceptualization must ultimately depend on the effective distinction between nondifferentiation and generalization, concepts that have a history of confusion in psychology. Generalization here may be considered in cross-modal terms. Let us construct a hypothetical experiment to test the issue. We will present a stimulus object haptically to a young infant, then present it visually and examine some indicator that will tell us whether the prior haptic experience affects the subsequent visual perception. Let us assume that it does have such an effect. What can we conclude? Bower would argue that the effect occurs because the haptic and visual experiences are simply equivalent aspects of an undifferentiated perceptual unity. That is, no cross-modal transfer need occur, because there are no modalities. An opponent would say that the effect occurs because the experience in one modality is available, via some cross-modal transfer mechanism, to the subsequent experience in the other modality.

Perhaps this is a pseudoargument. Certainly the data available to the two theorists are the same; perhaps their differences are more illusory than real. I suggest that the issue centers on the question, at what point is perception complete? If perception is complete within a modality, as a modern descendant of the specific nerve energy doctrine might hold, then a percept may be entirely visual or entirely haptic, and cross-modal situations must involve the comparison of completed intramodality percepts. Any softening of this position allows a significant foothold for the competing position. That is, if we agree that information initially chosen by one sensory system and that by another system interact at any point before the two percepts are completed, then the issue simply becomes a technical one of determining where the separate information channels (which even the primitive unity theorist readily recognizes) feed into a common processing mechanism.

The issue is not settled, despite the persuasive theoretical stance of Gibson (1966). We should be convinced only by data, and the critical data are not available. Perhaps we should hope that no one soon solves the difficult problems inherent in acquiring them. After all, the issue has given us decades, indeed centuries, of theoretical excitement, and perhaps we would feel lonely without it.

Childhood

After this work on infancy, which is primarily concerned with the nature of the developing relationships between haptic behavior and visual control, there is something of a developmental gap in the research literature until the age of 3 or 4 years. There then begins a literature that addresses a related but more elaborate set of issues. One such issue concerns developmental changes in the dimensions of information that are particularly salient, and the relationship between them and haptic exploratory behavior. A related issue concerns the way in which haptically perceived information is encoded and stored in memory. The availability of haptically perceived information for visual comparison (and vice versa) has been extensively studied and provides a useful picture of the role of the haptic modality in relation to other modalities.

General developmental trends

We may begin again with a presentation of Piaget's (Piaget & Inhelder, 1956) views. Based on observation of children in a simple haptic perception experiment, Piaget and Inhelder suggest a series of stages and substages, not so much of haptic development as of the growth of spatial representation. The situation involved having children feel and manually explore one of various objects and shapes, without vision, and then naming or choosing it in a collection of alternatives. (Note that this is really a haptic–visual comparison task, as typified in later research, and that the question can be raised of whether any failure is due to haptic inadequacies or to the inability to transfer information from haptic intake to visual or verbal matching. This confounding is probably not a problem in Piaget's task, given its extremely simple nature and the general finding that cross-modal translation occurs readily at even very young ages.) On the basis of findings with an age range from about 2 to 7 years, Piaget and Inhelder formulated the following rough stages.

Stage I is characterized by a relatively passive type of haptic exposure in which the child responds to chance discoveries, whereas in Stage II, more regular and organized search patterns develop. These are not yet, however, governed by general rules, or "operations." More specifically, during Stage II the child still fails to link the contact with various elements of the form to a point of reference. The search may be regular and trace the outlines of the form, but the elements are not placed with respect to a point of reference.

Thus Stage I is characterized by the absence of regular exploration (i.e., running fingers regularly over the object), despite the presence of the contour in direct activity. Piaget asks the difficult question, why does regular exploration not occur? His answer involves the concepts of centration: Each momentary contact becomes important, so that the child is centrated on that momentary relation and does not attend peripherally to other aspects of the form. "Being incomplete, each centration must lead to the over-emphasis of the part contacted at the expense of parts peripheral to the area of centration" (1956, p. 24). The transition from this kind of sporadic contact (including sometimes the accidental discovery of important features) to a more regular search involves decentration, or the decreasing relative importance of a fragmentary perceptual act, so that several such acts can be put together, directed by the external stimulus, to form "perceptual activity."

During Stage II, children gradually acquire this ability to decentrate, and by about 6 years, they can encounter serially the various information points on a shape. What is lacking in Stage II is exploration for the purpose of constructing a shape that can be abstracted and compared with others. The exploration is said to lack operational guidance: "The child explores everything but keeps moving ahead all the time, never returning systematically to obtain a stable point of reference" (p. 35). That is, the search is organized in a linear rather than a spatial fashion. Features are regularly contacted but are not combined into a spatial whole.

It is this operational direction that characterizes the mature Stage III, beginning around 6 years of age. An operation is "an action which can return to its starting point, and which can be integrated with other actions also possessing this feature of reversibility" (p. 36). So, the operational method involves "grouping the elements perceived in terms of a general plan, and starting from a fixed point of reference to which the child can always return" (p. 37).

The relation between haptic and visual progress is of interest. According to Piaget, regular visual progress occurs earlier: "Visual shapes are more rapidly constructed than tactile ones" (pp. 24–25). But he argues that the developmental process is the same in both modalities, the difference in timing being due to two factors: (1) the relative clumsiness of hand as opposed to eye movements and (2) the presence of a relatively effective peripheral field in the case of vision, allowing a simultaneous intake of spatial relations as opposed to the sequential characteristic of haptic search.

The Russian work presents some similarities with and some contrasts to that of Piaget. Generally, the similarity is in the concentration on activity as a vital component of perception (both views reject the notion of a passive or receptive perception), holding that activity is necessary to the construction of percepts. The major difference is that the Russian work concentrates less on the conceptual bases that Piaget stresses, for example, the notion that operations come to provide a cognitive direction for perceptual activity. The Russian school does not reject the concept of cognitive direction; it simply does not consider it. Zaporozhets (1965) presents the general position:

> We shall try to show here that the increasing effectiveness of solving various sensory problems depends upon the development of children's perceptive activity, that is, upon the degree to which they acquire more perfect means of acquainting themselves with the objects they perceive . . . The function of these orienting–exploratory movements is to investigate its features or forming a "likeness." (p. 82)

Zaporozhets cites excerpts from Ginevskaya's work: 3- to 4.5-year-olds (Piaget's Stage I) used movements that involved rolling, playing with, and pushing the objects rather than exploring them. Later, by 6.5 to 7 years, the child traces the outline of a form, examining it systematically for information. Zaporozhets also describes the research of Zinchenko and Ruzskaya. They used two-dimensional irregular forms, examining the exploratory movements of the hands. Children 3 years old pushed with a palmar action "more like catching than touching." They played with the object rather than examining it. Children 4 to 5 years old showed some new elements, involving more fingertip exploration, rather than just contacting the object. But the fingertips were relatively passive and usually involved only one hand. Children 5 and 6 years old tended to use two hands but still did not engage in systematic exploration. They showed exploration of a feature or two but "without correlating them or locating their position on the whole figure" (p. 85). The similarity to Piaget's Stage II is evident, in that the child still does not explore for the purpose of constructing a whole shape. Describing 6-year-olds, Zinchenko and Ruzskaya note a "systematic tracing of the whole outline of the figure with the fingertips, as if the children were reproducing the form of the figure with their tactile movements by modeling its form" (p. 85). These shifts in search, involving more regular tactual contact, were related to increasing success in visually identifying the touched object from among several alternatives.

Zinchenko and Ruzskaya also examined the role of eye movements in visual exploration and found a similar developmental progression, again occurring somewhat earlier than in the haptic case. Note again the similarity to Piaget's account. Errors in visual recognition decreased earlier than errors in haptic recognition, and haptic + visual search resembled visual search, as if the addition of the haptic information were inconsequential.

Dimensions of haptic perception

A series of studies on the relative salience of texture and shape attributes illustrates aspects of these developmental trends in haptic activity. Gliner, Pick, Pick, and Hales (1969) evaluated the preference of kindergarteners and third graders, in a matching task, for texture as opposed to shape. They used a discrimination learning task in which the subject was given both shape and texture information. Kindergarteners tended to use texture as the basis for discrimination (64 percent), whereas third graders tended to use shape (67 percent). This is the sort of result that one would expect based on the exploration patterns described by Piaget and the Russian workers: The texture covered the entire shape (sandpaper grits were used to vary the texture), so the children gained the texture information even if they encountered just a part of the stimulus, whereas a more regular and complete search, characteristic of older children, was necessary to discriminate the varying elliptical shapes. The situation is more complex than this, though. As texture differences were made smaller in the Gliner et al. work, even the kindergarten children moved toward a tendency to discriminate on the basis of shape, whereas the third graders tended to use shape regardless of the discriminability of the two dimensions. Thus it is not simply that texture is always more salient for younger children; their performance varies with the relative discriminability of the two dimensions available. (Interestingly, when a visual variation of the task was used, kindergarteners used shape as the basis for discrimination more than they did in the haptic task, illustrating again the general lag of haptic behind visual development.)

Subsequent work has also drawn attention to the interrelations of various factors in the dimensional choice paradigm. Abravanel (1970) noted that the Gliner et al. stimuli were effectively two-dimensional (masonite cutouts mounted on a tray) and were thus not conducive to effective manual exploration. Abravanel hypothesized that making the forms three-dimensional would facilitate effective exploration and thus increase the relative salience of shape. In his work, the shapes were highly discriminable (cylinders vs. rectangular figures), as were the textures (felt cloth vs. smooth paper). The task involved presenting a standard form, available for exploration by both hands, then a pair of comparisons, one the same as the standard in shape and the other the same in texture. When the comparisons were presented haptically (and simultaneously), a group of 4- to 5.3-year-olds showed matching primarily based on shape (62 percent), whereas a group of 5.5- to 6.5-year-olds matched even more predominantly on shape (79 percent). Thus the younger children showed more shape matching with the three-dimensional stimuli than Gliner et al. had found with flat stimuli.

In a similar approach, Siegel and Vance (1970) used three-dimensional stimuli that were discriminable in shape and texture as well as in size. The method involved the simultaneous presentation of three stimuli, with the subject required to judge which two were the same. There was a distinct preference for shape in kindergarten, first-grade, and third-grade groups. A preschool group showed somewhat more attention to texture, but still less than to form. Size was not a salient dimension at any age. The results for a visual condition using shape and color showed a similar developmental pattern, with color playing a role equivalent to that of texture. In a subsequent study, Siegel and Barber (1973) used two-dimensional stimuli and found the preference for form over color to emerge earlier with visual presentation. With haptic presentation, form preference was slower to emerge. The possibility of manipulating three-dimensional objects presumably allows form to become salient earlier, compared to two-dimensional objects, in which texture remains more salient.

This picture seems reasonably clear. Haptic exploratory activity interacts with stimulus characteristics in determining relative dimensional salience. The haptic developmental pattern is similar to that found with vision, but restricting haptic exploration, as with two-dimensional forms, interferes with the emergence of form as a salient dimension.

A study by Abravanel (1968a) gives further information about the sensitivity of younger children to various haptic dimensions, including texture and shape, and spatial relations such as up–down, inside–outside, and rightside up–upside down. Two matching procedures were used, both requiring a visual match to a haptically presented standard. One procedure involved making a same–different judgment. The other involved the choice between two visually presented comparison objects, one identical to the haptic standard and one with the spatial attribute reversed. Children were in 3-, 4-, 5-, and 6-year-old groups. Performance was virtually random for the 3- and 4-year-olds, indicating that the younger children had difficulty with the haptic perception of the spatial attribute, whereas by 5 or 6 years, they had considerable success with these tasks. A group of 3.5- to 4.5-year-olds performed successfully on visual–

visual same–different judgments, indicating that the spatial attributes themselves were understood and that the concept of same–different did not pose a problem. Apparently the difficulty for the younger subjects lay either in the haptic discrimination of spatial relations or in their inability to translate spatial information gained haptically into a form suitable for visual comparison. Abravanel cited work by others (e.g., Blank & Bridger, 1964) showing that the difficulty was not in cross-modal transfer. Thus he concluded that the problem was with the haptic perception of spatial attributes.

The perception of spatial relationships is a more difficult haptic task than that of discriminating shape or texture. The discrimination of texture does not require sophisticated exploration, the discrimination of shape requires regular exploration, and the comparison of spatial attributes requires an operational approach in which each part is somehow abstracted or represented for comparison with the other. Thus Abravanel's results fit nicely into a logical developmental pattern. Pick and Pick (1966) report a haptic discrimination study whose results also fit this formulation. Haptic versions of the letterlike forms used visually by Gibson, Gibson, Pick, and Osser (1962) were used with children from 6 to 13 years and with adults. The forms are not letters; they are constructed of elements such as lines, curves, and angles, which commonly occur in letters. Each form also had a series of transformations involving various features. The transformations used by Pick and Pick were changing a line to a curve, rotating or reversing the form, changing size or perspective, and break and close, having to do with the continuity or discontinuity of various segments. The subject felt a standard form and one of its transformations, one with each hand, and judged whether they were the same or different. (The standard was also used as a comparison, of course.) Perspective and size transformations were the most difficult at all ages, and in fact there was no improvement from 6-year-olds to adults. Line-to-curve transformations were the next most difficult and showed significant improvement with age, whereas rotations and reversals and breaks and closes were quite similar, showing a gradual improvement from ages 6 to 11. The relative difficulty of these haptic discriminations may be interpreted as follows. The perspective and size judgments are difficult in that they involve the entire form; they cannot be easily made by attending simply to individual features. Breaks and closes, though, may be discriminated on the basis of a single feature, although the key feature must be located by the child. Line-to-curve transformations are intermediate in that there is a figural component to the discrimination between a curve and a straight line, but the discrimination does not

102

involve the whole figure. The ease of the rotations and reversals would seem confusing, because these are transformations of the whole figure rather than of selected features. However, the whole figure need not be explored in order to perceive, for example, that a particular angle is not in the same place on the two stimuli. Thus, although appearing to require figural analysis, the rotations and reversals may be performed on the basis of features, and the developmental results suggest that they were. Thus the Pick and Pick results fit with the developmental progression, constructed from other evidence, from featural to figural sensitivity, based on the development of appropriate exploration strategies.

Interestingly, the relative order of difficulty of the various transformations was similar to that found for visual performance by Gibson et al. (1962), with the exception of the rotations and reversals, which were intermediate in difficulty in that study. Although strict comparison could not be made between the relative difficulty of the haptic results of Pick and Pick and the visual results of Gibson et al., it is clear that the haptic task was considerably more difficult. Older children and adults made numerous haptic errors, whereas very good performance was found for 8-year-olds in the visual task.

The use of haptic information

Earlier, several infancy studies were discussed that concerned the usefulness of haptic information, given the apparent developmental leading of haptic by visual perception. There is a corresponding literature using children as subjects. The issue has practical as well as theoretical implications. On the theoretical side, the questions center on the role of vision in educating touch, or vice versa. As will become evident, much of the evidence does not support the "touch teaches vision" formulation (cf. Pick, Pick, & Klein, 1967, for a review of the evidence). There is nevertheless the Russian emphasis on the role of motor activity in the formation of "motor copies," the closest Russian equivalent to the schema or image.

The issue is also potentially important from a practical point of view. In education, for example, if visual perception can be aided by related tactual information, then it might make sense to allow young children, when they are learning to discriminate letters visually, to explore letter forms tactually at the same time, in hopes of aiding visual discrimination. In fact, more than one educator has advanced this notion vigorously (e.g., Fernald, 1943; Gillingham & Stillman, 1966; Orton, 1966). The question, then, is this: What, if anything, does haptic perception add to visual perception? Although visual perception seems, based on observational and experimental evidence, to develop earlier than haptic perception, might it be facilitated by the addition of a haptic component?

A study with ambiguous results, but one that sparked a good deal of interest, was reported by Denner and Cashdan (1967). The subjects were 3- and 4-year-old nursery-school children. Three groups of eight performed in different conditions. In a visual + haptic condition, the subject inspected the form (a hexagon) visually in addition to handling it; in a visual + manual condition, the object was enclosed in a clear plastic ball, so that the subject could handle the ball manually and see the object but could not gain haptic information about the object; and in a visual condition, the subject could only see the object, with no manual activity at all. All groups were also required to learn the name of the object, calling it a "hex." Two days later, the children were tested to see if they could point to the test object from among a set of four objects. All of the children in the visual + haptic and visual + manual groups identified the test object correctly, whereas only five of eight did so in the visual condition. The results suggest that visual exposure may be facilitated by some manual activity. Within the constraints of the simple task, though, it was not possible to decide whether motor activity increased visual attentiveness, whether the haptic contact with the object or the ball was the key to facilitation, or whether the motor activity, which was common to both tasks, was involved. Further, it is undetermined whether haptic contact with the object itself (in the visual + haptic group) was especially beneficial, because both the visual + haptic and visual + manual groups performed perfectly. The naming requirement during the initial exposure complicates the situation somewhat. It turned out that few children in any group could remember the name of the object, though, so it is likely that the procedure had little effect and probably no differential effect between groups.

In a methodological variation on this theme, DeLeon, Raskin, and Gruen (1970) had 3- and 4-year-old subjects match a standard from a set of three comparisons. The stimuli were random shapes with 4, 8, 12, or 16 sides. Each subject performed in four conditions, only two of which are relevant to this section. They were a visual condition, in which the subject viewed the standard, presented above the three comparisons, and a visual + haptic condition, in which the array was the same but the subject was able to see and handle the forms. Thus there were no memory demands, in contrast to the Denner and Cashdan task. The older children performed significantly better than the younger ones. There was no difference between the two conditions and no interaction with age.

Performance was very good in both conditions, though, and a ceiling effect is possible. Exploration times were recorded and were equivalent for the two conditions, indicating that additional time was not taken to process haptic information. (In a haptic condition with no vision, exploration time was greater and performance substantially worse.)

Abravanel (1972a) observed the nature of manual activity in a visual + haptic condition, thinking that the developmental changes in haptic exploration, discussed earlier, might interact with the task to determine performance. Four tasks were used, two of which are relevant here. One used a visual standard with visual comparison and the other a visual + haptic standard with visual comparison. In addition, two levels of discriminative difficulty were used. The easier stimuli were irregular, two-dimensional forms with obvious distinctive features, whereas the difficult stimuli were the irregular three-dimensional forms of Gibson (1963). The standard was presented for 10 sec; then the standard remained while two comparison forms were added. The subject was instructed to choose the comparison that was the same as the standard. The subjects averaged 4.3 years, roughly equivalent to the older group of DeLeon et al. (1970). The availability of haptic exploration did not facilitate performance for either difficulty level, although as in the previous studies, a ceiling level of performance is indicated. However, Abravanel noted that film analysis of the haptic activity revealed that the subjects "used their hands to orient and direct the shapes for visual regard, but rarely for purposes of exploration" (p. 173), even in the case of the more complex objects. He suggested that by the age of four, "the young child has created a division of labor between eye and hand in which visual perception is given the major role for shape differentiation" (p. 174). However, he noted that the situation might be different for the discrimination of texture or hardness. (Abravanel's qualifier, to which we will return, is a very important one.)

Similarly, Millar (1971) used a matching to standard procedure with four visual comparison alternatives, with 3- and 4-year-olds. There was a 15-sec delay between exploration of the standard stimulus and presentation of the comparison set. No ceiling effects were present, thus avoiding the difficulties in interpretation present in the DeLeon et al. (1970) and Abravanel (1972a) studies. In contrast to the division of labor noted by Abravanel for 4-year-olds, Millar noted that her 3-year-old subjects felt the test objects actively when haptic involvement was allowed: The hands were not used just for holding the object. Even with this more active haptic activity, performance in a haptic + visual condition did not surpass that in a visual-only condition, whereas both of these conditions were significantly better than a haptic-only condition for both age groups. (Other interesting results from this study involved intermodal transfer and will be discussed presently.)

Thus, although there are several studies on whether haptic experience facilitates visual experience, many of them are not too useful, primarily because of the existence of apparent ceiling effects. The significant exception is the study by Millar (1971), which showed no difference in performance as a result of adding haptic to visual exposure. Keeping in mind the danger of conclusions based on negative results, the tentative but appealing conclusion seems to be that the addition of haptic to visual information does not facilitate performance. This conclusion seems further justified, although only on inferential grounds, on the basis of observations by Piaget and Inhelder (1956), Zaporozhets (1965), and others that visual exploration in preschool children shows more maturity than haptic exploration.

The question may also be turned around, putting the burden on vision. That is, does the addition of visual to haptic exposure facilitate haptic performance? Despite its apparent simplicity, the question is not a straightforward one. Conditions have been tested in which presentation of the standard was purely haptic and the comparison either visual or haptic (e.g., DeLeon 1970; Millar, 1971). In such conditions, performance has been found routinely poorer than in those conditions in which visual information was available for examination of the standard, either alone or together with haptic information. These conditions, however, involve other factors, such as the use of the haptic response modality or a haptic-to-visual information transfer, and these factors complicate the situation. The key test is that involving a visual + haptic standard and visual + haptic comparison, a visual standard and visual comparison, and a haptic standard and haptic comparison. Millar (1971) found performance in the visual–visual condition to be better than that in the haptic–haptic condition but did not include the third condition. DeLeon et al. (1970) used the three key conditions and found the visual–visual and the visual + tactual–visual + tactual to be equivalent (although near the ceiling), with both significantly better than the tactual–tactual.

Schiff and Dytell (1971) studied the haptic identification of letters in an experiment that also bears on this issue. The stimulus letter was raised slightly from a flat background and was presented haptically with vision occluded. In one condition, subjects identified the letter verbally; in another, they had the printed alphabet available for visual inspection, simultaneous with the haptic presentation of the stimulus letter, and pointed to the appropriate letter on the page. Performance on both conditions improved substantially over the age range of 7 to 19 years. The visual response condition was performed better than the verbal condition across the entire age range, indicating that the presence of visual information facilitated haptic identification. With increasing age, the children were more clearly searching haptically for distinctive features, and it was also evident that the older children were examining the haptic and visual material simultaneously, rather than alternately. Thus the results suggest both improving haptic exploration strategies and increasing intermodal facility with age. Finally, an interesting result was that the errors indicated a confusion pattern for haptic stimuli that was very similar to that found for visually perceived letters (Gibson, Osser, Schiff, & Smith, 1963).

Thus, to the extent that these studies may be interpreted to bear on the question at hand, it may be tentatively concluded that haptic added to visual information does not play a facilitory role, whereas visual added to haptic information does.

Jessen and Kaess (1973) present a study that runs somewhat counter to this conclusion in showing an incremental benefit of haptic exposure to forms experienced visually compared to visual-only exposure. The paradigm involved a training session in which one group received visual exposure and another received visual + haptic exposure. The stimuli were the letterlike forms of Gibson et al. (1962). In the 18-trial training session, the subject placed or directed the experimenter to place forms in their indentations. One group was allowed haptic in addition to visual information, whereas the other received only visual information. Subsequently, a test was used in which each subject saw a standard form, then chose a match from three alternatives that were either seen or felt. The haptic test situation is not relevant here, because it involved cross-modal performance. In the visual test situation, 3.5-year-old subjects performed better after visual + haptic training than after visual-only training. Older subjects, averaging 5.5 years, showed no difference as a function of the training condition (but both groups, as well as a no-training control group, performed very accurately, suggesting a ceiling effect). For the younger group, then, where there was a significant number of errors, the addition of haptic exposure during training significantly facilitated performance, compared to visual-only training.

A study by Wolff (1972) corroborates the results of Jessen and Kaess and shows the importance of several variables. Using two-dimensional nonsense forms as standards, Wolff constructed three variations of each standard. The standard was presented for exploration; then it was covered and four alternatives were uncovered. The child was required to choose a match for the standard. Feedback was given: The correct choice had stars on its reverse side, and the child's choice was turned over on each trial to show whether or not it was correct. The criterion was two correct choices in a row. Three groups of children had average ages of 4.7, 5.6, and 6.7 years. Half of each group was restricted to visual exploration of the standard, whereas the other half was also allowed haptic exploration, being told: "You can do anything you want to with your hands." The response was made visually for all children. The nature of any haptic exploration in the optional group was noted. Most of the haptic activity was rudimentary, consisting at most of extended-finger tracing of the contour. Some children in the visual-only group attempted to use their hands but were prevented by the experimenter; nonetheless, a number of the visual-only subjects made tracings of the standard with their heads. On the basis of the activity actually present during inspection, subjects were classified into activity and nonactivity groups. The subjects who used haptic exploration, or who moved the head, reached the criterion more quickly than the visual-only subjects. Thus motor activity of the hand or head, termed *stimulus-correlated activity*, facilitated discrimination achievement. Analysis by age revealed that no significant change in stimulus-correlated activity occurred with age; however, the association of stimulus-correlated activity with better performance apparently decreased with age.

In this experiment, stimulus-correlated activity was at the subject's choice (even for the headmovers in the visual-only condition, as it turned out). In a second experiment, Wolff used essentially the same learning task but imposed exploration strategies experimentally. One group was restricted to visual exploration, a second was required to examine the standard both visually and haptically, and a third was required to touch two edges of the figure with the fingers of both hands but was not allowed true haptic exploration. The subjects were 4 to 5 years of age. Blocks of 12 trials were given, and the number of correct choices was recorded (in place of the trials-to-criterion measure). The visual + haptic group performed best, but there was no difference between the visual-only and the visual + limited touch groups. The performance of the latter group did not differ from chance.

Wolff (1972) offers a useful discussion of the critical differences between his experiments, which found added effectiveness of haptic exposure, and prior ones. First, in Wolff's study the comparison figures did not differ from the standard in perceptually salient features (such as angles vs. curves), but only in aspects of general configuration. (In this respect, though, Wolff's two-dimensional stimuli were analogous to the three-dimensional stimuli used by Abravanel, 1972, who found no haptic facilitation of vision.) Wolff reasoned that haptic exploration might facilitate the "construction of holistic percepts [more] than . . . detection of differences between values on feature dimensions which are already familiar to the child" (p. 438). As a second and closely related point, Wolff suggested that his procedure, involving repeated trials with the same stimulus forms, may have facilitated the gradual construction of a percept, in contrast to the typical single presentation and no-feedback procedure of most other research. The interesting phenomenon of the head movers suggests that it is not just the haptic or motor activity of the hand that contributes to such percept construction, but rather any stimulus-correlated activity of a "moving extremity." (Unfortunately, eye movements were not recorded.)

Wolff and Levin (1972) further explored the role of the child's haptic activity in facilitating paired-associate learning, using common toys as stimuli. In the first experiment, the subject could always see the paired toys. Simple visual exposure was less effective than a condition in which the child could also handle the pairs of toys in creating an interaction between them. (A condition in which the experimenter manipulated the toys in an interaction was also effective, whereas a condition in which the subject was instructed to imagine the stationary toys interacting was effective in facilitating performance for a group of third-grade children, but not for kindergarteners.) In a second experiment, kindergarten and first-grade children were required to manipulate the paired toys in an interaction, but the manipulation was performed in a box that prevented sight of the interaction. Compared with an imagined interaction, the unseen haptic manipulation condition was facilitory for both age groups. Thus sight of the manipulated interaction was not required for the effectiveness of the haptic involvement. In a subsequent study, Wolff, Levin, and Longobardi (1972) hypothesized that haptic manipulation helped to evoke images of the stimulus pairs. Again, tactual involvement in the manipulation facilitated paired-associate learning.

Taken as a group, this set of studies on the possibility of haptic facilitation of various kinds of performance is somewhat confusing. It seems reasonable to conclude that in simple discriminations, where vision can be used by young children, the addition of haptic information does not generally facilitate discrimination. In such cases, vision seems to play the leading role, with the hand perhaps serving primarily to orient objects for visual inspection. However, this conclusion may be applicable only when featural distinctions are readily available (although note the unresolved conflict between the finding of Abravanel, 1972, and Wolff, 1972, the latter finding haptic facilitation). Haptic involvement may also contribute significantly when the task requires improving discrimination over time or trials and when performance involves the creation of an image.

Herein may lie the resolution of the apparent conflict between the Russian work, citing the role of the motor copy in perception, and a body of American research that shows no apparent facilitory role of haptic involvement. The motor copy theory seems to apply best to the Wolff (1972) and Jessen and Kaess (1973) procedures, in which extended experience was gained with the stimulus materials, allowing the establishment of a schema or image of the objects. The use of procedures that allow only brief contact with the stimulus materials, as in the work by DeLeon et al. (1970), Abravanel (1972a), and Millar (1971), may not allow the potential facilitory effect of haptic exposure to occur. With respect to the applied issue of learning to discriminate useful shapes (e.g., letters), then, it still seems that haptic facilitation of vision is possible.

As noted earlier, Abravanel (1972a) concluded that by age 4, the child has created a division of labor between eye and hand, with the hand serving primarily to orient stimuli for visual inspection. He qualified this conclusion, however, noting that it may apply to shape perception but not to other stimulus qualities, such as texture and hardness, in which haptic perception may play a more integral role. Thus the specialization of modalities for various perceptual events may be more complex than is suggested by the body of evidence showing that vision matures earlier. The earlier discussion on the dimensions of haptic perception may be reinterpreted in this regard. Generally, this evidence shows that younger children tend to attend to texture information when it is available together with shape information, whereas older children are more likely to attend to shape. Findings of this sort have been typically interpreted to indicate the inadequacy of exploration of shape by the younger children (note that texture can be experienced even on an incompletely explored stimulus, whereas effective perception of shape requires fuller exploration). This conclusion is undoubtedly valid, but the earlier salience of texture may also indicate an emerging specialization of the haptic modality for texture information. Thus these data may indicate not only what younger children *cannot* do haptically with shape but what they *can* do haptically with texture. Research on this recasting of the issue may be very useful (see Chapter 4).

Cross-modality integration

There is a large literature on cross-modality integration of haptic and visual information. For the most part, this literature is concerned with integration itself, but there is also considerable information on the relative course of haptic and visual development. The issues are closely interrelated, and we shall discuss them together. A focal question, for the purpose of this chapter, is whether information gained haptically can immediately be compared with other kinds of information. This is clearly a question involving both haptic information processing and intermodality integration.

Birch and Lefford (1963) provided an early study on this issue. They studied children from 5 to 11 years of age, using three intermodality form-matching tasks. Stimulus shapes were from the Seguin Formboard, and thus were regular and relatively familiar. The procedure involved paired comparisons with simultaneous presentation, with same or different judgments. In the haptic presentation, subjects explored the form with the active hand, using the fingers or palm at will. In the kinesthetic presentation, subjects held a stylus in their fingers and the experimenter moved the stylus around the outline of the shape. Thus three combinations of the three modalities were used: visual–haptic, visual–kinesthetic, and haptic–kinesthetic. On each trial, a form was presented to each of the two modalities and the subject judged them the same or different. The visual–haptic integration task was done best at all ages, showing a low error rate even at 5 years and a gradual improvement up to age 8. The ability to match visual with haptic information by age 5 is not surprising in view of the evidence that we have already reviewed suggesting cross-modal transfer in infants. Both combinations that involved kinesthetic presentation were substantially worse, but both showed a gradual improvement with age, roughly fitting a logarithmic function. Birch and Lefford concluded that the period from 6 to 8 years, in which most of the kinesthetically related success was gained, represented a "period of rapid change in functional organization and capacity" (p. 40). The combinations involving kinesthesis may have lagged as a result of the more gradual development of intermodality function involving kinesthetically presented information, as Birch and Lefford suggest, but it seems more likely that the poorer performance in these conditions was due to the artificiality of the kinesthetic condition, involving passive movement of the hand and the interposed stylus.

Blank and Bridger (1964), in another early study, assessed the ability of 3-, 4-, and 5-year-olds to feel a familiar shape (triangle, circle, etc.) and select one of two visually presented objects to match the haptic standard. The 3-year-olds performed at a level (68 percent correct) not significantly better than chance, whereas the 4- and 5-year-olds approached perfect performance. Although the difficulty experienced by the youngest group was attributed to a failure of cross-modal transfer of information, this conclusion is not strictly defensible because the results might have been due to poor haptic discrimination of the standard object rather than (or in addition) to poor cross-modal transfer.

Other studies have attempted to solve this problem by comparing intramodal and cross-modal tasks. For example, Rudel and Teuber (1964) used visual–visual, visual–haptic, haptic–visual, and haptic–haptic tasks, in which the first modality named refers to the presentation of the standard stimulus and the second to the presentation of the comparison objects. The standard form was presented for a 5-sec inspection period, and then five comparison forms were presented in succession. The results for 5-year-olds showed clearly that the haptic–haptic task was the most difficult, whereas the other three tasks were roughly equal in difficulty. Cross-modal transfer was clearly not the limiting factor, because the two cross-modal tasks were done better than the haptic–haptic task. Rather, reliance on haptic information about both standard and comparison stimuli produced poor performance. The work also demonstrated clearly the necessity of choosing task difficulty carefully. The procedure using five comparison objects presented successively was too difficult for 3- and 4-year-olds, whereas 4-year-olds performed somewhat better when the five objects were presented for simultaneous inspection. Subsequent research thus sought to use somewhat easier tasks. A study that successfully evaluated the relationships among the four conditions in 4-year-olds was reported by Bryant and Raz (1975). Their procedure involved presenting the standard simultaneously with two choice shapes, one the same as the standard. The visual–visual condition was performed best, and significantly better than any of the others. The fact that the visual–visual condition was better than either of the two cross-modality conditions suggests that either there is difficulty in cross-modal matching or that the haptic modality is less useful in shape discrimination than the visual modality. The relatively poor performance in the haptic–haptic condition suggests that at least the latter conclusion is justified: Whether there is also cross-modal matching difficulty is not resolved by the data. The pattern of results reported by Bryant and Raz has, with minor variations, been found in the bulk of the research using this paradigm. Thus a tentative conclusion seems justified: For shape perception, the haptic modality is generally less effective than the visual modality.

This is not the end of the story, however, because this conclusion is too general. Researchers have studied two categories of variables and their effects on performance on such tasks; exploration strategies and memory and encoding characteristics.

Exploration strategies

Exploration strategy is an important issue. It is necessary to separate haptic sensory abilities from the strategies used to direct haptic activity, because it may be in the strategy area that the younger child's weakness lies, rather than in haptic sensitivity itself. Strategies may indeed be susceptible to training, whereas it seems unlikely that sensitivity itself can be substantially improved.

Abravanel (1968b) studied matching of length, concentrating on the manner of haptic exploration and its relation to performance. The two conditions of primary interest here involved adjustments of the length of a bar. When the standard bar was presented visually, the child haptically adjusted a stop on it to match the length without seeing the response bar. When the standard bar was presented haptically, the subject felt it and instructed the experimenter to adjust a visual length to match the haptic standard. Subjects would use both hands for the haptic components. Generally, the age trends showed the visual–haptic task to improve earlier than the haptic–visual task, with equivalence achieved at about age 9. Some interesting age-related changes in haptic strategies were noted. Children 3 and 4 years old seemed to be more inclined to feel the *shape* of the bar than its length, whereas the 5-year-olds tended to assess length by holding the ends of the bar. By contrast, 7- and 8-year-olds engaged in a more systematic exploration of the length of the bar, spanning its extent or moving the fingers along its length. The younger children tended to use the palms, whereas the older ones tended to use the fingers. The relationship between strategy and accuracy was unfortunately not analyzed within each age group, but an examination of the data across age groups showed that the more regular scanning strategies were related to more accurate performance. It is possible that the poor performance of the younger children may have been due to lesser haptic ability, but it also seems possible that they used inappropriate strategies because they were, in effect, doing a different task from the one set by the experimenter. Certainly their strategies suggest this interpretation. It would be interesting to know how well they would have done if they had been directed to use the more appropriate haptic scanning techniques.

Abravanel (1972b) used a relatively easy task to investigate cross-modal shape matching in 4-year-old children. In each condition, a standard form was presented for a 10-sec inspection period. Then two comparisons, one the same as the standard, were added, so that comparisons and standard were available simultaneously. Three conditions are of interest here. One used a haptic standard with a visual comparison, a second allowed haptic + visual exposure to the standard with a visual comparison, and the third allowed haptic + visual exposure to the standard with a haptic comparison. The visual + haptic condition was performed very accurately. In this condition, most of the children used their hands only to orient the standard for visual inspection. The haptic–visual and visual + haptic–haptic conditions were performed equally and significantly, although not much, better than chance. Both of these conditions required the use of haptic information, and the lack of appropriate haptic exploration strategies undoubtedly restricted performance. A group of adults tested subsequently on the visual + haptic–haptic condition performed much better than the children (Abravanel, 1973), and it was noted that the adults showed substantial haptic exploration of the standard. Thus the haptic strategy is clearly related to matching success, although again the question remains of whether children would match more successfully if they were required to engage in real haptic exploration of the standard.

There is some evidence on the possibility of training strategies that are not spontaneously used. Davidson (1972), working with adults, found congenitally blind subjects to be better at judging curvature than sighted subjects performing blindfolded. Analysis of videotaped scanning behaviors revealed that the blind subjects tended to use scanning strategies that encompassed the whole stimulus, whereas the sighted subjects tended to scan more locally. When they were required to use the more holistic strategies of the blind, the sighted subjects' performance was comparable to that of the blind. The work of Berlá and his colleagues is also of interest. Berlá and Murr (1974) examined the effectiveness of various scanning strategies and found, for example, that a vertical scan using two hands is more effective than various horizontal strategies. The training issued was also explored: Visually impaired children in the early grades benefited from training in the vertical scan strategy. High school students were disadvantaged by the training. In another study, Berlá and Butterfield (1977) found that children who scanned haptically in a regular way and who attended to distinctive features of the shapes were relatively good at finding tactual shapes on a map. Further, they found that map search was improved by training that emphasized regular scanning and attention to distinctive features. The work of Berlá and of Davidson is important in exploring the relationships between spontaneous strategies and the training question. Further, the work is encouraging in finding that performance is sensitive to strategies and strategies to training. Although this work has been primarily oriented to visually impaired samples, the issues are also of importance and interest for the sighted population, particularly if one wishes to explore the full range of capabilities of the various perceptual systems.

From a variety of observational and experimental evidence, it is clear that haptic perception improves substantially during the early childhood years. Part of the improvement may be a result of increasing haptic discrimination, but evidence suggests that improvement in haptic exploration strategies is the key to development. Piaget and Inhelder (1956), Zaporozhets (1965), and others present observational evidence for such developmental progression, and in more experimental work, performance on haptic tasks has been found to vary with the exploration strategy spontaneously used (Abravanel, 1972b, 1973; Wolff, 1972). Further, the strategies that are spontaneously used vary both within developmental level (Berlá & Murr, 1974) and across development (Abravanel, 1968b, 1972b). The strategy training question has two aspects. First, can children who do not use the optimal strategies available to their developmental level be trained to do so? Second, can strategies that are characteristic of a higher developmental level be induced at a lower level? There is little evidence on the latter question, although it is of considerable interest given the relationship between experience and development. On the former question, existing evidence suggests that inadequate strategies are susceptible to training (e.g., Berlá & Butterfield, 1977; Berlá & Murr, 1974).

Several writers (e.g., Piaget & Inhelder, 1956; Zaporozhets, 1965) have noted that the development in haptic exploratory characteristics is similar to that in visual exploration, with haptic development following a timetable that is comparatively delayed. Much of this delay may be related to the characteristics of the receptors for the two modalities. Two important differences are obvious: First, the hand and its fingers are more cumbersome than the eye, and it is evident that the visual system is thus better, and earlier, prepared to make the fine muscular adjustments needed for regular and rapid exploration of stimuli. Second, the spatial distribution of receptors in the eye is more conducive than that on the hand to the simultaneous registry of spatially distributed stimulus arrays. Certainly some direction of search by tactual information may occur in a manner analogous to the peripheral reception of visual information that helps to direct eye movements in stimulus exploration, but this matter has not been addressed directly in the literature. These two differences may account for the apparent developmental lag in organized haptic search.

It is important to note that significant similarities are also described in the development of haptic and visual exploration strategies, and it is useful to consider what the basis for these commonalities might be. Piaget and Inhelder (1956) and Uzgiris (1967) argue that exploration in both modalities gradually comes under the direction of cognitive operations, so that the momentary activity becomes controlled by an overall operation rather than by the immediate nature of the stimulus element being contacted. Wright and Vlietstra (1975) provide an excellent review and analysis of a wide variety of literature that illustrates such trends. They find it useful to distinguish between exploration and search. Exploration is characteristic of younger children, is more stimulus commanded and playful, and is less task related. Search involves a more cognitively controlled behavior that may be applied to the performance of a specific task. Being cognitively controlled, it is less dominated by particularly salient stimulus elements. This is an important developmental progression, because the emerging regularity of search allows more effective contact with the stimulus world, thereby facilitating the course of cognitive growth. Thus cognitive control emerges, and as it emerges and directs search, it allows more regularly organized information to be acquired, thus facilitating the child's "generalized competence to acquire useful and orderly information from his environment" (p. 234). Wright and Vlietstra cite evidence from a variety of experimental and observational paradigms in support of their developmental hypothesis. In doing so, they illustrate the need to consider superordinate factors, in addition to modality-specific factors, in explaining development.

Memory and encoding

Several studies have explored the possibility that haptic information is less useful in matching tasks because it is less well retained than visual information. Rose, Blank, and Bridger (1972) use visual–visual, visual–haptic, haptic–visual, and haptic–haptic matching tasks, comparing simultaneous exposure to standard and (two) comparisons with successive exposure under no-delay and 15-sec delay conditions. The subjects averaged just under 4 years. The discriminations were relatively easy, involving regular three-dimensional geometric figures in one series and discriminable textures in another. The texture series was generally more difficult than the form series. Generally, the visual–visual condition was performed best, but there was a significant statistical interaction for condition delay. With simultaneous presentation of the standard and the comparisons, all conditions were performed equally well (but few errors were made, and there was a possible ceiling effect). In the successive condition with no delay (comparisons presented immediately upon removal of the standard), performance deteriorated in all tasks but significantly more in the conditions involving a haptic component. The fact that the simultaneous haptic–haptic condition was performed very well indicates that the problem with haptic information is not intake but retention. Thus when a successive condition is used, the information is presumably discriminated, but performance deteriorates because of poor retention. The decrement under successive conditions when the standard was presented visually and the comparisons haptically cannot be accounted for by this notion alone, however, and some difficulty in cross-modal transfer of information must also be postulated. The authors suggested that visual–visual performance under successive conditions must have been facilitated by visual images; by implication, they suggest that effective images of haptically presented standards did not occur.

Goodnow (1971) similarly concluded that haptic information is less well retained than visual information. Her task involved the presentation of five standard stimuli, explored one by one either haptically or visually. Then a comparison set of 10 forms was presented, containing the five standards plus five other similar forms (the forms were cut-out Greek and Russian letters). The child had to identify the forms that had been in the standard set. Kindergarten children performing a visual–visual task did very well, but the younger kindergarteners (5–5.4 years) performed "chaotically" on the haptic–haptic task, averaging only a random 5.5 correct out of 10. Older kindergarten children (5.5–6.7 years) showed better haptic performance, averaging 7.6 correct. With a fourth-grade group (9–10 years), Goodnow administered cross-modal tasks in addition to the two intramodal tasks. Visual–visual performance was still best (9.9), with haptic–haptic (8.2) performance improving over the older kindergarteners. The visual–haptic task (8.8) was performed better than the haptic–visual one (7.1). Goodnow concluded that visual memory was better than haptic, particularly in this task which makes relatively great memory demands. The difficulty of the task did, in fact, differentiate between the two cross-modal tasks: The haptically exposed standard was less well retained for visual comparison (7.1) than the visually exposed standard was for haptic comparison (8.8).

Davidson, Cambardella, Stenerson, and Carney (1974) explored the effects of task difficulty in a similar study. The usual four tasks were used

117

in a successive format. After the presentation of the standard for 4 sec, either one, three, or five comparison objects were presented successively, each for 4 sec and with a 1-sec interstimulus interval. Thus difficulty was varied with the size of the comparison set, and memory for the standard was clearly involved. The stimuli were the Gibson three-dimensional free forms. The subjects were second (7.9 years) and fifth (11 years) graders. The main effects of age, task, and difficulty level were found, with no significant interactions. The visual–visual task was performed best, followed by equivalent haptic–haptic and visual–haptic tasks, with the haptic–visual task worst. Thus the pattern of results was quite similar to that of Goodnow (1971). The difficulty of the haptic-visual task may be explained by the joint effects of poor memory for the haptic standard and the demand for cross-modal transfer of information. The latter variable is suggested by the poorer performance on the haptic-visual task than on the haptic–haptic one, which also involved the haptic standard but no cross-modal transfer.

The issue of memory for various kinds of information leads naturally to the question of how information is encoded and what is stored. Various approaches, none of them wholly satisfactory, have been used in studying these issues. They include specific instructions to "image" or otherwise encode in various ways (e.g., Hertz, 1971); postperformance interviews to assess the nature of the coding approach (Ford, 1973); experimental procedures designed to interfere selectively with possible kinds of coding (Millar, 1972, 1974); and comparison of groups with certain kinds of coding (McKinney, 1964). This literature will not be reviewed exhaustively, but examples will be provided with some comment on the conclusions, advantages, and disadvantages of the various approaches.

The study by Ford (1973) is an example of evaluating coding of haptic information by asking for subjective reports. The subjects were fourth-grade boys (9.2 years). The task involved presenting a standard stimulus (a raised geometric form) for two-hand haptic exploration and then four visual comparison forms in succession, with the subject required to choose a match for the standards. When asked how they did the task, most subjects reported a combination of strategies, such as "felt and pictured," "pictured and described," and "felt and described." The largest category of subjects reported that they pictured and described (50 percent). Fully 80 percent of the children reported that they pictured the standard, usually in conjunction with another operation, whereas 62 percent reported that they described it, again typically together with another operation. These two categories of coding operation represent the two types most commonly found in other studies of coding of haptic information, typically referred to as *imagery* (usually visual imagery) and *verbalization*. In contrast to the frequent reporting of picturing and describing, Ford found only 28 percent of the group reporting that they felt the standard (although, of course, all actually did); five subjects (10 percent of the total) reported that they only felt the standard, and they performed below the group mean in matching performance. Thus Ford's results suggest that fourth graders rely heavily on coding strategies that are not restricted to haptic coding. Several qualifications must be expressed, however. First, the visual presentation of the comparison forms may have induced more use of nonhaptic strategies than would have occurred if the comparisons had been presented haptically. Second, it may not be safe to assume that fourth graders (or adults, for that matter) are able to report coding strategies reliably (the question asked of the subjects was not specified) or that their use of the various terms is consistent with the experimenter's interpretation of them. The use of verbal report would seem to have limited potential, particularly to investigate developmental changes, in which the problems with cross-age equivalence of verbal responses must be seriously considered. Nonetheless, taken at face value, Ford's results may be taken as evidence that the tendency to non-haptic coding of haptic information is strong in this age group.

A study by Hertz (1971) exemplified the use of instructions to attempt to influence coding of haptically gained information. Second- and sixth-grade children were studied. The stimuli were cylinders covered with various textures. They were explored haptically under instructions either to visualize them or to concentrate on how they felt. Recognition was then tested visually. There were no striking differences in performance, but the paradigm is illustrated by the experiment. The approach suffers, as Hertz noted, from the absence of an independent assessment of whether effective visualization actually occurred.

Two studies by Millar (1972, 1974) exemplify the experimental interference with coding by means of various interventions during a retention interval between stimulus presentation and response. Generally, both studies produced results that do not provide support for the visual coding hypothesis. Millar (1972) presented a standard (a nonsense shape) either haptically or visually and three comparisons, again either haptically or visually. Thus the four modality combinations were used, although only the haptic–haptic and haptic–visual ones are of relevance here. Each task was performed under four conditions, one involving simultaneous presentation of standard and comparisons and three involving successive presentations, with a 9-sec delay before presentation of the comparisons. During the delay, the subject either (1) did nothing,

(2) performed a verbal digit span task, or (3) performed a visual memory task with figures unrelated to the relevant stimulus materials. Subjects consisted of three groups of children, averaging 8.4, 6.0 and 3.9 years. The youngest group performed at chance levels on the conditions of interest to us here. The oldest group performed better than the middle group, but there were no interactions of age with the modality combination or delay condition variables. Consider first the haptic–haptic task. If the haptic standard were visually encoded, then the interposed visual task should interfere more with performance than the interposed verbal task or the unfilled interval. In fact, though, there were no differences among the four conditions for either age group; that is none of the delay conditions was performed significantly worse than the simultaneous condition. Consider now the haptic–visual task. Because the comparison forms were presented visually, the tendency to encode the haptically presented standard visually might be enhanced if visual coding were available. (The subjects were in set conditions, so that they knew the nature of the response task. They could, therefore, have selected a visual coding approach if this alternative had been available.) Again, though, the results indicated that no such coding occurred: There were no differences among the three delay conditions for each age group. The results suggest simply that visual encoding of the haptically presented standard did not spontaneously occur and, furthermore, was not induced by the visual comparison requirement in the haptic–visual task. We are left with some question about the negative results, though, and with the possibility that visual encoding did occur but was not effectively interfered with by the visual task in the visual interference condition.

Another operation that is suggested by this approach involves the interpolation of a distraction task with haptic demands. Millar (1974) used such an approach, with conditions involving (1) unfilled delay, (2) delay with a verbal distraction task, (3) delay with a hand movement distractor, and (4) delay with hand movement rehearsal, in which the subject was instructed to finger-trace the shape of the (now absent) standard stimulus during the delay. The standard was presented haptically, and a same–different judgment was required with a single comparison object. The stimuli were three-dimensional irregular shapes with a high degree of discriminability. A group of 9- to 10-year-olds showed very low error rates that did not apparently differentiate among conditions. A subsequent experiment with 5- to 7-year-olds was then conducted, and error rates suitable for analysis were found. Three delay intervals of 5, 10, and 30 sec were used, but the results may safely be generalized across intervals. Briefly summarized, the error rates suggested equivalence of the unfilled delay and rehearsal conditions, with the two distractor conditions showing substantially more errors. The movement distractor condition, in which the subject had to manipulate and arrange a set of barrel-shaped objects, produced the worst matching performance, but the substantial deterioration of performance under the verbal distractor condition suggests that much of the distraction effect in even the movement condition was not specific to the haptic modality. Rehearsal apparently did not facilitate performance, compared to the unfilled delay condition. Millar's conclusion that rehearsal was ineffective, however, may be too hasty, because performance in the unfilled delay condition was quite good and may have represented a ceiling effect.

Millar concluded that a modality-specific encoding hypothesis was not supported by the data, because movement rehearsal had no effect compared to unfilled delay (and because verbal distractors were almost as effective as movement distractors). Rather, Millar suggested that "attentional rather than movement demands produced the response deficits" (p. 262) and, further, that "tactile short-term memory involves both decay of tactile impressions with time, and interference by attentional demands with a longer-term process" (p. 263).

The fourth approach to the coding issue involves the comparison of performance by groups that are assumed, a priori, to differ in the ability to perform a certain kind of coding. In the case of haptic information, particularly when spatial performance tasks are at issue, the kind of coding hypothesized is usually visual, and the groups compared are typically the sighted and the blind or severely visually impaired. (This is not the only possibility, however: Hearing-impaired subjects would, by the same logic, be expected to have difficulty with spatial or other tasks that required verbal coding of information, whether haptically gained or otherwise.) A prototypical experiment is reported by McKinney (1964), who investigated the ability of children to remember which of their fingers had been touched under various conditions. If the hand were turned over after stimulation but before response, McKinney reasoned that performance would deteriorate somewhat if a visual image was involved, whereas if the hand were turned over and then back to its original position before response, the physical position of the hand would again coincide with the image, and performance would not suffer. McKinney found this pattern of results with young sighted children. He then hypothesized that without an effective means of visually encoding the tactual information, congenitally blind children would show deteriorating performance as a function of the number of hand turns, rather than showing improved performance once the hand was turned back to its original position. The results supported this hypothesis, and McKinney concluded that the sighted subjects used a "visual schema" of the hand that was effective in mediating performance whenever the hand was in its original stimulated position.

Although the McKinney study did not involve haptic information as we have been using the term, it makes the logic of the paradigm clear: A hypothesis is formulated about the kind of information encoding involved, and two groups, one of which is assumed to have that kind of encoding unavailable, are compared. If their performance differs in the expected direction, then the coding hypothesis is supported. Although this paradigm is very widely used, and is probably not misleading in most cases, it should be noted that on two counts it rests on somewhat shaky grounds. First, it depends on the assumption that one group has the coding capability and the other does not. This assumption is typically not subject to independent empirical test. Second, the groups are, by the logic of the Method of Difference, assumed to be equivalent in all other respects but the availability of coding by one group. This is a risky assumption at best, as I have argued elsewhere for the specific case of blind versus sighted comparisons (Warren, 1978a,b).

The literature on the encoding and retention of haptic information, particularly as it might change with development, is far from conclusive. The last paradigms discussed, those directly concerned with encoding, are based on questionable assumptions and present a mixed picture. The subjective report approach is confounded with verbal usage patterns, and developmental comparability may not be lightly assumed. Nor do instructions to visualize or verbalize necessarily re-create the information-processing methods that children normally use, and again, developmental comparability is uncertain. The use of intervening tasks that are assumed to interfere selectively with different kinds of stored information seems to be a more promising approach, but it has not been used often enough with children to give a good indication of its potential. As with many so-called information-processing operations, many inferences about the precise nature of coding and the function of experimental operations must be made, and there is a great need for extensive converging operations before definitive conclusions may be drawn. Nonetheless, for the encoding and retention of haptic information, such approaches seem to hold the greatest promise, and it is hoped that they will receive research attention.

These issues clearly are concerned as much with the nature of intermodality organization as with the processing of haptic information. This area is far too large and complex to be discussed fully here, but several points of reference may be mentioned to demonstrate the range of factors that should be considered. The danger of overgeneralizing the notion that visual perception precedes haptic perception has already been mentioned: The perception of texture is certainly different from that of spatial relationships. The various modalities are differentially suited for the perception of different kinds of events (cf. the discussion by Warren, 1979): Vision seems to be better for the perception of spatial relationships, audition for temporal relationships, and perhaps haptics for textural qualities. Freides (1974) reviews much of this evidence, particularly on vision and audition, and proposes that for relatively simple perceptual tasks, the modalities function more or less equivalently, but that as the task becomes more complex, the relative advantages of one modality or another emerge. As complexity increases, therefore, information tends to be translated into a form suitable for processing by the most appropriate modality.

A related argument, again primarily concerned with vision and audition, is developed by Posner, Nissen, and Klein (1976). Noting that vision is typically dominant in situations in which two modalities are involved, they suggest that vision is a less adequate alerting system than audition, and that because of this relative weakness visual information is actively attended to. The attentional system is "tuned" to visual information; the auditory modality does not need such tuning because it is in a constantly alert state.

Haptic perception has been relatively underemphasized in these accounts, in comparison to vision and audition. It is clear, though, that a full account of haptic information processing will involve other modalities, particularly vision, and that such an account must include both the nature and the complexity of the perceptual event and the special characteristics and capabilities of the various modalities.

In general, then, there is much research to be done on the encoding and retention of haptically gained information. As with most developmental research, careful attention will have to be paid to the comparability of experimental tasks across age groups. Converging operations, in which the same issue is approached from several experimental paradigms, will be necessary before firm conclusions can be reached. At this point, although there is some indication that haptically gained information is less well retained than visually gained information, we do not have a good picture of the differences or of the extent to which they may depend on different ways of encoding and storing visual and haptic information. Nor do we have a clear picture of the developmental changes that may occur. Perhaps the most important issue concerns encoding and how encoding of haptic information may change with development. Until these issues are fully understood, there will be little significant progress on the other questions.

Concluding comments

Conclusions have been drawn throughout this chapter, and only the most important of them will be reviewed here. In infancy, the most significant unresolved issue is the theoretical question of intermodality organization. Although many writers are in basic agreement about much of development, noting that vision gradually assumes control over the perceptual activity of the hands about midway through the first year, there is a fundamental disagreement about the earliest phases of intermodality organization. Piaget and others maintain that the visual and haptic modalities are initially separate systems that gradually become organized under the leadership of vision by about 6 months of age. Bower, on the other hand, argues that there is a primitive unity of the senses, so that initially there is no functional distinction between the haptic and visual modalities. When both are in use, the visual and haptic receptor systems deliver to the infant two types of information about an event, but the infant makes no distinction between them and, in fact, becomes upset when experimental conditions lead the sources to signify spatially separate events. As a result of various pressures, haptic and visual perception become differentiated and then organized, with vision playing a leading role. This issue involves little apparent practical application, but its theoretical importance is substantial. As was earlier suggested, however, the issue will be extremely difficult, if not impossible, to resolve.

An important trend in infancy is from the subjective to the objective role of the haptic sense. Very early in infancy, the child apparently engages in haptic activity purely for the stimulation it affords. Gradually, and perhaps as cognitive mediating processes mature, the infant engages in haptic activity for the sake of the information that it can deliver about the physical world. This shift in the role of haptic perception is striking. Piaget (1953) describes infant development through about 2 years of age and emphasizes, as does Uzgiris (1967), the role of emerging cognitive control as an influential factor. For the preschool child, Wright and Vlietstra (1975) provide an analysis that is quite similar to that of Piaget. As cognitive development proceeds, it provides more and more direction to haptic as well as visual activity. (The developmental lag of haptic as compared with visual activity, documented by Wright and Vlietstra and others, may be accounted for largely if not completely by characteristics of the receptor systems themselves.) The result is that whereas the younger child engages in sporadic but stimulus-directed exploration of objects, the older child searches them in a cognitively directed, regular way to gain original information about the world.

This issue leads naturally to another, one that represents a large gap in our knowledge about haptic perception: the role of strategies of haptic exploration. Although there is very good observational evidence suggesting that exploration becomes more regular, particularly as it comes under cognitive guidance, there is far less information on individual differences. Why do some children of a given age show more or less mature strategies of haptic (or visual) exploration and search than others? How are less mature strategies related to cognitive development? Might the training of more effective learning strategies lead to the availability of better information for the developing cognitive system to feed on? Or is the nature of the information-acquiring strategy constrained by cognitive level? Or, as Wright and Vlietstra have suggested, are the two developments closely interrelated? This suggestion seems reasonable. If it is true, though, precisely how are learning strategies and cognitive level interrelated?

This gap is related to another. Although much research has been done (with little of it, though, truly developmental), there is little real understanding of information encoding and storage for the haptic modality. Various methodologies, none of them wholly satisfactory, have been used, and various suggestions have been made. One common hypothesis is that haptic information is somehow encoded in a visual format. Problems exist with this suggestion, though. What does it mean to say that haptic information is visually encoded and stored? This conclusion is typically based on data showing that haptic information decays in the same way as visual information, or that a visual task intervening between haptic exposure and response demand interferes more with performance than an amodal or a haptic task. Even if there were no contradictory data (which there are), such patterns of results do not clearly demonstrate that haptic information is visually encoded: They simply demonstrate a parallel between process characteristics. As discussed here, the visual encoding hypothesis is just an example. If visual encoding is the answer, it is undoubtedly more so for some kinds of perception (e.g., spatial location, shape) than for others (e.g., texture).

However the data may be interpreted for any given perceptual task, it is clear that we do not understand how haptic information is encoded at any given developmental level, let alone how this encoding may change from one level to another. No one methodology will answer such questions. The procedures associated with information-processing research seem attractive, but they lend themselves to model building, with the attendant danger that the model may be internally consistent but have little external validity. Models must be used in conjunction with other approaches, each of which has its own faults.

It should be obvious, then, that there are some important unanswered questions in the development of haptic perception. The questions are both theoretical and practical. Vigorous focal research is needed to answer them.

References

Abravanel, E. Intersensory integration of spatial position during early childhood. *Perceptual & Motor Skills*, 1968, 26, 251–256. (a)

The development of intersensory patterning with regard to selected spatial dimensions. *Monographs of the Society for Research in Child Development*, 1968, 33, 1–52. (b)

Choice for shape vs. textural matching by young children. *Perceptual & Motor Skills*, 1970, 31, 527–533.

How children combine vision and touch when perceiving the shape of objects. *Perception & Psychophysics*, 1972, 12, 171–175. (a)

Short-term memory for shape information processed intra- and intermodally at three ages. *Perceptual & Motor Skills*, 1972, 35, 419–425. (b)

Division of labor between hand and eye when perceiving shape. *Neuropsychologia*, 1973, 11, 207–211.

Berlá, E. P., & Butterfield, L. H. Tactual distinctive features analysis: training blind students in shape recognition and in locating shapes on a map. *Journal of Special Education*, 1977, 11, 335–346.

Berlá, E. P., & Murr, M. J. Searching tactual space. *Education of the Visually Handicapped*, 1974, 6, 49–58.

Birch, H. G., & Lefford, A. Intersensory development in children. *Monographs of the Society for Research in Child Development*, 1963, 28, 1–48.

Blank, J., & Bridger, W. H. Cross-modal transfer in nursery school children. *Journal of Comparative and Physiological Psychology*, 1964, 58, 277–282.

Bower, T. G. R. Object perception in infants. *Perception*, 1972, 1, 15–30.

The development of reaching in infants. Unpublished monograph, 1973. Cited in T. G. R. Bower, *Development in infancy*, 1974.

Development in infancy, San Francisco: W. H. Freeman, 1974. (a)

The evolution of sensory systems. In R. B. MacLeod & H. L. Pick, Jr. (Eds.), *Perception: essays in honor of James J. Gibson*, Ithaca, N.Y.: Cornell University Press, 1974. (b)

A primer of infant development. San Francisco: W. H. Freeman, 1977.

Bower, T. G. R., Broughton, J. M., & Moore, M. K. The coordination of visual and tactual input in infants. *Perception & Psychophysics*, 1970, 8, 51–53.

Bruner, J. S., & Koslowski, B. Visually preadapted constituents of manipulatory action. *Perception*, 1972, 1, 3–14.

Bryant, P. E., & Raz, I. Visual and tactual perception of shape by young children. *Developmental Psychology*, 1975, 11, 525–526.

Davidson, P. W. The role of exploratory activity in haptic perception: some issues, data, and hypotheses. *Research Bulletin of the American Foundation for the Blind*, 1972, 24, 21–27.

Davidson, P. W., Cambardella, P., Stenerson, S., & Carney, G. Influences of age and task's memory-demand on matching shapes within and across vision and touch. *Perceptual & Motor Skills*, 1974, *39*, 187–192.

DeLeon, J. L., Raskin, L. M., & Gruen, G. E. Sensory–modality effects on shape perception in preschool children. *Developmental Psychology*, 1970, *3*, 358–362.

Denner, B., & Cashdan, S. Sensory processing and the recognition of forms in nursery school children. *British Journal of Psychology*, 1967, *58*, 101–104.

Fernald, G. *Remedial techniques in basic school subjects.* New York: McGraw-Hill, 1943.

Ford, M. P. Imagery and verbalization as mediators in tactual–visual information processing. *Perceptual & Motor Skills*, 1973, *36*, 815–822.

Freides, D. Human information processing and sensory modality: cross-modal functions, information complexity, memory, and deficit. *Psychological Bulletin*, 1974, *81*, 284–310.

Gesell, A., Ilg, F., & Bullis, G. F, *Vision: its development in infant and child.* New York: Hoeber, 1949.

Gibson, E. J., Gibson, J. J., Pick, A. D., & Osser, H. A. A developmental study of the discrimination of letter-like forms. *Journal of Comparative and Physiological Psychology*, 1962, *55*, 897–906.

Gibson, E. J., Osser, H. A., Schiff, W., & Smith, J. An analysis of critical features of letters, tested by a confusion matrix. In final report: *A basic research program on reading.* Cooperative Research Project No. 639, Cornell University and U.S. Office of Education, 1963.

Gibson, J. J. The useful dimensions of sensitivity. *American Psychologist*, 1963, *18*, 1–15.

The senses considered as perceptual systems. Boston: Houghton Mifflin, 1966.

Gillingham, A., & Stillman, B. W. *Remedial training for children with specific difficulty in reading, spelling, and penmanshp,* (ed. 7). Cambridge, Mass.: Educators Publishing Service, 1966.

Gliner, C. R., Pick, A. D., Pick, H. L., Jr., & Hales, J. J. A developmental investigation of visual and haptic preferences for shape and texture. *Monographs of the Society for Research in Child Development*, 1969, *34*, 1–40.

Goodnow, J. J. Eye and hand: differential memory and its effect on matching. *Neuropsychologia*, 1971, *9*, 89–95.

Gottfried, A. W., Rose, S. A., & Bridger, W. H. Cross-modal transfer in human infants. *Child Development*, 1977, *48*, 118–123.

Gratch, G. A study of the relative dominance of vision and touch in six-month-old infants. *Child Development*, 1972, *43*, 615–623.

Gratch, G., & Landers, W. F. Stage IV of Piaget's theory of infant's object concepts: a longitudinal study. *Child Development*, 1971, *42*, 359–372.

Harris, P. L. Examination and search in infants. *British Journal of Psychology*, 1971, *62*, 469–473.

Infants' visual and tactual inspection of objects. *Perception*, 1972, *1*, 141–146.

Hertz, T. W. A developmental study of the role of visual imagery in crossmodal transfer in children. Unpublished doctoral thesis, University of Minnesota, 1971.

Jessen, B. L., & Kaess, D. W. Effects of training on intersensory communication by three- and five-year-olds. *Journal of Genetic Psychology*, 1973, *123*, 115–122.

McDonnell, P. M. The development of visually guided reaching. *Perception & Psychophysics*, 1975, *18*, 181–185.

McKinney, J. P. Hand schema in children. *Psychonomic Science*, 1964, *1*, 99–100.

Millar, S. Visual and haptic cue utilization by preschool children: the recognition of visual and haptic stimuli presented separately and together. *Journal of Experimental Child Psychology*, 1971, *12*, 88–94

Effects of interpolated tasks on latency and accuracy of intramodal and cross-modal shape recognition by children. *Journal of Experimental Psychology*, 1972, *96*, 170–175.

Tactile short-term memory by blind and sighted children, *British Journal of Psychology*, 1974, *65*, 253–263.

Orton, J. L. The Orton–Gillingham approach. In J. Money (Ed.), *The disabled reader: education of the dyslexic child*, Baltimore: Johns Hopkins University Press, 1966.

Piaget, J. *The origin of intelligence in the child*. London: Routledge & Kegan Paul, 1953.

Piaget, J., & Inhelder, B. *The child's conception of space*. London: Routledge & Kegan Paul, 1956.

Pick, A. D., & Pick, H. L., Jr. A developmental study of tactual discrimination in blind and sighted children and adults. *Psychonomic Science*, 1966, *6*, 367–368.

Pick, H. L., Jr., Pick, A. D., & Klein, R. E. Perceptual integration in children. In L. E. Lipsett & C. G. Spiker (Eds.), *Advances in child development and behavior*, vol. 3. New York: Academic Press 1967, pp. 192–220.

Posner, M. I., Nissen, M. J., & Klein, R. M. Visual dominance: an information-processing account of its origins and significance. *Psychological Review*, 1976, *83* 157–171.

Rose, S. A., Blank, M. S., & Bridger, W. H. Intermodal and intramodal retention of visual and tactual information in young children. *Developmental Psychology*, 1972, *6*, 482–486.

Rudel, R. G., & Teuber, H. L. Cross-modal transfer of shape discrimination by children. *Neuropsychologia*, 1964, *2*, 1–8.

Schaffer, H. R., & Parry, M. H. The effects of short-term familiarization on infants' perceptual–motor co-ordination in a simultaneous discrimination situation. *British Journal of Psychology*, 1970, *61*, 559–569.

Schiff, W., & Dytell, R. S. Tactile identification of letters: a comparison of deaf and hearing children's performances. *Journal of Experimental Child Psychology*, 1971, *11*, 150–164.

Siegel, A. W., & Barber, J. C. Visual and haptic dimensional preference for planometric stimuli. *Perceptual & Motor Skills*, 1973, *36*, 383–390.

Siegel, A. W., & Vance, B. J. Visual and haptic dimensional preference: a developmental study. *Developmental Psychology*, 1970, *3*, 264–266.

Uzgiris, I. C. Ordinality in the development of schemas. In J. Hellmuth (Ed.), *Exceptional infant*, vol. 1. Seattle: Special Child Publications, 1967.

Warren, D. H. Childhood visual impairment: perspectives on research design and methodology. *Journal of Visual Impairment and Blindness*, 1978, *72*, 404–411. (a)

Perception by the blind. In E. C. Carterette & M. P. Friedman (Eds.), *Handbook of perception*, Vol. 10 New York: Academic Press, 1978. (b)

Spatial localization under conflict conditions: is there a single explanation? *Perception*, 1979, *8*, 323–337.

White, B. L. *Human infants*. Englewood Cliffs, N.J.: Prentice-Hall, 1971.

Wolff, P. The role of stimulus-correlated activity in children's recognition of nonsense forms. *Journal of Experimental Child Psychology*, 1972, *14*, 427–441.

Wolff, P., & Levin, J. R. The role of overt activity in children's imagery production. *Child Development*, 1972, *43*, 537–547.

Wolff, P., Levin, J. R., & Longobardi, E. T. Motoric mediation in children's paired-associate learning: effects of visual and tactual contact. *Journal of Experimental Child Psychology*, 1972, *14*, 176–183.

Wright, J. C., & Vlietstra, A. G. The development of selective attention: from perceptual exploration to logical search. In H. W. Reese (Ed.), *Advances in child development and behavior,* vol. 10. New York: Academic Press, 1975, pp. 195–239.

Zaporozhets, A. V. The development of perception in the preschool child. *Monographs of the Society for Research in Child Development,* 1965, *30,* 82–92.

4. The perception of texture by touch

SUSAN J. LEDERMAN

In Chapter 4, Susan Lederman conceptualizes the domain of texture perception as including a number of ostensibly different, although related, surface qualities. These include roughness, hardness, stickiness, slipperiness, coarseness, and others. Texture, she points out, offers the perceptual investigator an opportunity to study the integrated and independent functioning of sensory–perceptual systems as well as a means of examining a wide range of perceptual phenomena, such as pattern recognition, masking, and lateralization. In Lederman's view, texture includes the stimulus dimensions par excellence for touch. She points out that textural judgments are a far more ecologically valid task for the skin and hands than are form or orientation-judging tasks, which psychologists frequently provide observers for haptic examination.

Following a thorough analysis of the interplay of several sources of textural information, Lederman reviews studies by David Katz as well as by herself and her colleagues, seeking to tease apart the effective stimulus information for judgments about textural dimensions. An important determiner of perceived roughness is groove width, whereas (perhaps surprisingly) fundamental spatial frequency does not seem a promising candidate. This interpretation could grate on some theorists. The role of shear forces in tactual texture perception is given considerable attention in this review chapter. Lederman then reviews some possibilities regarding peripheral and more central neural coding mechanisms that may mediate texture perception and judgment. This discussion is followed by an examination of the intersensory equivalence issues (visual or acoustical vs. tactual, for example) involved with textural perception. In the area of texture, vision appears *not* to dominate touch, unless factors such as lighting direction are optimal. Generally, Lederman thinks one is as good as the other. Note that this finding counters the general belief that vision is superior to touch. Clearly, one must consider the stimulus dimension as well as the task demands and modality when evaluating such general statements.

Finally, Lederman examines the implications of our knowledge about texture perception for braille reading and tactual graphics for visually impaired persons. This integration is a most useful one for those concerned with creating optimally useful tactual displays.

WILLIAM SCHIFF

130

Introduction

The perception of texture by touch is a task with which we are all familiar. We frequently reach out to feel the roughness of sandpaper, the smoothness of a baby's skin, the softness of cashmere, the rubberiness of elastic, even the slipperiness of fresh ice. These examples indicate the breadth of the term *texture perception* as it will be used in this chapter. By *texture perception,* I mean the experience of any of a number of surface qualities, for example, roughness, smoothness, hardness, stickiness, slipperiness, oiliness, coarseness, and graininess.

Texture perception is an interesting area of study in its own right, and it serves several other functions as well. Perceiving the texture of a surface by touch is a multimodal task in which information from several different sensory channels is available. In addition to cutaneous and thermal input, kinesthetic, auditory, and visual cues may be used when texture is perceived by touching a surface. Texture perception by touch, therefore, offers an excellent opportunity to study both the integrated and independent actions of sensory systems. Furthermore, it can be used to investigate many other traditional perceptual functions, such as lateralization, sensory dominance and integration, masking, figural aftereffects, and pattern recognition. The perception of texture may be thought of as a microcosm of the entire spectrum of perceptual activities.

In Neisser's (1976) terms, texture perception is an "ecologically valid" judgment for touch to make; we are both comfortable with and accustomed to doing so. The perception of texture, therefore, is a task that we can validly use to examine many of the limitations and capabilities of the tactual system.

Most of the tactual research in the past 2 decades, however, has used tasks involving the perception of form, size, orientation, and spatial localization. Such tasks are performed relatively infrequently by touch; they are more suited to the simultaneous processing capabilities of vision than to the sequential ones of touch. Not surprisingly, then, studies abound showing that vision dominates (or strongly biases) and is more accurate than touch (Bryant & Raz, 1975; Cashdan, 1968; Milner & Bryant, 1970; Rock & Victor, 1964). Such studies can certainly document some of the limitations of tactual processing, but of course, they overlook those perceptual activities for which the tactual system is better designed, including texture perception.

A final reason for studying texture perception is the possibility that such research may be used to facilitate braille reading and to improve the design of tangible graphics for the visually impaired. We will consider this area in greater detail later in the chapter.

Right now, feel the texture of a surface near you. What kinds of sensory information are at least potentially available? You have visual information about the surface's texture, and about where your fingers are in relation to those visual patterns, even if the object is moving. You know through kinesthetic feedback how your hand is moving. You know kinesthetically, and possibly through cutaneous cues as well, what forces you are applying, both normal and lateral to the skin surface. As you move your hand, your fingertips are grossly squashed inward and sideways. Your skin also deforms to follow, in part, the tiny irregularities on the surface of the object. These small-scale deformations may be sensed as vibrations of the tiny areas of the fingertips because the moving hand changes the spatial patterns of deformation to temporal ones at any given point on the finger. Vibration has many characteristics, such as temporal pulse frequency, energy, skin deformation, and rate of displacement. Any of these may contribute to the perception of different components of the surface texture. Moreover, you can sometimes hear the vibrations produced by touching a surface; what role, if any, do these touch-produced sounds play in texture perception? And finally, you can sense the transfer of heat between finger and object; this may tell you something about the temperature and physical characteristics of the object.

This brief description suggests that there is a wealth of sensory information potentially available for judging texture. At this time, however, we know relatively little about which physical effects contribute to which aspects of the texture percept.

Early research on tactual perception of texture

With the notable exception of David Katz (1925), few researchers studied the tactual perception of texture prior to about 1960. Because Katz's monograph *The world of touch* is not yet available in English translation, the present discussion of his work is taken from commentaries by Zigler (1926) and Krueger (1970 and Chapter 1).

Katz was very interested in surface texture, or "modifications" of the surface, as he described it. He argued strongly for the necessity of vibration. When the finger is stationary on a surface, there is no vibration and no perception of texture. Vibrations are set up in the skin by relative movement between hand and object, and with movement comes the perception of a texture. Test this yourself; rest your hand very gently on a surface. You definitely experience the *presence* of a surface, but you feel the surface's texture only fleetingly, if at all. When the hand remains on a surface without relative motion, it becomes impossible to determine the qualities of the surface.

Katz suggested that lateral motion is required for the perception of roughness and smoothness and vertical motion for hardness and softness. The pressure sense, for Katz, was quite separate from that of vibration and played almost no role in his speculations concerning texture. The only concession he made to the role of the pressure sense, as opposed to vibration, was his observation that on occasions "when the bumps are high on the surface, pressure sensations may influence judgments on roughness to a large extent" (Krueger, 1970, p. 341). Pressure, for Katz, seems to be a static quality, whereas vibration is interpreted as any sufficiently rapid change of pressure, or motion of the skin. It does not seem necessarily to mean regular oscillation or rhythmic movement.

Katz offered the results of several demonstrations in support of the importance of vibration for texture perception. For example, he discussed the observation that the global resistance felt in moving the hand had no effect on perceived roughness. He glued a pair of different-textured surfaces back to back, and then moved one hand across the two textures simultaneously, the thumb along one side and the index and middle fingers along the other. Two distinct textures were experienced at the same time, despite the presumed constancy of felt resistance to movement of the hand. Katz argued that the differences in perceived texture could be due only to the different vibratory patterns set up under the thumb versus the index and middle fingers.

In another demonstration used to support his case for vibration, Katz reported that paper surfaces feel very smooth when sticky glue is applied to the fingers. He argued that this experience results from the elimination of vibrations. Recently however, Lederman (1978b,c) has suggested that lateral "shearing" forces on the fingertips may mask whatever stimuli give rise to the perception of roughness. If this is the case, then the glue might have increased these lateral forces and thus masked further the sensation of roughness.

The masking effect of the lateral force might also account for the results of another of Katz's demonstrations. When their fingers were covered with a 0.1-mm layer of collodion or a 0.2-mm layer of leukoplastin, subjects showed better discrimination of pairs of surfaces felt by the two hands when both hands or neither were coated than when only one hand was coated. Katz suggested that "the collodion fills in irregularities on the skin surface, thus perhaps excluding the pressure sense, yet only slightly dampening the vibrations" (Krueger, 1970, p. 340). Katz expected that if the pressure sense played a major role, discrimination should have been much poorer when the skin was covered. However, the covering might have reduced the lateral force acting on the skin. Such an effect might have altered the perception of surface texture but would have done so *equally* when collodion was on both hands. Only when it was on one hand would it have altered the experience of one surface relative to another in such a way as to increase the number of errors (for further discussion, see the section "Psychophysical studies"). Thus again, there are alternatives to Katz's explanation.

Katz also considered the contribution to texture perception of another kind of information, the thermal properties of both skin and surface. His subjects used heat conductance to identify different materials, such as wood and metal. Cooling their fingers resulted in an inability to discriminate between some otherwise discriminable paper surfaces. Moreover, surfaces felt smoother to the cooled skin; cooling the skin might reduce skin flexibility. If reduced flexibility did occur, the skin might not be able to follow the contours of the surface as well. Alternatively, or in addition, cooling may have caused a reduction in activity of the temperature-sensitive mechanoreceptors that likely code for texture (Djalali, 1977; Inman & Peruzzi, 1961). Finally, vasomotor factors could also play a role in the tactual perception of texture. Katz also emphasized the importance of touch-produced sounds for the recognition of different materials. However, he did not systematically investigate the role of such cues in the perception of surface texture (see Lederman, 1979, and the section "Equivalence and bias in intersensory function").

Given Katz's emphasis on motion, it is not surprising that his studies also examined the effects of hand speed and force on the perception of surface texture. He found, for example, that perceived roughness increases with increasing force when the surfaces are moved across the stationary fingers. The mode of touching just described is referred to as *passive touch* by J. J. Gibson (1962): Contact with the observer's skin is effected by some external agent. In contrast, *active touch* refers to the observer's initiation and execution of the movements required to effect skin–object contact. The same effect of increasing vertical finger force on texture perception has been obtained using active touch (Lederman & Taylor, 1972). However, Katz also found that discrimination of roughness and smoothness is slightly impaired when passive touch is used, even at the optimal rate of movement, that is, 15 cm per second. The roughness perceived as well as the consistency of such judgments is unaffected by the mode of touch (Lederman, in press).

In one study on the effect of hand speed, Katz used a surface that consisted of a long strand of wire wrapped tightly around a pencil to form a set of ridges. Subjects moved their hands over the ridges at different speeds varying from 1 to 10 cm per second. The fact that judgments of roughness remained unchanged may indicate a form of roughness constancy in which subjects compensate for the alterations in vibratory frequency resulting from variation in hand speed. This finding contrasts to the results of another experiment in which paper surfaces were moved across an observer's stationary fingers at speeds of 3, 15, and 60 cm per second. At the highest speed, all papers seemed much smoother and less discriminable than at the medium speed; at the lowest speed, the smoother papers seemed to become less smooth than with the middle speed, and again were less discriminable. In summary, Katz considered (directly or indirectly) most of the sources of sensory information concerning texture that were discussed in the "Introduction."

Apart from the work of Katz, few studies have considered tactual texture perception. Passive touch was used in two experiments that followed the introspective tradition. Meenes and Zigler (1923) investigated the perceived roughness of objects, whereas Sullivan (1927) studied the perception of hardness and softness. Meenes and Zigler, in particular, provided some interesting findings on the perception of surfaces of different roughness, on the contribution of relative motion between hand and object, and on the effect of varying the force of the object against the skin. Sullivan discussed differences in the perception of hardness and softness and the effects on these percepts of varying the object's temperature. A clear perception of hardness required a cool object.

Finally, Binns (1934, 1937) conducted a series of experiments in the textile industry. Using both trained and naive judges, he examined visual and tactual judgments of the fineness, softness, and value of wool. He found that experience improved visual judgments but had little effect on tactual skill. His research did not attempt to deal with the stimulus parameters underlying the subjects' judgments.

Current research on tactual perception of texture

Psychophysical studies

Texture perception by touch still remains relatively unexplored today. This section will examine the literature available from about 1960 to the present. Virtually all of the recent psychophysical studies deal with roughness or smoothness.

Lederman and her associates have carried out a systematic series of studies that provides the data base for a sensory model of tactual perception of roughness. These studies used as stimuli aluminum plates with linear gratings of rectangular cross section cut into the surface. The earliest experiments (Lederman, 1974; Lederman & Taylor, 1972) showed that perceived roughness depends strongly on the width of the groove cuts, increasing with spacing. Apparent roughness depends much less, if at all, on the width of the ridges, decreasing slightly as ridge width increases. The ratio of groove to ridge width does not affect the perceived roughness. Neither apparently does the fundamental spatial frequency of the stimulus grating (Lederman, 1973; see also Lederman & Taylor, 1972).

In addition to the role of surface structure, the effects of hand speed and force have been considered systematically. In the experiments mentioned above, subjects used several forces to examine each surface. Overall, finger force proved to be the second most influential factor, perceived roughness increasing with increases in the force applied perpendicular to the surface. It will be recalled that this finding replicates an earlier observation by Katz. At first glance, this result suggests a failure in roughness constancy. However, *constancy* is probably an inappropriate term to use. Normally we use it to refer to the assignment of the same response to the same distal object. In the experiments above, however, the grooves were deep enough to prevent the finger from "bottoming out"; subjects, therefore, could not have known from touch alone that they were feeling the same plate with different forces. For all intents, the surface geometry (a distal property) was different for each force applied. This change in perceived roughness as a function of finger force, incidentally, occurred whether the subjects moved their fingers across a stationary plate or the plate was moved across their stationary fingers (Lederman, in press.; see also Katz, 1925). To describe the overall effects of groove width (G) and finger force (F), it may be said that roughness increases approximately as $f(FG)^4$ for grooves over 0.375 mm, where f is the function k^4FG, (i.e., $k(FG^4)$) and k is an arbitrary constant.

Hand speed also has a consistent effect on perceived roughness, decreasing slightly with increasing speed (Lederman, 1974). But it is negligible relative to groove width and force effects for a 25-fold change in hand speed. This finding, therefore, supports what was observed earlier by Katz. Current researchers, however, considered only changes in the magnitude of roughness sensations; unlike Katz, they did not consider possible changes in discriminative ability.

In 1975 Taylor and Lederman proposed a sensory model for perceived roughness that accounted for the major features of the data described above; it was also shown by extension to account qualitatively for the more subtle effects (involving the effects of the ridge width and speed, etc.) in the data. The irrelevance of hand speed led to the assumption that the actual movements of the skin in assuming its various deformations are unimportant. Thus, factors such as temporal pulse frequency and rate of skin displacement[1] should play no role in the perception of roughness. Vibration (produced by movement) per se is crucial for perceiving roughness only in that it prevents the receptors from adapting out and, perhaps, as Katz might have argued, because it provides multiple exposures to the stimulus, a requirement in any perception task. What actually matters is the deformation of the skin at any moment. The results of the above studies therefore favor an interpretation of roughness perception based on *spatial/intensive* aspects of skin deformation. Three skin deformation parameters predicted apparent roughness as a function of the two most influential factors, groove width and force, quite well. They were the depth to which the skin penetrates a groove and two aspects of the cross-sectional area (i.e., volume, because the grooves were linear) of the fingertip pressed into the grooves.

One test of the value of a model is whether it can make correct but counterintuitive predictions. Many people think that roughness depends on the coefficient of friction[2], μ between the skin and the surface being evaluated. More specifically, roughness might decrease with decreases in μ. Ekman, Hosman, and Lindstrom (1965) have published an experiment that supports this intuition. But the Taylor and Lederman model of roughness is insensitive to changes in the coefficient of friction over a wide range. In fact, a very large decrease in the coefficient of friction should cause a negligibly small *increase* in the predicted values of perceived roughness. In an experimental test, μ was altered by a factor of at least 6; however, the perceived roughness remained essentially unchanged (Taylor & Lederman, 1975). The discrepancy between the two friction experiments may be due to differences in the authors' definitions of the coefficient of friction (for further discussion, see Taylor & Lederman, 1975).

Also following directly from the model is the prediction that the degree of callus, that is the thickened keratin layer of the epidermis, on the fingertip should influence the perceived roughness of grooved surfaces. As the skin becomes less pliable, its coefficient of elasticity should decrease, and the skin should become less capable of penetrating the surface grooves. Hence, perceived roughness should also decrease. An experimental test of this prediction (Lederman, 1976) required subjects to judge the roughness of various grooved plates with different fingers of the writing hand. Most people would agree that the index finger is used most frequently and is likely to have the largest buildup of callus. A subsequent survey indicated that people would rank their fingers index, middle, then ring in order of decreasing frequency of use. At this stage, the ordering of the fingers in terms of degree of callus must be based on everyday knowledge of the frequency with which the fingers of the writing hand are used. To the extent that this ordering is correct, surfaces should feel least rough with the index finger, somewhat rougher with the middle finger, and roughest of all when the ring finger is used. The results of the experiment confirmed this prediction. Check it yourself by using in turn the index, middle, and ring fingers of your writing hand to examine the texture of the skin on your thumb. It feels roughest with the ring finger and least rough with the index finger. However, the slope of the psychophysical function for the index finger was steeper than those for the middle and ring fingers. Such results were tentatively interpreted in terms of differences in discrimination by the fingers, but alternatively they could be discussed in terms of low-frequency recruitment. Regardless of the single finger used, however, the consistency of response was about the same.

More recently, Lederman (1978b,c) has described a heightened roughness phenomenon that demands modification of the current model of roughness to include the effect of skin shear as a result of relative motion between skin and surface. This recent work derived from a simple but intriguing result reported by Gordon and Cooper (1975). When a thin intermediate paper was moved with the fingers over a surface, the orientation of a slight undulation on that surface was detected more accurately than when the bare fingers were used. Similarly, surfaces feel *rougher* when the intermediate paper is used than when it is not (Lederman, 1978c). People were presented with textured surfaces consisting of various grades of sandpaper, each covered with a piece of writing paper to prevent particles from being dislodged. This paper was always present. On half of the trials, the surfaces were felt with the bare fingers; on the other half of the trials, they were examined through an additional piece of paper[3] that was moved with the fingers. With all surfaces, magnitude estimates of roughness were significantly greater when the intermediate paper was used. In interpreting this effect, the importance of relative motion between skin and surface for judging roughness was emphasized, as was done earlier by Katz. This motion means that as the hand is moved, both downward (normal) and lateral (shear) forces are applied to the skin of the fingertips. Earlier experimental and theoretical work pointed to the importance of vertical forces in the perception of roughness: Roughness grows as a function of increases in the normal force.

The effect of shear was not evaluated. The presence of the intermediate paper, however, does reduce the shear force acting on the skin. It was suggested, therefore, that in general, shear might interfere with or mask the effects of the relevant normal forces on perceived roughness. By reducing the shear force, the intermediate paper might also reduce the amount by which the roughness signal is masked.

There are two additional tests of the reduced-shear interpretation that you may try yourself. Place a thin piece of paper over a surface. Move your fingers across the paper, but without displacing it. The surface will feel smoother than if you were to move both paper *and* fingers across the surface. The perception is to be expected because now shear has been increased, and this in turn increases the masking of the effects caused by normal force. Next, move your fingers back and forth across the surface, again with the piece of paper underneath. This time, move the intermediate paper, but in a direction other than the one in which you are moving your fingers. The surface feels a little smoother than when you feel the surface moving *with* the fingers. This experience would also be predicted by the reduced-shear interpretation, because shearing of the skin has been increased when the fingers move relative to the paper. In a subsequent study, shear was experimentally reduced in an attempt to test directly the postulated masking effect of shear forces on the perception of roughness. As predicted, the perceived roughness increased as the shearing force was reduced.[3,4]

Returning now to the heightened roughness phenomenon, there are at least two other explanations of the paper effect that seem intuitively plausible. The intermediate paper might serve as an amplifier, the edges catching on the surface irregularities, thereby producing traveling waves that add their effects to the vibratory signal directly under the fingertips. Alternatively, the paper may serve as a low-pass filter, passing only energy in the low-frequency range (involving the larger, more widely spaced bumps). This last interpretation must also show that tactual roughness is dependent upon temporal pulse frequency and, more specifically, that roughness increases as pulse frequency decreases, an idea that was challenged above. However, the Lederman and Taylor (1972) and Lederman (1974) studies did not specifically deal with the effect on perceived roughness of the relative distribution of pulse frequencies present. Such a factor may therefore play a role in the paper phenomenon, and it is worth considering at greater length vis-à-vis roughness perception in general. It remains possible that surfaces with predominantly lower-frequency components feel rougher than surfaces with the same fundamental frequency and more of the higher harmonics. This is a counterintuitive idea and would be interesting, if true. It would run counter to the "intensive" interpretation of roughness proposed above.

Such research with the paper handcovering is reminiscent of work by David Katz that was discussed earlier. Katz found that subjects discriminated among surfaces more poorly when only one hand (as opposed to both or neither) was coated with collodion. The current findings (Lederman, 1978 b,c) provide a tentative interpretation of this observation.

It is possible that the layer of collodion, like the intermediate paper, alters the shear force acting on the skin as it moves across a surface. Provided the collodion is on *both* hands, there should be no impairment (relative to the use of two bare hands). Whatever alterations in perceived texture (e.g., roughness) occur with one hand should occur similarly with the other. The situation is quite different, however, when only one hand is coated. First, consider the condition in which a pair of identical stimuli are felt simultaneously using one hand to examine each surface. If the collodion alters the feel of only one of the surfaces, the pair of identical surfaces will be perceived as different. When two truly different surfaces are presented, they should feel either more or less discrepant. When the collodion is on the hand that feels the rougher surface, the difference between the two surfaces will be exaggerated; subjects should show increased discrimination. But when the collodion is on the hand that examines the smoother of the two surfaces, the perceived difference will be reduced; subjects will be more likely mistakenly to identify the pair of stimuli as the same. Because sufficient methodological information is not available to make such exact predictions for Katz's experiment, this interpretation can be offered only tentatively. However, a recent experiment by Lederman and Kinch (unpublished) provides support for this interpretation, particularly as it relates to roughness discrimination. When both hands were either bare or covered with a thin piece of paper, roughness discrimination remained about the same. A same–different judgment task was used. When only one hand used the paper, however, roughness discrimination was either heightened or impaired as predicted above, depending upon (1) whether the members of the texture pair were the same or different and (2) in the case of the different pairs whether the "paper" hand was feeling the rougher or smoother of the two surfaces. Such results indicate that an intermediate paper moved with the fingers over a surface will affect not only the magnitude of the roughness perceived but also roughness discrimination.

Finally, we may consider the role of *thermal* effects in the tactual perception of texture. In an unpublished study by R. H. Gibson and A. Sztepa, it was found that the exponent of a perceived roughness function was not influenced by the temperature (within 10°c of room temperature) of the textured surface. With a warm hand on a warm textured surface, the whole function was the same as that found with stimuli and hands at normal room temperature. But when the stimuli and hands were cooled 10°c, the function was substantially lowered with no change in exponent. Cold textured surfaces felt smoother than neutral or warm ones. Because skin and object temperatures were varied simultaneously, it is not possible to assess the effects independently.

More recently, Green, Lederman, and Stevens (1979) altered skin temperature between 10°c and 40°c while leaving constant at 32°c (normal skin temperature) a set of grooved metal plates varying in groove width. Subjects made magnitude estimates of felt roughness. The overall effect of skin temperature can be summarized as follows. Cooling below normal skin temperature consistently degrades the perception of roughness; the greatest effect was for the smoothest plates. Warming above normal skin temperature either enhances perceived roughness (primarily for the smoothest plates) or leaves it unchanged (mainly for the roughest plates).

The research discussed so far has varied the parameters of hand force and speed, surface geometry, and skin and object temperature. Most of this psychophysical research on tactual perception of texture has used metal gratings as stimuli. To what extent can we relate these findings to other surfaces and expect the same results?

LaMotte (1977) has performed a simple experiment on the apparent roughness of various fabric surfaces. His subjects were asked to rank several fabrics numerically according to the magnitude of perceived roughness. He found that perceived roughness decreased with increases in weave density, that is, fundamental spatial frequency. It is possible, however, that weave density has been confounded with the spacing between the yarn, and that the roughness of fabrics (much like that of grooved metal plates) is in fact determined by the spacing, not the spatial frequency, of the pattern. LaMotte's other speculations concerning the effects of yarn diameter, and the force and speed of relative motions between skin and fabric, are supported by the data obtained with grooved plates.

Stevens and Harris (1962) have shown that perceived roughness decreases with increases in the grit value of abrasive surfaces. *Grit* refers to the number of openings per 2.54 cm in the sieves used to produce the sandpapers. Once again, fundamental spatial frequency may not be the crucial factor affecting roughness perception. As grit value increases, particle diameter, particle spacing, and particle density (i.e., fundamental spatial

141

frequency) change. The results of the studies by Lederman and Taylor (1972) and Lederman (1973, 1974) question whether either particle size or density determines the decreasing roughness function; such studies strongly implicate element spacing in the tactual perception of roughness.

The exponent of the psychophysical function for roughness varies considerably depending upon the surfaces used, for example, grooved metal plates or uncovered and paper-covered sandpapers. However, there is little value to such comparisons when the surfaces vary along so many different dimensions. For example, Vierck (1978) notes that sandpaper produces an additional experience of "sharpness" due to the jagged particles on the surface. The analysis of roughness based on grooved metal plates has not yet considered this aspect, but it is likely to prove an important component of the roughness percept. Moreover, power functions vary considerably across individuals; Ekman, Hosman, and Lindstrom (1965), for example, reported exponents within a single experiment that ranged from 0.8 to 3.5.

This section has focused on data concerning the *magnitude* of roughness percepts. Other studies that examine texture *discrimination* will be presented later in the chapter. They relate primarily to the use of texture in tangible graphics for the visually impaired.

In summary, most current psychophysical work has dealt with the tactual perception of roughness, one of the most prominent aspects of texture. Research has either shown or suggested that the perception of roughness (and smoothness) is controlled not only by surface microstructure (e.g., spacing between the ridges) but also by surface temperature and skin properties, such as the degree of callus and skin temperature. It has been suggested that together with the forces (lateral and normal to the skin) used to explore a surface, the factors just mentioned alter the shape of the skin deformation, which in turn strongly affects the perception of roughness. Vibratory pulse frequency, as determined by fundamental spatial frequency and hand speed, does not appear to play a significant role. For this reason, Taylor and Lederman (1975) have suggested that dynamic aspects of vibration are not important in the perception of roughness by touch. Vibration serves only to prevent adaptation of the receptors and to provide the observer with multiple "looks" at the relevant skin deformation information.

Neurophysiological mechanisms

A different approach to the study of tactual perception of texture involves determining the peripheral and central neural mechanisms that underlie the processing of textural properties. As will become obvious, very little work has been done in this field.

Peripheral mechanisms. Knibestol and Vallbo (1970) first demonstrated that there are four different types of low-threshold, mechanoreceptive units in the glabrous skin of the human hand. These units are usually differentiated by their responses to steady indentation and by their receptive field properties.

Two of the four types respond to skin indentation only while the stimulus is changing (i.e., transients); they show no reponse to sustained indentation. Accordingly, they have been described as rapidly adapting. The other two types do show a sustained discharge during steady indentation of the skin, and have been described as slowly adapting.

Although it is somewhat confusing, only those rapidly adapting units with small, distinct receptive fields have been labeled *RA* units. It has been tentatively suggested that primate RA units end in Meissner corpuscles found high in the dermal ridges of the skin. Talbot, Darian-Smith, Kornhuber, and Mountcastle (1968) found that RA units coded low frequency (5- to 40-Hz) mechanical sinusoids delivered to the hand of a monkey. Given the strong similarity between the neural events in the monkey and the sensory measures in human response to similar stimuli (Mountcastle, Talbot, Sakata, and Hyvarinen, 1969; Talbot et al., 1968), it is believed that such units code the human sensation "flutter."

The other rapidly adapting mechanoreceptors are known as *PC* units because they have as end organs the Pacinian corpuscles found in subcutaneous tissues. PC units have very large receptive fields, and in the monkey (Talbot et al., 1968) they code mechanical sinusoids in the range of 40 to 400 Hz. Verrillo and his colleagues (e.g., Gescheider & Verrillo, 1979; Verrillo, 1968; Verrillo & Gescheider, 1979) have provided impressive psychophysical data to support the notion of at least a duplex theory of vibration, with the PCs presumed to code high-frequency vibration and one (or more) populations (of which the RAs are likely ones) for coding low-frequency vibration.

Of the two kinds of slowly adapting units, the SA I fibers have small, distinct receptive fields (as do RA units), indicating again the potential for coding spatial details. They respond to steady indentation but show low sensitivity to stretch. The end organs of the SA I units are believed to be the Merkel cell complexes, located on the deep aspect of the intermediate ridges (large epidermal folds that project into the dermis).

Finally, the SA II units respond to sustained indentation (like SA I units), and have large receptive fields (like the PCs). The fibers are believed to end in Ruffini endings, which are located more deeply within the dermis. SA II units tend to be very sensitive to tangential forces on the skin (Johansson, 1976).

Given the complexity of the sensations subsumed under the general heading of "texture," it is likely that all of the mechanoreceptive populations described above will play a role.

Only LaMotte (1977) has provided empirical information concerning single unit responses to texture *per se*. He recorded the responses of Meissner afferents in monkeys when textured surfaces (nylon filament fabrics of varying yarn counts, i.e., number of weft plus number of warp per centimeter) were moved across receptive fields on the fingertip. The cumulative nerve impulse count in one Meissner afferent unit that La-Motte presented was higher for the factor with the lower-weave density and increased as a function of the pressure of stroking. The pattern of these data was similar to that obtained from human psychophysical judgments of the roughness of some of the same fabrics used in the single unit monkey recordings. LaMotte's data suggest that RA units might peripherally code fabric roughness in terms of an inverse relationship between nerve impulse count (or perceived roughness) and weave density. As pointed out earlier, however, weave density is confounded with yarn spacing; therefore it is still unclear which physical value of the fabric surface is the more important. LaMotte also recorded activity in several SA I units. Unfortunately, some of these afferents adapted to the continual pressure applied to the skin for several minutes prior to lateral movement of the fabric across the skin and would not respond to each successive stimulus. One unit that did not adapt showed only a slight increase in activity as pressure was increased; there were only slight differences in response profile as a function of the particular weaves presented. Given the limited data on SA I response, we cannot exclude them in the coding of roughness. LaMotte has speculated that sensations of softness may correlate with activity in SA I fibers because their rate of firing is determined by the amount of sustained deformation.

Lederman (1978b) has speculated very tentatively on the role of SA I units in the heightened roughness phenomenon. The suggestion derives from the structural properties of the skin, in particular the downward and lateral micromovements of the intermediate ridges in response to normal and shear forces, respectively. Because the SA I units lie at the deep end of the intermediate ridges, it was proposed that SA I units might code both normal and shear forces, the effects of shear interfering with the simultaneous coding of normal force and hence with perceived roughness. According to such an analysis, when shear is decreased by the intermediate paper, the lateral bias in the motion of the intermediate ridge would be lessened. This, in turn, would result in a relatively larger roughness signal. However, evidence by Johansson (1976) seems to question the validity of this interpretation; participation by the SA II units that code shear is more strongly implicated at this time.

It is clear that the peripheral coding mechanisms for roughness, and more generally for texture, remain an open question as yet.

Central mechanisms. Other investigators have studied the function of the most direct somatosensory pathways to the cerebral cortex (i.e., the dorsal column–lemniscothalamic, or dorsal column, system; the spinocervical–lemniscothalamic, or spinocervical, system; and the spinothalamic tract) and of the cortex in roughness discrimination by a variety of species (rat, cat, monkey, human). As advocated by Brown and Gordon (1977), the lemniscal–extralemniscal (or anterolateral) system distinction used in much of the early somatosensory literature will be avoided. Such a distinction seemed valid when the medial lemniscus was believed to be uniform in function; however, we now know that this view is false (Brown, Gordon, & Kay, 1974).

Recently, Vierck (1978) has emphasized the role the dorsal columns may play in coding spatiotemporal information. In view of this analysis, it is somewhat surprising that investigators have reported little if any deficit in roughness discrimination following dorsal column lesions in cats and monkeys (Dobry & Casey, 1972; Kitai & Weinberg, 1968; Schwartz, Eidelberg, Marchok, & Azulay, 1972). Dobry and Casey did find, however, that more than 90 percent of the dorsal column fibers had to be sectioned before cats showed deficits in the postoperative learning and retention of a difficult roughness discrimination task. Studies that report no deficit (e.g., Kitai and Weinberg's cats and Schwartz et al.'s monkeys) may have sectioned a smaller preparation of the dorsal columns. This suggests that there may exist considerable functional redundancy within the dorsal columns. Alternatively, other pathways, for example, in the spinocervical or spinothalamic system, might carry roughness information, either regularly or as a consequence of injury to the dorsal column system. The spinocervical system in cats has certainly been implicated because lesions restricted to this system have resulted in impaired performance in roughness discrimination tasks of varying difficulty (Kitai & Weinberg, 1968). Moreover, Semmes and Mishkin (1965) have demonstrated ipsilateral impairment of roughness discrimination thresholds in monkeys with unilateral cortical ablation of the sensorimotor cortex. Because almost all projections in the dorsal column and spinocervical system are contralateral, one interpretation of this deficit is that some other system with ipsilateral projections is involved. As Semmes and Mishkin point out, the deficit in their animals was unlikely due to the loss of motor-related functions of the sensorimotor cortex, because the use of the ipsilateral limbs in normal behavior and motor control related to the discrimination task was unaffected. They also argue against the impairment's being caused by a disruption of the efferent regulation of activity in the other hemisphere via subcortical mechanisms. Kohn and Dennis (1974) have argued in favor of a role for uncrossed somatosensory pathways in the tactile matching of texture by four human subjects with infantile hemiplegia (hemidecortication was performed some 9 to 14 years later). Subjects performed significantly better with the hand ipsilateral to hemidecortication than with the contralateral hand. However, when the texture matching was executed intermanually (regardless of which hand felt the standard and which did the matching), subjects performed better than when the contralateral hand alone was used. Kohn and Dennis suggest that such intermanual improvement in texture matching argues for the summation of input from *two* somatosensory systems, one involving crossed pathways (probably the dorsal column system in humans) from one limb, the other involving uncrossed pathways from the other limb.

Other studies contribute to our knowledge of cortical localization of function in roughness discrimination. Tactile maps of the body surface are represented at least twice in the cerebral cortex of most mammals. Somatosensory area I (S I) lies in the postcentral gyrus behind the central sulcus, whereas somatosensory area II (S II) lies below and behind S I, so that the two areas representing the face lie nearest each other.

In general, investigators have demonstrated the importance of the somatosensory cortex for roughness discrimination (e.g., rat: Finger & Frommer, 1968; Zubek, 1951, 1952b; cat: Benjamin & Thompson, 1958; Zubek, 1952a; monkey: Semmes & Mishkin, 1965; humans: Weinstein, Semmes, Ghent, & Teuber, 1958). Removal of both S I and S II in adult animals leads to severe impairment of retention and postoperative learning of roughness discrimination tasks. Ablation of S I generally results in greater deficits than S II, although combined S I and S II lesions cause greater impairment than removal of S I alone. However, when S I and S II were removed in newborn kittens (Benjamin & Thompson, 1958), their performance on all but the most difficult roughness discrimination tasks was indistinguishable from that of unoperated controls. In contrast, when the operation was performed on mature cats, the latter were unable

146

to learn any of the tasks. The differences in performance argue once again for the tremendous flexibility of the infant nervous system.

Semmes and Mishkin (1965) have compared the performance of monkeys on a number of tactual discrimination tasks as a consequence of removing either the sensorimotor region or the rest of the hemisphere, leaving the sensorimotor region intact. We have already discussed the ipsilateral deficits on roughness thresholds that result when the sensorimotor region is removed. When the complementary nonsensorimotor cortex was ablated, the group did not differ from the nonoperated controls with respect to the *ipsilateral* roughness threshold; the nonsensorimotor tissue removed did not seem to affect performance. Semmes, Mishkin, and Cole (1969) also examined the role of the nonsensorimotor cortex in *contralateral* performance using the same set of tasks as Semmes and Mishkin. Ablation of the contralateral nonsensorimotor region resulted in contralateral elevations of roughness thresholds. The deficit was somewhat less severe than that caused by removal of the sensorimotor cortex and was attributed to the ablation of areas receiving information via pathways from both contralateral and ipsilateral limbs.

However, subsequent analysis with modified lesions indicated that deficits found in preliminary hardness–softness discriminations were due both to the tissue removed and to the unintended cutting of the corpus callosum. The impairment in the preliminary discriminations was interpreted as a more general problem in developing basic tactile discrimination strategies. It is probably a "parietal lobe neglect" syndrome that fits the recent data of Mountcastle et al. (1975), Sakata, Takaoka, Kawarasaki, and Shibutani (1973), and Hyvarinen and Poranen (1974).

One final study should be mentioned to conclude this survey of neural mechanisms that underlie the perception of texture by touch. Myers and Ebner (1975) have recently shown that in juvenile monkeys, the posterior portion of the corpus callosum plays a crucial role in the transfer of information concerning tactual roughness discrimination.

We can see that what little work there is deals primarily with tactual perception of roughness (as does the psychophysical literature) and remains highly speculative. There has been no direct peripheral (with the exception of LaMotte, 1977) or central neural recording of single-unit response to textured surfaces in any species. The results of human psychophysical studies such as those reported in the section "Psychophysical studies" may provide the sensory physiologist with a better idea of what kinds of mechanisms to look for. The information we do have concerning neural mechanisms underlying the tactual perception of tex-

ture derives from the study of a variety of species. As the neural organization is not the same for all mammals, extreme care should be exercised when extrapolating from one species to another (especially to humans) and when assuming similar functions for differently located sensory systems, or for similar anatomic structures in different species
(Brown, 1973).

Equivalence and bias in intersensory function

Intersensory equivalence. At the beginning of this chapter, it was pointed
out that the tactual perception of texture is a multimodal task involving
not only cutaneous and kinesthetic channels but, at least potentially,
visual and auditory inputs as well. In the previous section, we dealt with
the role of cutaneous and kinesthetic cues in texture perception. In the
present section, we will consider the potential contribution of the accompanying visual and acoustic cues.

Visual texture provides important information for depth and distance
perception, for figure–ground distinctions, and for form recognition (Gibson, 1950). Nevertheless, the perception of visual texture per se has received relatively little attention until the recent work of Julesz. He (1975)
adopted a statistical approach to the production and analysis of texture
that has not yet been used in the tactual field. In considering the nature of
the processing involved in "preattentive" texture perception, Julesz originally suggested that a Fourier transform of the input image is taken, with
the phase (position) spectra ignored by the preattentive perceptual system. In more recent work (Julesz & Caelli, 1979), however, this has been
revised to take into account evidence for local, nonlinear feature extrac-
tors. If this type of analysis were to hold for tactual perception of texture as
well, the early work of Lederman (e.g., Lederman, 1973; Lederman &
Taylor, 1972) showing the relative unimportance of spatial frequency suggests nonlinearities must occur at an even earlier stage of processing.

More directly in line with research reported in the section "Psychophysical studies," Lederman and Abbott (1981) demonstrated that using
vision, touch, or vision and touch, subjects performed a magnitude estimation task similarly, in terms of the magnitude estimates of roughness,
the rates of growth of perceived roughness, and response precision. Moreover, using the same three modes, subjects performed a roughness identification task (also using abrasive papers) with equivalent matching accuracy and precision.

The similarity in visual versus tactual performance of textural tasks was
likewise demonstrated in an earlier study by Bjorkman (1967), although

the task was different again from those used above. He had subjects make "equal" or "different" judgments of abrasive papers presented sequentially, either intramodally or intermodally. Intramodal matching was again similar for vision and touch, although the linear fits of the data were slightly better for vision. Intermodal matching data were best fit by power functions. Unfortunately, it is difficult to interpret these results any further because Bjorkman did not specify the dimension (e.g., roughness) along which the stimulus pairs were to be compared; subjects may well have chosen to use entirely different kinds and/or numbers of dimensions visually and tactually.

Brown (1960) examined the ability of both skilled and unskilled subjects to judge the roughness of a set of flat, wooden surfaces worked to different degrees of roughness. Brown, like Binns (1934, 1937) before him, was concerned with the quality of the texture judgments that must be made by human observers in the textile (and woodworking) industries. Skilled operators use both visual and tactual cues to judge surface qualities. Brown was therefore interested in assessing the relative superiority of the two modalities under normal industrial conditions. He also evaluated two new inspection conditions that used oblique lighting and compared the performance of skilled operators with that of unskilled observers. Subjects selected the rougher of each pair of surfaces under five inspection conditions: vision only (oblique lighting), vision only (normal direct lighting), touch only, vision (oblique) + touch, and vision (normal) + touch. The skilled group was about equally sensitive in the vision (oblique) and touch conditions; vision (normal) resulted in considerably poorer performance. The unskilled group was not as sensitive in their tactual as opposed to visual (oblique) judgments; once again, however, the vision (normal) condition resulted in poor discrimination. Although the skilled group was more discriminating than the unskilled group in the three conditions commonly used in industry (i.e., vision [direct lighting], touch, and vision [direct lighting] and touch), the superiority was eliminated by the oblique lighting of the surfaces. When both modalities were used together, discrimination was somewhat reduced compared to the "superior" modality alone, though not significantly so.

A set of studies by Walker (1967) has demonstrated corresponding visual and tactual texture aftereffects. A visual display consisting of fine and coarse pieces of sandpaper on either side of a fixation point was fixated for several seconds. A patch of intermediate texture that replaced the fine texture appeared more coarse visually than the intermediate texture that replaced the coarse texture. Similarly, when a fine piece of sandpaper was stroked for several seconds with one hand, and a coarse piece simultaneously with the other, an intermediate texture felt more coarse to the former hand than to the latter. No intermodal aftereffects were found. Other work on intermodal transfer of texture information is considered in the section "Developmental studies."

Other research (Lederman, 1979) has examined the role of touch-produced sounds in the perception of roughness. The sounds a person produces when touching vary considerably with the materials being touched, the mechanical state of the skin, and the various hand speeds and forces used during exploration. Katz certainly recognized the importance of such sounds for identifying the material composition of objects. Can and, more importantly, *do* people use such cues to evaluate surface texture? Subjects made magnitude estimates of the perceived roughness of grooved metal plates varying in groove and ridge width using only the sounds the experimenter produced by touching the surfaces. The auditory judgments of plates that varied in surface geometry were similar to, but not as discriminating as, those made on the basis of (subject-produced) tactual cues alone. Hand speed and force also altered auditory judgments of roughness, but not in a manner that was entirely consistent with corresponding tactual estimates. Moreover, under certain conditions, auditory judgments were more discriminating than those of touch. Nevertheless, whenever both tactual and auditory sources of information were available, subjects tended to use the tactual cues.

The studies in this section indicate that people are indeed capable of judging texture (usually roughness) using any of several channels of information. Generally speaking, the various sensory systems provide corroborative information, although sometimes one system proves better, that is, more discriminating or more reliable, in judging roughness than another.

Intersensory bias. We may also ask whether one modality can be dominated or biased by another modality. Intersensory bias has been evaluated experimentally by examining how subjects resolve a discrepancy in the information presented to two sensory systems (e.g., Pick, Warren, & Hay, 1969). Logically, they may handle intersensory discrepancy by ignoring information from one channel or by using the information from both channels in some form of compromise judgment. In the latter situation, the compromise might favor one modality or weight information from all senses equally.

It is still commonly and generally asserted, especially in textbooks (e.g., Schiffman, 1976, p. 155), that "vision is the dominant sensory system"; people speak of the priority of vision over touch. Such imprecise statements should be avoided. We must qualify them by specifying the particular tasks used to evaluate the relative dominance of one system over another. It is quite likely that the degree and even the direction of intersensory dominance can be shifted by changing the particular demands imposed upon the sensory system (e.g., see Warren, 1979).

In the literature, most of the intersensory discrepancies that involve touch also involve vision. And almost all of these studies have used macro-spatial tasks, such as form, size, extent, orientation, or spatial localization (e.g., Hay, Pick, & Ikeda, 1965; Power & Graham, 1976; Rock & Victor, 1964; Teghtsoonian & Teghtsoonian, 1970). Such tasks usually produce strong visual dominance. But because vision performs these tasks markedly better than touch, visual dominance is not particularly surprising. The superiority of vision in these macro-spatial tasks may relate to the benefits that result from the simultaneous processing strategies typically used by vision but not by touch.

Abbott (1979; Lederman & Abbott, 1981) recently examined the resolution of a discrepancy between visual and tactual information concerning surface texture. The experimental design was very similar to that used by Rock and Victor (1964), but the task was not. Texture perception, unlike shape perception, is performed frequently and easily by *both* vision and touch. In keeping with this observation, subjects tended to resolve the discrepancy by using information from both modalities about equally.

The relative superiority of one modality over another in a given task may also account for the reason subjects appeared to ignore auditory cues to texture when tactual information was simultaneously available (Lederman, 1979). It might be because touch was generally superior to audition in the judgment of surface roughness.

In addition to a modality-superiority analysis of intersensory bias, one may also adopt an "ecological" approach. Such an approach is suggested by the additional results from Lederman's auditory–tactual texture study. Although touch usually differentiated roughness better than audition, there were certain occasions when the reverse was true. At such times, when both tactual and acoustic information was present, why was the latter still ignored? In ecological terms, it may be that touch-produced sounds are frequently unavailable to us. Outside the experimental soundproof room, extraneous sounds often mask the potentially useful auditory cues to surface roughness, but the tactual cues still remain. People may have simply learned to ignore the auditory information at all times, therefore, in favor of the more reliable tactual information.

Studies of intersensory discrepancy further our understanding of the nature of intersensory organization and of the relative capabilities and limitations of the sensory–perceptual systems involved.

Developmental studies

Dimensional preferences. Several investigators have used the dimension of texture to study the development of tactual preference as well as the nature of intra- and intermodal integration.

A number of studies have demonstrated that young children show preferences for particular dimensions of information available in a complex situation. In vision, for example, preschool children attend more to an object's color than to its form (e.g., Brian & Goodenough, 1929). In touch, Klein (1963) observed that before the age of 8 (and especially before 6.5) years, children tend to match on the basis of textural similarity; however, by the age of 8, they prefer to match on the basis of a common tactual form. Such a trend has been compared to the color-to-form transition in vision, texture being to touch what color is to vision. Gliner (1967) argued that previous studies failed to control for relative differences in discriminability of the stimulus dimensions used. She suggested that the shape preference obtained with touch might be due to nothing more than differences in discriminability among the stimuli. However, this interpretation proved insufficient. Gliner found that shape discrimination thresholds remained unchanged for kindergarten and third-grade children; in fact it was the texture thresholds that decreased with age. In a continuing series of studies, Gliner, Pick, Pick and Hales (1969) compared tactual and visual preferences with discriminable differences in the stimulus values equated. Kindergarten children still preferred to match tactually on the basis of texture, whereas third-grade children preferred to use form cues; form was preferred visually by children in both age groups. Gliner et al. also found that when the perceived difference in texture was increased, third-grade children persisted in their choice of shape; when the difference in shape was increased, kindergarten children switched to a shape match. The investigators suggested that with touch, the shape preference might be due to the fact that as children become older, they learn that shape provides a better cue for identifying objects than does texture. Children therefore give up the earlier preference for texture, because it is usually more important that one identify an object than know about its surface qualities. The developmental shift from texture to shape preference has been further supported by Siegel and Vance (1970). More recently, Gliner (publishing under the name of Margolin, 1976) considered the effect of pretraining kindergarten and third-grade children on only one of the two dimensions used in a subsequent test of preference for shape or texture. She also examined the effect of preference on the subsequent learning of a discrimination task. These studies therefore asked (1) whether new experiences could alter the nature (or degree) of the tactual preference and (2) whether such preferences might help or hinder the child's ability to handle a discrimination problem when the preferred dimension was relevant or irrelevant. The results provided little support for Margolin's specific predictions. She concluded that pretraining can alter the tactual preference of children and that initial preference affects discrimination learning; but she failed to consider the reasons why the results for various sex-by-age-group combinations, though significant, were not always in the direction predicted by her previous research.

Abravanel (1970) suggested that the early preference for texture over shape found by Klein and Gliner et al. may be due to their use of planometric stimuli. Because young children have been observed to use mainly holding, grasping, clutching, and palpating movements (Zaporozhets, 1965; Zinchenko & Lomov, 1960) during haptic exploration, Abravanel argued that they may be at a disadvantage when exploring the shape (compared with the texture) of flat objects. However, the salience of shape should increase for solid three-dimensional objects, because the latter lend themselves more readily than do two-dimensional objects to the exploratory motions used by very young children. Abravanel predicted and found that shape preference would occur at an earlier age than found previously if *solid* stimulus shapes were used. This finding was further supported by Siegel and Barber (1973). This body of research points to complicated interactions among the preferred mode of haptic exploration, observer age, the nature of the stimulus materials, and the perceptual task required.

Intersensory and intrasensory function. Abravanel's findings also relate to the questions concerning inter- and intrasensory function. It can be suggested that the difficulties reported in intermodal matching and transfer tasks (Blank & Bridger, 1964; Milner & Bryant, 1970) may be due to the need for more advanced processing than in intramodal tasks. However, Abravanel found that intra- (tactual–tactual) and intermodal (tactual–visual) choice matches involving texture and shape were similar by the ages of 4 and 5. Rose, Blank and Bridger (1972) argued that the difficulty may not necessarily be in the intermodal demands per se. It could also be in the initial processing and/or subsequent retention of tactual information. As most of the research on intermodal matching and transfer has used the dimension of form, the investigators chose to examine intra- (visual–visual, tactual–tactual) and intermodal matching of shapes and textures by 3-year-olds. When there was no memory load, that is, simultaneous stimulus presentation, performance was equally good in all conditions of examination (unfortunately, the task may have been too easy). When stimulus presentation was successive, or when a delay was imposed between the initial stimulus presentation and the following matching condition, performance was impaired in all three conditions involving tactual examination. The authors concluded that the deficit young children frequently show in intersensory integration tasks is likely due to the difficulty in *retaining* tactual information. However, this explanation cannot fully account for the decrement in performance when a visual standard and tactual comparisons were used. Presumably, there must have been some deficit in intermodal transfer as well. However, Abravanel's intermodal finding supports the retention explanation by Rose et al. because his tactual–visual condition involved simultaneous presentation of stimuli.

Studies by Blank and Klig (1970) and more recently Tyrrell (1977) have demonstrated transfer of dimensional (texture and shape) information between vision and touch. Both studies also showed that intradimensional problems were learned more quickly than extradimensional problems. The fact that there were no differences between Blank and Klig's visual–visual and tactual–visual modes, or between Tyrrell's visual–tactual and tactual–visual conditions, further supports Rose et al's. emphasis on tactual storage difficulties, because there was no memory load imposed in conditions that involved the tactual system.

The preceding developmental studies provide information concerning dimensional preferences in children. In addition, they provide valuable information concerning inter- and intrasensory function, and in so doing force us to consider the nature and limitations of tactual processing (for further details, see Chapter 3).

Braille and tangible graphics for the visually impaired

Given the technological advances and the recent legislation mandating equal access to education for the handicapped in the United States, it is becoming increasingly possible to provide educational materials for the visually impaired. However, given the heterogeneity of this population, producing such materials is far from easy. They could benefit substantially from a successful union of basic and applied research, each providing questions and possible approaches for the other. The present section, therefore, will consider both basic and applied research on the presentation of written and graphic information through the skin.

Braille

Let us consider braille first. Braille is a tactual reading and writing system that uses as characters rectangular arrays of raised dots, three rows high and two columns wide. As patterns of raised dots, it seems not unreasonable to ask whether they are also perceived as textures (Millar, 1978; Nolan & Morris, 1960, 1965). For example, Nolan and Morris (1960, 1965) developed a roughness discrimination test to serve as a predictor of braille reading readiness in very young children. And Millar (1978) has recently suggested that texture plays a role in tactual pattern recognition, although it is a complex one. One experiment she performed indicated that young children (blindfolded) recognized differences in unfamiliar raised dot patterns better when discrimination was based on textural cues (differences in the number of dots forming a shape) as compared to differences in spatial features (symmetry vs. asymmetry). Millar suggests that when there are no spatial referents available with which to condense spatial information (e.g., as when exploring unfamiliar tactual dot patterns), crude differences in texture may be coded instead. Texture differences could be used effectively in the task above. Normally, however, textural codes are considerably less efficient in condensing spatial information than spatial codes that focus on spatial configuration or spatial features. The multiplicity of texture codes required in spatial tasks would quickly overload the system; such codes, therefore, cannot be used as easily as the spatial codes mentioned in attentional strategies. On the basis of her interpretation, Millar (pers. comm., July 1977) has speculated that poor braille readers may code braille patterns inappropriately in terms of texture rather than spatial configuration or spatial features.

Also relevant to the hypothesized link between braille reading and the perception of texture is some of Lederman's earlier work on the effect of finger force. In the section "Psychophysical studies," it was mentioned that increasing finger force causes perceived roughness to grow in magnitude. If the perceived texture (i.e., roughness) of the braille patterns could not be ignored by a poor blind reader, *and* if the reader was unable to maintain a steady force while examining the braille letters, reading could be hampered by the perception of a constantly changing texture. Work by Kusajima (1974) lends some initial support to this idea by showing that poor braille readers are indeed more variable than good braille readers in the force they apply when reading.

Tangible graphics

Maps, charts, graphs, and so on are important sources of information in books and journals for the sighted. Unfortunately, they are rarely included in braille translations.[5] *Tangible graphics* is the general term for such informational displays. Most of the available research on this topic deals with tactual maps, which may be used to provide political and geographical information about towns, regions, and the world. In addition, they potentially offer visually handicapped pedestrians the opportunity for independent travel. However, maps are used infrequently. Many persons with visual impairments have never encountered a tactual map; moreover, those individuals who have used them have often been discouraged by the poor quality of the maps available. Evaluation and advancement of map design are further hampered by the lack of map-reading skills (Nolan & Morris, 1971). And knowledge of basic geographical concepts, both concrete and abstract, is still rather limited in those people for whom the maps are intended (Franks & Nolan, 1971).

In this section, I will consider the role of texture mainly in tactual map design; however, the discussion is relevant to all forms of tangible graphics (see Hanninen, 1971; Lederman & Kinch, 1979). Research on map design focuses primarily on the choice of a legible tactual symbology. Three different sets of tactual symbols are typically used: areal (texture), line, and point. Areal symbols are used to represent a particular space; lines represent a boundary or continuous connection between two locations; and point symbols represent a single landmark or place. As texture perception is a task we perform relatively easily and well, texture is, at least potentially, an effective symbol to choose for any tactual graphics display.

A number of studies have attempted to determine a set of legible texture symbols for presenting nominal (and occasionally ordinal; see Schiff, 1966) information on a tactual display; the subjects in most of these studies were legally blind school children. As the research is discussed more thoroughly in Chapter 11, I will only reference the studies here: Bauer (1952), Culbert and Stellwagen (1963), Heath (1958), James and Gill (1975), Morris and Nolan (1961, 1963), Nolan and Morris (1963, 1971), Schiff (1967), Stellwagen and Culbert (1963), and Wiedel and Groves (1972). The textures were created from sandpapers (of different coarseness) and patterns that varied along a number of dimensions, for example, continuous versus interrupted, regular versus irregular, pattern density, size of elements, and sharpness of elements (Nolan & Morris, 1971; Schiff, 1967). Most often these patterns were reproduced in plastic using a vacuum-forming process. Success has been very limited. At best, Nolan and Morris have found no more than eight highly discriminable symbols (according to their criteria for legibility). They believe that this limit is inherent in the processing of texture; however, they may be somewhat premature in drawing this conclusion.

The choice of areal patterns to date has been somewhat arbitrary, with visual criteria for apparent discriminability often determining the items selected. Items have therefore differed along more than one dimension at a time. To which dimension(s) can we attribute the high discriminability? Conversely, why do two physically dissimilar patterns feel so similar in texture? It could be that although the dimension(s) sampled may be relevant, the *values* arbitrarily selected from the dimension(s) are confusable. Could we therefore choose other values along that same dimension(s) that might prove more distinct to the observer? Only systematic alteration of the stimuli along a number of dimensions will permit us to determine which of them are relevant, as well as what values are appropriate for each dimension chosen. When the intention is to reproduce the "master" display in multiple copies, one is of course limited to using discriminable dimensions within a single material (usually a heat-sensitive plastic known as Brailon). However, there is also considerable need for single-copy displays, for example, orientation and mobility maps. In such instances, more than one material may be used so as to exploit distinctive differences in the physical characteristics of the materials, for example, resilience, coefficient of friction, and heat conductance and capacity.

Multivariate designs and analyses may be used to determine the dimensions relevant for the perception of texture. Such methodologies allow the investigator to determine how a set of items clusters perceptually, and to begin to understand the dimension(s) that underlie the clustering. Following this initial broad attack, one could determine a set of textures that were judged as very dissimilar on the most important dimensions. Using these items in a paired comparison (same–different) or matching task would allow one to evaluate legibility according to criteria such as those used by Nolan and Morris. Furthermore, knowing somewhat better what dimensions were relevant to the tactual perception of texture, one could attempt to expand the set of legible symbols by systematically extending the range of values used.

The psychophysical work by Lederman also bears on the issue of tactual dimensions of texture. In the discrimination studies above, same–different judgments of textures might have been based, at least in part, on the evaluation of roughness. Her research suggests that the spacing between elements may be crucial in same–different judgments, and not, as some have suggested, pattern density or size of element. The mechanical analysis of skin deformation that Taylor and Lederman (1975) proposed could theoretically determine for a variety of areal patterns values of the several skin deformation qualities believed to underlie the tactual perception of roughness. Models such as this permit the investigator to make predictions about potentially discriminable stimuli and to evaluate subsequently their effectiveness as symbols in tactual displays. Jansson (1972) has referred to the value of such theoretical analyses for the development of a tactual symbology.

Line symbols typically used in studies of legibility also possess a degree of perceived roughness. Is it possible that confusions among line symbols are due in part to their similarity along roughness dimensions? Should this be confirmed, one can again use the dimensions of perceived roughness already isolated to develop additional line symbols for testing.

A psychophysical approach would further permit the construction of a discriminable texture symbology for presenting ordinal (rank) as well as nominal (class) information on a tactual map. To date, only Schiff (1967) and Ogrosky (1973) have considered the potential of ordinal symbol-scaling studies in representing more complex spatial relationships.

The texture discrimination experiments in this section have all used pairs of surfaces in isolation. In considering the use of texture (or any other symbol class) in maps and other tactual displays, one must not ignore the possibility that legibility will be further affected by the presence of other symbols. This leads to consideration of one problem examined in signal detection theory (see McNicol, 1972), that of detecting a "signal" in the presence of background "noise" (i.e., nonsignals). Three different kinds of symbols are used in tangible graphics. Identifying or tracking a given symbol requires the user to ignore all others, both within and across these three symbol classes. Whatever the target symbol is for the moment becomes a signal; nontargets, by definition, must be noise.

Does the nature of the background alter the speed or accuracy with which a user may identify a target or its spatial representation on a map? Texture symbols could aid or hinder the accurate detection of another texture symbol. I know of no work that relates to this suggestion. Or they may interfere with the reader's ability to pick out line and point target symbols. Berlá and Murr (1975) investigated this issue by having young braille readers locate instances of a given point symbol and trace a dotted line on a tactual pseudomap with either a noise-free or noisy background

158

(i.e, irrelevant areal symbols were present). It was found that irrelevant textures interfered with the encoding of point and line symbols on the map.

How can one eliminate or at least reduce the interfering effects of texture? Nolan and Morris (1971) used differences in the height of line, point, and areal symbols to reduce error. It may well be that information coded by areal symbols can be presented even more effectively when necessary, in underlays, as Kidwell and Greer (1972) and Gill (1973) have done. Such a technique would provide the noise-free environment Berlá and Murr found desirable by keeping areal symbol information physically separate from line and point symbols.

In the Nolan and Morris study, height was used effectively as a source of redundant information concerning symbol class; that is, different heights were associated with areal, point, and line symbols. The value of using redundant information on a tactual display supports earlier work by Schiff and Isikow (1966). They showed that if texture is used in a redundant manner, its presence can improve the accuracy of performance of legally blind high school students using a bar graph. Information about the length of the bars was presented in five different ways: raised outline only, bars represented by different grades of sandpaper, bars represented by different heights, outlines plus corresponding changes in texture, and corresponding changes in texture *and* height. The mode of presentation thus varied in terms of the amount of correlated or redundant information about tactual length, as well as in the quality of redundant information. Briefly, the results of this part of the study indicated that the maximum amount of redundancy (texture + height) produced the fewest errors.

Corsini and Pick (1969) demonstrated (in college students) a natural interaction between texture and perceived length; fine-textured stimuli were perceived as being longer than coarse-textured stimuli of physically equal lengths. Hanninen (1970) was unable to show the same biasing effect of texture on length perception in children, either sighted or blind. However, he did find some texture facilitation and interference in length discrimination among the sighted subjects. Interpreting Hanninen's findings meaningfully is somewhat difficult. However, interactions of texture with length, area, shape, and so forth warrant further careful consideration because they may potentially but substantially alter the readability of tactual displays. Should such interactions be found, one ought to build upon these natural redundancies, much as Schiff, Kaufer, and Mosak (1966) have done in the design of their "tactual arrow." This symbol is a sawtooth pattern that feels smooth when the hand moves over it in the direction the symbol is intended to represent; when the hand moves in the opposite direction, the symbol feels rough. With no initial training, Schiff et al.'s subjects automatically picked the "smooth" direction as the one the symbol was meant to represent.

Few studies have actually evaluated the accuracy with which symbols (including texture) are identified *within the context of a map*. The only relevant study I have found is one by Berlá and Murr (1976), which was designed for another purpose. They required young braille readers to locate on a tactual pseudomap as many of 16 (identical) point and 6 (identical) areal symbols as possible within a 5-min period. There were four different kinds of point, five line, and five areal symbols in all. Generally speaking, symbol recognition was a good deal lower than should be acceptable. Unfortunately, it is impossible to isolate the reasons for the poor performance because of the design of the experiment. Poor symbol recognition may have been due to any of a number of factors, such as poor map-reading strategies, complexity of map design (e.g., noise added by background and other target symbols), and/or heavy memory demands (especially with respect to the numerous point targets).

Another meaningful way of assessing symbols in map displays is to use matching tasks in which a standard is presented and subsequently chosen from among a set of comparison stimuli. Such a task is difficult to perform by touch alone because of the heavy memory load imposed by the serial order of stimulus presentation (Rose et al., 1972). However, it does correspond more closely to the map-reading task of examining a symbol key followed by a variety of symbols on the map itself. We must properly assess the limitations involved in presenting graphical information through the tactual system.

Legibility of texture symbols could be affected by other aspects of the tactual exploration process, such as force and speed of hand motion (see the section "Psychophysical studies"). As early as 1952, Bauer mentioned that accuracy of texture discrimination was altered by variations in force, but he gave no data to support his claim. As mentioned earlier, some of Lederman's work shows that estimates of the magnitude of apparent roughness increase substantially with increases in finger force. Because roughness is a prominent component of texture, it is reasonable to predict that variation in finger force might interfere with the proper discrimination of surface textures on a map. It may well be necessary, therefore, to teach the maintenance of a relatively constant force in any map-reading program. Because roughness is not strongly affected by changes in hand speed, however, speed can probably be safely ignored.

Summary

In this chapter I have attempted to integrate the body of literature that relates directly and indirectly to the tactual perception of texture. There is still relatively little systematic research in the field, although there are several important functions such work can provide (see "Introduction"). The section "Early research on tactual perception of texture" (mainly) documents the major features of David Katz's work on texture perception, a primary concern in his classic monograph, *The world of touch* (for further details, see Chapter 1). The section "Current research on tactual perception of texture" examines the more current literature in this area; its subsections cover the four major approaches or issues: psychophysics, neural coding mechanisms, equivalence and bias in intersensory function, and developmental issues. The last section examines "Braille and tangible graphics for the visually impaired." For clarity, I categorized the research on the tactual perception of texture. There is considerable overlap across sections. Wherever relevant, therefore, I have attempted to draw parallels and make obvious connections (e.g., as between Katz's work and the more recent psychophysical literature). Finally, where research has been particularly scanty, I have offered my own somewhat liberal speculations and interpretations.

Acknowledgments

I would like to thank a number of people for their very helpful comments on an earlier draft of this chapter: Frances Aboud, Lester Krueger, Jack Loomis, Bill Schiff, Martin Taylor, Chuck Vierck, and Michael von Grunau.

Notes

1 The rate of displacement should not matter provided the skin is not deformed so slowly as to result in adaptation of the receptors.
2 To a fairly good approximation, the coefficient of friction, μ, may be empirically defined as the ratio of the force needed to overcome friction (F) to the normal force (i.e., perpendicular to the surface) between the two surfaces that are in contact (N); that is, $\mu \approx F/N$ (Feynman, Leighton, & Sands, 1963).
3 In the 1979 article that appeared in *Perception and Psychophysics*, the thicknesses of intermediate papers were incorrectly reported. They are actually 0.001 cm (0.0004 in) and 0.0005 cm (0.0002 in).
4 There clearly must be some lower, nonzero limit to the range of shearing forces over which this masking is believed to occur. Otherwise perceived roughness should be greatest when there is no motion between skin and object. As mentioned before, however, roughness is not perceived at all when relative motion does not occur.
5 Recording for the Blind supplies tactual drawings with their recorded textbooks. The address is: Recording for the Blind, 121 East 58th Street, New York, NY 10022.

References

Abbott, S. Sensory dominance in texture perception. Honors psychology thesis, Queens University, Ontario. Canada, 1979.

Abravanel, E. Choice for shape vs. textural matching by young children. *Perceptual & Motor Skills*, 1970, *31*, 527–533.

Bauer, H. Discrimination of tactual stimuli. *Journal of Experimental Psychology*, 1952, *44*, 455–459.

Benjamin, R., & Thompson, R. Differential effects of cortical lesions in infant and adult cats on roughness discrimination. *Experimental Neurology*, 1959, *1*, 305–321.

Berlá, E. P., & Murr, M. The effects of noise on the location of point symbols and tracking a line on a tactile pseudomap. *Journal of Special Education*, 1975, *9*, 183–190.

Locating symbols on a tactile pseudomap by braille readers operating under different frames of reference. In C. Y. Nolan (Ed.), *Facilitating the education of the visually handicapped through research in communications*. Part 3, Louisville, Ky.: American Printing House for the Blind, 1976, pp 25–37.

Binns, H. A visual and tactile analysis of typical Bradford wool-tops. *Journal of Textile Industry*, 1934, No. 21.

Visual and tactual "judgment" as illustrated in a practical experiment. *British Journal of Psychology*, 1937, *27*, 404–410.

Bjorkman, M. Relations between intra-modal and cross-modal matching. *Scandinavian Journal of Psychology*, 1967, *8*, 65–76.

Blank, M., & Bridger, W. Crossmodal transfer in nursery school children. *Journal of Comparative and Physiological Psychology*, 1964, *58*, 272–282.

Blank, M., & Klig, S. Dimensional learning across sensory modalities in nursery school children. *Journal of Experimental and Child Psychology*, 1970, *9*, 166–173.

Brian, C., & Goodenough, E. The relative potency of color and form perception at various ages. *Journal of Experimental Psychology*, 1929, *12*, 197–213.

Brown, A. G. Ascending and long spinal pathways: dorsal columns, spinocervical tract and spinothalamic tract. In A. Iggo (Ed.), *Handbook of sensory physiology*, vol. 2. Berlin: Springer-Verlag, 1973, pp 315–338.

Brown, A. G., & Gordon, G. Subcortical mechanisms concerned in somatic sensation. *British Medical Bulletin*, 1977, *33*, 121–128.

Brown, A. G., Gordon, G., & Kay, R. H. A study of single axons in the cat's medial lemniscus. *Journal of Physiology*, 1974, *236*, 225–246.

Brown, I. D. Visual and tactual judgments of surface roughness. *Ergonomics*, 1960, *3*, 51–61.

Bryant, P., & Raz, I. Visual and tactual perception of shape by young children. *Developmental Psychology*, 1975, *11*, 525–526.

Burgess, P., & Perl, E. Cutaneous mechanoreceptors and nociceptors. In A. Iggo (Ed.)., *Handbook of sensory physiology*, vol. 2. Berlin: Springer-Verlag, 1973, pp. 29–78.

Cashdan, S. Visual and haptic form discrimination under conditions of successive stimulation. *Journal of Experimental Psychology*, 1968, *76*, 221–224.

Corsini, D., & Pick, H. L., Jr. The effect of texture on tactually perceived length. *Perception & Psychophysics*, 1969, *5*, 352–356.

Culbert, S., & Stellwagen, W. T. Tactual discrimination of textures. *Perceptual & Motor Skills*, 1963, *16*, 545–552.

Djalali, E. Depression of cutaneous mechanoreceptor response to mechanical stimulation by skin cooling. *Society for Neuroscience Abstracts*, 1977, *3*, 455.

Dobry, P. J., & Casey, K. L. Roughness discrimination in cats with dorsal column lesions. *Brain Research,* 1972, *44,* 385–397.

Ekman, G., Hosman, J., & Lindstrom, B. Roughness, smoothness and preference: a study of quantitative relations in individual subjects. *Journal of Experimental Psychology,* 1965, *70,* 18–26.

Feynman, R., Leighton, R., & Sands, M. *The Feynman lectures on physics.* London: Addison-Wesley, 1963.

Finger, S., & Frommer, G. P. Effects of cortical lesions on tactile discriminations graded in difficulty. *Life Science,* 1968, *7,* 897–904.

Franks, F. & Nolan, C. Y. Development of geographic concepts in blind children. *Exceptional Children,* 1971, *38,* 321–324. (a)
Measuring geographical concept attainment in visually handicapped students. *Education of the Visually Handicapped,* 1971, *3,* 11–16. (b)

Gescheider, G., & Verrillo, R. T. Vibrotactile frequency characteristics as determined by adaptation and masking procedures. In D. Kenshalo (Ed.), *Sensory functions of the skin of humans.* New York: Plenum Press, 1979.

Gibson, J J. *The perception of the visual world.* Boston: Houghton Mifflin, 1950.
Observations on active touch. *Psychological Review,* 1962, *62,* 477–491.

Gill, J. M. Design, production and evaluation of tactual maps for the blind. Unpublished doctoral thesis, University of Warwick, England, 1973.

Gliner, C. R. Tactual discrimination thresholds for shape and texture in young children. *Journal of Experimental and Child Psychology,* 1967, *5,* 536–547.

Gliner, C., Pick, A., Pick, H. L.,, & Hales, J. A developmental investigation of visual and haptic preferences for shape and texture. *Monographs of the Society for Research in Child Development,* 1969, *34,* no. 6 (serial no. 130), 1–40.

Gordon, G. (Ed). *Active touch. The mechanisms of recognition of objects by manipulation: a multidisciplinary approach.* Oxford: Pergamon Press, 1978.

Gordon, I., & Cooper, C. Improving one's touch. *Nature,* 1975, *256,* 203–204.

Green, B., Lederman, S. J., & Stevens, J. C. The effect of skin temperature on the perception of roughness. *Sensory Processes,* 1979, *3* 327–333.

Hanninen, K. A. The effect of texture on tactual perception of length. *Exceptional Children,* 1970, *36,* 655–659.
Review of the educational potential of texture and tactually discriminable patterns. *Journal of Special Education,* 1971, *5,* 133–141.

Hay, J. C., Pick, H. L., & Ikeda, K. Visual capture produced by prism spectacles. *Psychonomic Science,* 1965, *2,* 215–216.

Heath, W. R. Maps and graphics for the blind: some aspects of the discriminability of textual surfaces for use in areal differentiation. Unpublished doctoral thesis, University of Washington, 1958.

Hyvarinen, J., & Poranen, A. Function of the parietal associative area 7 as revealed from cellular discharges in alert monkeys. *Brain,* 1974, *97,* 673–692.

Inman, D. P., & Peruzzi, P. The effect of temperature on the response of Pacinian corpuscles. *Journal of Physiology,* 1961, *155,* 280–301.

James, G., & Gill, J. M. A pilot study on the discriminability of tactile areal and line symbols for the blind. *American Foundation for the Blind Research Bulletin,* 1975, *29,* 23–31.

Jansson, G. Symbols for tactile maps. In B. Lindquist & N. Trowald (Eds.), *European conference on educational research for the visually handicapped,* Lararhogskolan and Uppsala: Pedagogiska Institutionen, Report No. 31, 1972.

Johansson, R. Skin mechanoreceptors in the human hand: receptive field characteristics. In Y. Zotterman (Ed.), *Sensory functions of the skin in primates (with special reference to man).* New York: Pergamon Press, 1976.

Julesz, B. Experiments in the visual perception of texture. *Scientific American,* 1975, *232,* 34–43.

Julesz, B., & Caelli, T. On the limits of Fourier decomposition in visual texture perception. *Perception.* 1979, *8,* 69–73.

Katz, D. Der Aufbau Der Tastwelt. *Zeitschrift für Psychologie,* 1925, *11,* 270 pp. Leipzig: Barth.

Kidwell, A., & Greer, P. The environmental perceptions of blind persons and their haptic representation. *New Outlook for the Blind,* 1972, *66,* 256–276.

Kitai, S., & Weinberg, J. Tactile discrimination study of the dorsal column–medial lemniscal system and spino-cervical-thalamic tract in the cat. *Experimental Brain Research,* 1968, *6,* 234–246.

Klein, S. D. A developmental study of tactual perception. Unpublished doctoral thesis, Clark University, 1963.

Knibestol, M., & Vallbo, A. Single unit analyses of mechanoreceptor activity from the human glabrous skin. *Acta Physiologia Scandinavia,* 1970, *80,* 178–195.

Kohn, B., & Dennis, M. Somatosensory functions after cerebral hemicortication for infantile hemiplegia. *Neuropsychologia,* 1974, *12,* 119–130.

Krueger, L. David Katz' Der Aufbau der Tastwelt (The world of touch): a synopsis. *Perception & Psychophysics,* 1970, *7,* 337–341.

Kusajima, T. *Visual reading and braille reading: an experimental investigation of the physiology and psychology of visual and tactual reading.* New York: American Foundation for the Blind, 1974.

LaMotte, R. H. Psychophysical and neurophysiological studies of tactile sensibility. In N. Hollies & R. Goldman (Eds.), *Clothing comfort: interaction of thermal, ventilation, construction and assessment factors.* Ann Arbor, Mich.: Science Publishers, 1977.

Lederman, S. J. The perception of roughness by touch. Unpublished doctoral thesis, University of Toronto, 1973.

Tactile roughness of grooved surfaces: the touching process and effects of macro- and microsurface structure. *Perception & Psychophysics,* 1974, *16,* 385–395.

The "callus-thenics" of touching. *Canadian Journal of Psychology,* 1976, *30,* 82–89.

Tactile texture perception. Address to the Lake Ontario Visionary Establishment, Niagara Falls, Canada, February 1978. (a)

Heightening tactile impressions of surface texture. In G. Gordon (Ed.), *Active touch. The mechanisms of recognition of objects by manipulation: a multidisciplinary approach.* Oxford: Pergamon Press, 1978, pp. 205–214. (b)

"Improving one's touch" . . . and more. *Perception & Psychophysics,* 1978, *24,* 154–160. (c)

Auditory texture perception. *Perception,* 1979, *8,* 93–103.

The perception of surface roughness by active and passive touch. *Bulletin of the Psychonomic Society,* in press.

Lederman, S. J., & Abbott, S. G. Texture perception: studies of intersensory organization using a discrepancy paradigm and visual vs. tactual psychophysics. *Journal of Experimental Psychology: Human Perception Performance,* 1981, *7,* 902–915.

Lederman, S. J., & Kinch, D. Texture in tactual maps and graphics for the visually handicapped. *Journal of Visual Impairment and Blindness,* 1979, *73,* 217–227.

Lederman, S. J., & Taylor, M. M. Fingertip force, surface geometry and the perception of roughness by active touch. *Perception & Psychophysics,* 1972, *12,* 401–408.

McNicol, D. *A primer of signal detection theory.* London: Allen & Unwin, Sydney: Australasian Publishing, 1972.

Margolin, C. R. Modifications and influences of tactual preferences for shape and texture. *Perceptual & Motor Skills,* 1976, *43,* 1123–1133.

Meenes, M., & Zigler, M. J. An experimental study of perceptions: roughness and smoothness. *American Journal of Psychology,* 1923, *34,* 542–549.

Millar, S. Aspects of memory for information from touch and movement. In G. Gordon (Ed.), *Active touch. The mechanisms of recognition of objects by manipulation: a multidisciplinary approach.* Oxford: Pergamon Press, 1978, pp. 215–227.

Milner, A., & Bryant, P. Cross-modal matching by young children. *Journal of Comparative and Physiological Psychology,* 1970, *71,* 453–458.

Morris, J. E., & Nolan, C. Y. Discriminability of tactual patterns. *International Journal for the Education of the Blind,* 1961, *11,* 50–54.

Minimum sizes for areal type tactual symbols. *International Journal for the Education of the Blind,* 1963, *13,* 48–51.

Mountcastle, V. B., Lynch, J. C., Georgopoulos, A., Sakata, H., & Acuna, C. Posterior parietal association cortex of the monkey: command functions for operations within extrapersonal space. *Journal of Neurophysiology,* 1975, *38,* 871–908.

Mountcastle, V. B., Talbot, W. H., & Kornhuber, H. H. The neural transformation of mechanical stimuli delivered to the monkey's hand. In A. deReuck & J. Knight (Eds.), *Touch, heat and pain.* Boston: Little, Brown, 1966.

Mountcastle, V. B., Talbot, W. H., Sakata, H., & Hyvarinen, J. Cortical neuronal mechanisms in flutter vibration studied in unanesthetized monkeys. Neuronal periodicity and frequency discrimination. *Journal of Neurophysiology,* 1969, *32,* 452–484.

Myers, R., & Ebner, F. Localization of function in corpus callosum: tactual information transmission in macaca mulatta. *Brain Research,* 1976, *103,* 455–462.

Neisser, U. *Cognition and reality.* San Francisco: W. H. Freeman, 1976.

Nolan, C. Y. *Facilitating the education of the visually handicapped through research in communications,* Part 3: *Facilitating tactile map reading.* Louisville, Ky.: American Printing House for the Blind, 1976.

Nolan, C. Y., & Morris, J. E. Further results in the development of a test of roughness discrimination. *International Journal for the Education of the Blind,* 1960, *10,* 48–50.

Tactual symbols for the blind (Final report OVR-RD-587 [unpublished]). Louisville, Ky.: American Printing House for the Blind, 1963.

Development and validation of the roughness discrimination test. *International Journal for the Education of the Blind,* 1965, *15,* 1–6.

Improvement of tactual symbols for blind children (Final report, Project 5-0421, Grant OEG-32-27-0000-1012). Washington, D.C.: Dept. of Health, Education and Welfare, U.S. Office of Education, Bureau of Education for the Handicapped, 1971.

Ogrosky, C. E. The ordinal scaling of point and linear symbols for tactual maps. Unpublished doctoral thesis, University of Washington, 1973.

Pick, H., Warren, D. H., & Hay, J. C. Sensory conflict in judgments of spatial direction. *Perception & Psychophysics,* 1969, *6,* 203–205.

Power, R. P., & Graham, A. Dominance of touch by vision: generalization of the hypothesis to a tactually experienced population. *Perception,* 1976, *5,* 161–166.

Rock, I., & Victor, J. Vision and touch: an experimentally created conflict between the two senses. *Science,* 1964, *143,* 594–596.

Rose, S. A., Blank, M. S., & Bridger, W. H. Intermodal and intramodal retention

165

of visual and tactual information in young children. *Developmental Psychology*, 1972, *6*, 482–486.

Sakata, H., Takaoka, Y., Kawarasaki, A., & Shibutani, H. Somatosensory properties of neurons in the superior parietal cortex (area 5) of the rhesus monkey. *Brain Research*, 1973, *64*, 85–102.

Schiff, W. *Using raised line drawings as tactual supplements to recorded books for the blind*. Final Report (No. RD-1571-S). Washington, D.C.: Vocational Rehabilitation Administration, 1967.

Schiff, W., & Isikow, H. Stimulus redundancy in the tactile perception of histograms. *International Journal for the Education of the Blind*, 1966, *16*, 1–11.

Schiff, W., Kaufer, L., & Mosak, S. Informative tactile stimuli in the perception of direction. *Perceptual & Motor Skills*, 1966, *23*, 1315–1335.

Schiffman, H. R. *Sensation and perception: an integrated approach*. New York: Wiley, 1976.

Schwartz, A., Eidelberg, E., Marchok, P., & Azulay, A. Tactile discrimination in the monkey after section of the dorsal funiculus and lateral lemniscus. *Experimental Neurology*, 1972, *37*, 582–596.

Semmes, J., & Mishkin, M. Somatosensory loss in monkeys after ipsilateral cortical ablation. *Journal of Neurophysiology*, 1965, *28*, 473–485.

Semmes, J., Mishkin, M., & Cole, M. Effects of isolating sensorimotor cortex in monkeys. *Cortex*, 1969, *4*, 301–327.

Siegel, A. W., & Barber, J. Visual and haptic dimensional preference of planometric stimuli. *Perceptual & Motor Skills*, 1973, *36*, 383–390.

Siegel, A. W., & Vance, B. J. Visual and haptic dimensional preference: a developmental study. *Developmental Psychology*, 1970, *3*, 264–266.

Stellwagen, T., & Culbert, S. S. Comparison of blind and sighted subjects in the discrimination of texture. *Perceptual & Motor Skills*, 1963, *17*, 61–62.

Stevens, S. S., & Harris, J. R. The scaling of subjective roughness and smoothness. *Journal of Experimental Psychology*, 1962, *64*, 489–494.

Sullivan, A. The cutaneous perceptions of softness and hardness. *Journal of Experimental Psychology*, 1927, *10*, 447–462.

Talbot, W., Darian-Smith, I., Kornhuber, H., & Mountcastle, V. The sense of flutter-vibration: comparison of the human capacity with response patterns of mechanoreceptive afferents from the monkey hand. *Journal of Neurophysiology*, 1968, *31*, 301–334.

Taylor, M. M., & Lederman, S. J. Tactile roughness of grooved surfaces: a model and the effect of friction. *Perception & Psychophysics*, 1975, *17*, 28–36.

Teghtsoonian, R., & Teghtsoonian, M. Two varieties of perceived length. *Perception & Psychophysics*, 1970, *8*, 389–392.

Tyrrell, D. Dimensional effects in cross-modal transfer of discrimination learning in children. *Child Development*, 1977, *48*, 625–629.

Verrillo, R. T. A duplex mechanism of mechanoreception. In D. Kenshalo (Ed.), *The skin senses*. Springfield, Ill.: Charles C. Thomas, 1968.

Verrillo, R. T., & Gescheider, G. Psychophysical measurements of enhancement, suppression and surface gradient effects in vibration. In D. Kenshalo (Ed.) *Sensory functions of the skin of humans*. New York: Plenum Press, 1979.

Vierck, C. J. Interpretations of the sensory and motor consequences of dorsal column lesions. In G. Gordon (Ed.), *Active touch. the mechanisms of recognition of objects by manipulation: a multidisciplinary approach*. Oxford: Pergamon Press, 1978, pp. 139–159.

Walker, J. Textural aftereffects: tactual and visual. Unpublished doctoral thesis, University of Colorado, 1967.

Warren, D. H. Spatial localization under conflict conditions: is there a single explanation? *Perception*, 1979, *8*, 323–337.

Weinstein, S., Semmes, J., Ghent, L., & Teuber, H. L. Roughness discrimination after penetrating brain injury in man: analyses according to locus of lesion. *Journal of Comparative & Physiological Psychology*, 1958, *51*, 269–275.

Wiedel, J., & Groves, P. Tactual mapping: design, reproduction, reading and interpretation. *Occasional papers in geography*, No. 2. Baltimore: University of Maryland, 1972.

Zaporozhets, A. V. The development of perception in the preschool child. In P. H. Mussen (Ed.), *European research in cognitive development. Monographs of the Society for Research in Child Development*, 1965, *30*, 82–101.

Zigler, M. L. David Katz's *Der Aufbau der Tastwelt. Psychological Bulletin*, 1926, *23*, 326–336.

Zinchenko, V. P., & Lomov, B. F. The functions of hand and eye movements in the processes of perception. *Voprosy Psikhologi*, 1960, *1*, 12 25.

Zubek, J. Studies in somesthesis. I. Role of the somesthetic cortex in roughness discrimination in the rat. *Journal of Comparative Physiology*, 1951, *44*, 339–353.

Studies in somesthesis. II. Role of somatic sensory areas I and II in roughness discrimination in the cat. *Neurophysiology*, 1952, *15*, 401–408. (a)

Studies in somesthesis. III. Role of somatic areas I and II in the acquisition of roughness discrimination in the rat. *Canadian Journal of Psychology*, 1952, *6*, 183–193. (b)

5. Reading braille

EMERSON FOULKE

Emerson Foulke carefully considers major differences between the printed and braille codes of language. He explores several reasons why the processes involved in reading via these displays may be similar or different. The skin and fingers simply do not permit the same sort of processing that occurs in the visual system, although both systems yield information that ultimately is mapped onto the same linguistic system.

The history of braille in the United States is reviewed, and Foulke examines the literature on factors involved in braille reading performance. Display factors, haptic–tactual strategies, scan or presentation rate, and discrimination factors are all explored for their relevance to reading braille. Foulke then discusses the possibility of increasing the relatively slow rate of braille reading typically achieved by experienced blind readers, including changing the display or changing the code. Foulke's discussion suggests a possible solution to problems of slow braille reading in terms of manipulating temporal scale parameters (e.g., see Shaw & Pittenger, 1978, p. 202). If the piecemeal process of character-by-character braille reading might be circumvented by time-lapsing the tactual display, braille readers might be induced to perceive larger units of language, reading larger language "events" in a brief time period. This chapter provides a wealth of information needed by anyone concerned with tactually perceived patterns in general or the coded patterns of written language in particular.

WILLIAM SCHIFF

Introduction

The symbols in the print code are displayed spatially. The visual system is ideally suited for the acquisition of spatially distributed information. This high compatibility between the display and the perceptual system that observes it accounts for the efficiency of visual reading. The patterns used as symbols in the print code take effective advantage of the ability of the visual system to perceive spatial organization. The relatively high acuity of the visual system makes possible the discrimination and identification of the relatively small patterns that serve as symbols, and the relatively large field of view of the visual system makes possible the observation, at one time, of a relatively large number of symbols. The information content of individual symbols is low, but with reading experience, symbols can be combined to form spatially extended patterns such as syllables, words, and phrases, the information content of which is high. Because these spatially extended patterns can be perceived as quickly as their component symbols (Cattell, 1886), the print code can be read at an impressively fast rate (Gallo, 1972; Harris, 1947; Taylor, 1966).

The symbols in the braille code are also displayed spatially. However, the tactual perceptual system is not as well suited as the visual perceptual system for the acquisition of spatially distributed information. Tactual acuity is much poorer than visual acuity, and the tactual field of view is much smaller than the visual field of view. A pattern that can be resolved visually may not be resolvable by touch, and so the patterns that serve as symbols in the braille code must be simpler than those in the print code. Because the tactual field of view is smaller, not much more than one symbol can be observed at one time, and so the symbol patterns in the braille code must be observed sequentially. The braille reading rate is typically much slower than the print reading rate, and this difference may be a consequence of differences in the perceptual systems employed.

On the other hand, a few braille readers read two to three times faster than average. This increased rate is not convincingly explained by a process in which characters are identified one at a time. It may be that their reading experience has taught them to integrate patterns that are low in information content to form temporally extended patterns that are high in information content.

This chapter has been written with two purposes in mind. The first is to examine the experimental data that permit inferences concerning the perceptual basis for reading braille. The second is to consider some possibilities for improving the reading rate of the typical braille reader.

The history of braille in the United States

Long experience has indicated that dot patterns are much more discriminable by touch than other kinds of embossed patterns. Before braille came into general use, several alphabets of embossed characters exemplifying different simplifications of print letters were contending for acceptance. When Louis Braille introduced his alphabet, it was rejected out of hand by the educational establishment of the time. It was pointed out that if braille characters were used, sighted teachers would not be able to read the books read by blind students. Furthermore, it was maintained that the dot patterns standing for letters in Braille's alphabet, unlike the linear symbols standing for letters in the print alphabet, were wholly arbitrary. Apparently, these educators believed that print letter shapes exist in the human mind as Cartesian innate ideas.

Fortunately, blind readers did not take the advice of these pedagogues seriously. Braille made rapid gains in popularity among blind readers for obvious reasons. The intellectual climate in pedagogical circles was not then conducive to the arbitration of dispute by experiment, but it was apparent to those who knew how to read both braille and embossed print that they could read braille much faster. Furthermore, because dot patterns can easily be embossed at a useful rate with simple and inexpensive tools, it was possible for blind readers both to write and to read braille; it was not possible for blind readers of embossed print to write, because there was no practical way for them to emboss print letters.

After many years of acrimonious dispute over the relative advantages and disadvantages of braille and embossed print, it occurred to William Wait (1869) that a simple experiment might settle the issue. Accordingly, he observed the reading rates of braille readers and readers of embossed print. It was apparent from his results that whereas most of the readers of embossed print could scarcely be said to be reading at all, most of the readers of braille were fluent. As such evidence accumulated, opposition to the use of braille dissipated, and it rapidly gained acceptance among blind readers and their educators.

The braille code

The characters in the braille code are patterns of dots to which meanings have been assigned. The code consists of those patterns that can be formed in a matrix with three rows and two columns of possible dot positions. In the parlance of braille producers and users, the term *cell* designates the matrix in which patterns are formed, and I will follow this practice. In the braille cell, it is possible to form 64 discrete patterns ($2^6 = 64$). One of these is the pattern in which no dots are present, and as in the print code, it is used to separate words. Figure 5.1 shows four dot patterns. The top pattern is the one that results when the cell is filled with dots. The remaining three are examples of other patterns that can be formed in such a cell.

The centers of vertically or horizontally adjacent dots in a cell are separated by 0.23 cm (0.090 in). The centers of dots at corresponding positions in adjacent cells in the same line of writing are separated by 0.64 cm (0.250 in). The centers of dots at corresponding positions in adjacent cells in adjacent lines of writing are separated by 1.02 cm (0.4 in). The

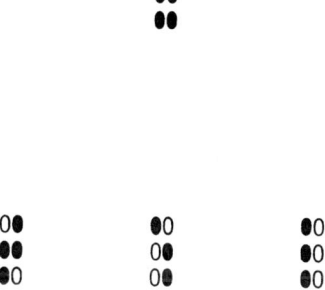

Figure 5.1. Four braille dot patterns.

height of a braille dot is between 0.02 and 0.05 cm (0.015 and 0.020 in). Though these spacing values were not determined by formal experiments, subsequent research (Ethington, 1956) has indicated that they were well chosen.

The meanings assigned to the 63 dot patterns in the braille code include the 26 letters of the alphabet and the punctuation marks. These assignments do not exhaust the supply of dot patterns, and the remaining patterns stand for frequently recurring letter groups. Such symbols are called *contractions,* and the supply of contractions is further increased by including those that require entries in two adjacent cells. Figure 5.2 compares the uncontracted and contracted forms of the word *understanding.* The contracted form includes a two-cell contraction.

The braille display

The display of braille characters is, in important ways, analogous to the display of print characters. Braille characters are displayed horizontally in lines that are read from left to right, and lines of characters are presented in an ordered sequence from the top of the page to the bottom. Because the two codes are displayed in the same manner, the braille code retains many of the advantages of the print code. Like the reader of print, the braille reader can vary the reading rate at will in order to adjust to the varying demands of reading matter and can retrace at will in order to clarify ambiguous material. Furthermore, because the information displayed on the braille page is spatially distributed, the braille reader, like the reader of print, can use features of the format, such as paragraph indentations, chapter headings, and page numbers to guide the search for information.

171

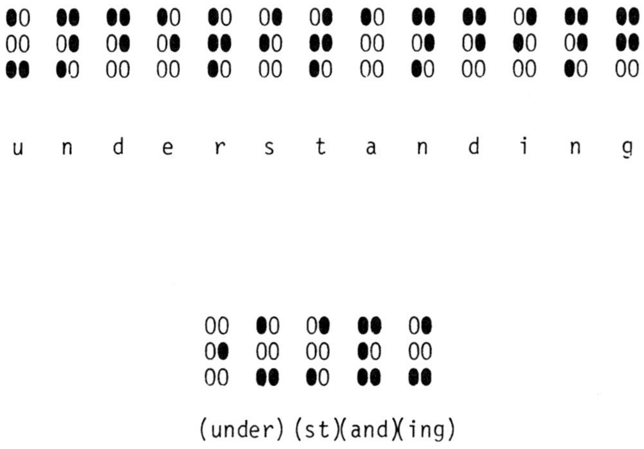

Figure 5.2. The word *understanding* written without and with contraction.

Braille reading performance

In spite of these advantages, the efficiency of braille reading is limited by a disadvantage of overriding importance – the rate at which it is generally read. Although braille can be read much faster by touch than embossed print, it is much slower than the visual reading of print. On the average, braille is read at 60 words per min (wpm) by junior high school students, 80 wpm by senior high school students (Meyers, Ethington, & Ashcroft, 1958; Nolan & Kederis, 1969), and 104 wpm by experienced adult braille readers (Foulke, 1964). To gauge the significance of these figures, consider the rate at which print is read visually. The average silent visual reading rate for high school students is between 250 and 300 wpm (Harris, 1947; Taylor, 1966), and reading rates two or three times as fast are occasionally observed. Just as there are exceptionally able readers of print, there are a few braille readers who can read about 250 wpm (Grunwald, 1966).

The usefulness of braille is seriously limited by the slow rate at which it is generally read. The student or practitioner of a profession, who must keep abreast of an enormous and rapidly expanding body of literature, simply does not have the time to read it at a rate of 100 wpm. Even the braille reader with leisure time, who reads only for recreation, usually prefers to encounter words at a faster rate that is more compatible with the rate of comprehension. Doubtless, if some way could be found to bring about a general and significant increase in the braille reading rate, it would offer the best perceptual alternative for those whose visual impairment prevents them from reading print.

Investigative approaches

A review of the research to date discloses three general approaches to the understanding of braille reading. In one approach, an effort is made to obtain a more careful and detailed description of the reading behavior of braille readers and to compare the behavior of good and poor readers. The second approach is concerned not with the behavior of readers but with the legibility of braille characters and the readability of words composed of them. The third approach calls for the manipulation of variables relating to the manner in which braille characters are displayed in order to observe their effects on reading behavior. Studies in this category frequently ascertain the effects of the same variables on the visual reading of print in order to acquire comparative data.

Braille reading behavior

A study reported by Eatman (1942) is a good example of the first approach. She made motion pictures of the hands of braille readers as they read. These films revealed that subjects read braille with only their index fingers, and that those who employed two index fingers usually read faster than those who employed only one. When two index fingers were employed, the best results were usually obtained by those who divided the reading task between them by searching for the beginning of the next line with the left index finger while reading to the end of the current line with the right. This strategy permits the reader to eliminate those intervals that would occur if the reader read to the end of the current line with both index fingers and then searched for the beginning of the next line.

It could be hypothesized that those braille readers who use two index fingers read faster because they have learned to involve both fingers cooperatively in the same perceptual process. For instance, the information acquired by the trailing index finger might be used to clarify and evaluate information acquired by the leading index finger (Heller, 1904, as cited in Bürklen, 1932). However, Eatman's (1942) findings suggest that faster reading is possible when two index fingers are employed independently, because the reader can utilize the time spent in reading more efficiently.

Eatman's camera also recorded the ineffective behavior of poor braille readers. These readers often engaged in scrubbing motions. They retraced frequently and often strayed from the line they were reading.

Eatman's technique provided a good molar description of what braille readers do, but her camera viewed the hands of braille readers from above, and because their hands were interposed between the camera and the braille they were reading, the camera could not look where the action was. This problem might be overcome by requiring readers to read braille written on a transparent sheet of plastic mounted on a glass reading surface. Their hands could then be photographed from beneath, and a clock could be placed in the camera's field of view. The film thus produced could be shown on a motion analysis projector in slow motion or a frame at a time. Each frame of this film would contain a record of the character(s) being observed, the fingertip(s) used, and the exact time of observation. With these data, in addition to the observations afforded by Eatman's technique, it would be possible to observe the time spent in reading each character, the time spent in reading each word, momentary variations in the speed of finger movement, the skipping of characters, syllables, and words that do not have to be read because they can be predicted, and so forth. With the detailed description of braille reading behavior obtained by this technique, it should be possible to extend the comparison afforded by Eatman's technique and to gain a better understanding of what fast braille readers do that slow braille readers must be taught to do.

In 1974, the American Foundation for the Blind published Kusajima's account of research he had conducted over a number of years concerning the perception of braille. To obtain a record of the reading behavior of blind children, he devised an apparatus that produced a tracing on the smoked paper chart of a kymograph when the finger(s) used in reading moved. In general, his results were similar to those reported by Eatman (1942).

In 1932, the American Foundation for the Blind published F. K. Merry's translation of a book by Karl Bürklen in which he reviewed the research and observations of others and reported a number of his own experiments with braille reading. Although his research was conducted in the early twentieth century, when there was little instrumentation for the quantitative measurement of behavior, he was quite ingenious in devising ways of obtaining behavioral records that could later be subjected to quantitative analysis. A good example of his ingenuity is the *Tastschreiber*, or touch writer. This was a simple clamp, one end of which was attached to the reading finger of a subject. A pencil, attached to the other end of this clamp, rested on the paper some distance above the line being read by the subject, and as the subject's reading finger moved, the pencil moved. Thus, it traced a record of the subject's finger movements. When Bürklen wished to study the finger movements of subjects who read with both index fingers, he placed *Tastschreibers* on both index fingers and used different colored pencils so that he could distinguish the tracings produced by these readers. In general, the results obtained by Bürklen are in close agreement with those reported by Eatman and Kusajima.

Legibility of braille characters

The second approach is directly concerned with the legibility of braille characters and the readability of words formed with them. In studying the legibility of dot patterns, one may obtain evidence regarding the speed and accuracy with which subjects can identify them absolutely, discriminate them from one another, or reproduce them from memory.

Absolute identification of dot patterns. The speed and accuracy with which braille characters can be identified absolutely would appear to be a satisfactory test of their legibility. An early attempt to assess the legibility of braille characters in this way was reported by the Uniform Type Committee (1913). The procedure they devised required the subject to read aloud, as rapidly as possible, a list of 160 braille letters. The list included 4 instances of each of the 25 letters not under test and 60 instances of the letter under test. Letters were presented in a random order that was changed from trial to trial. The time spent by subjects in reading the list was measured on the assumption that reading time would be a function of the time needed to identify the letter under test. By comparing reading times of lists with different test letters, the letters of the braille alphabet could be arranged along what would probably qualify as an interval scale of legibility.

The experiment conducted by the Uniform Type Committee lacked the sophistication of subsequent experiments, in which instruments were used for the controlled presentation of letters and the precise measurement of identification times. Nevertheless, their findings concerning the legibility of braille letters and their inferences concerning the characteristics of a dot pattern that make it more or less legible than other dot patterns have generally been corroborated by better-controlled experiments conducted in recent years. The experiments of the Uniform Type Committee should remind us that it is often possible to conduct useful research in the absence of elaborate instrumentation.

Nolan and Kederis (1969, Study 1) initiated their investigation of the perceptual basis for braille word recognition by determining the legibility of 55 of the 63 characters in the braille code. In their experimental

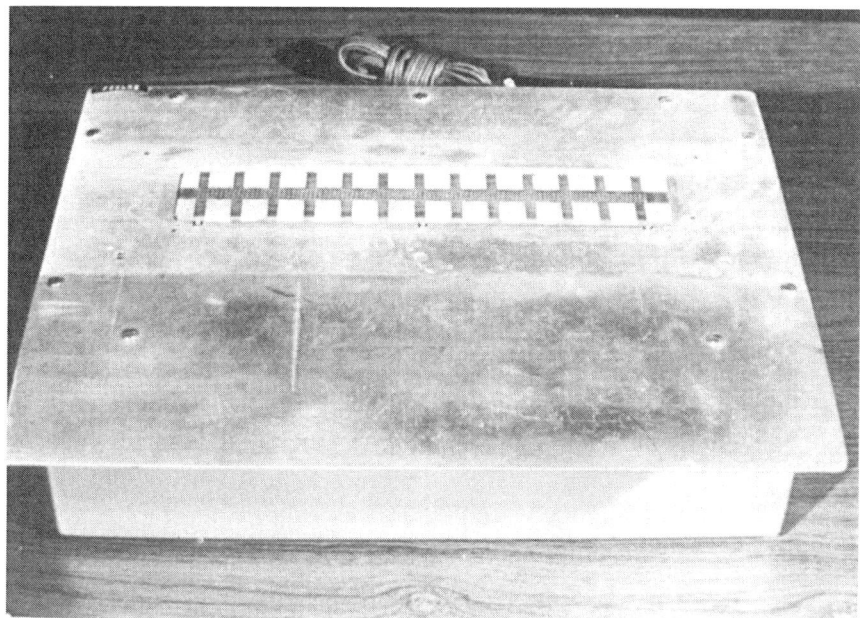

Figure 5.3. The tachistotactometer.

task, subjects were required to make absolute identifications of those 55 characters. The dot patterns that can be formed in the right-hand column of the braille cell were excluded. These dot patterns are used in conjunction with other characters to form the two-cell contractions mentioned earlier and have no meaning when they stand alone. In order to qualify for an experiment that required absolute identification of braille characters, subjects must have learned the dot patterns used as stimuli, the names assigned to those dot patterns, and the associations between names and dot patterns. The subjects tested by Nolan and Kederis were blind children in grades four through twelve at residential schools for the blind. Although they exhibited considerable variability in braille reading experience, the least experienced ones, those in the fourth grade, had 4 years of experience in reading braille. Nolan and Kederis could safely assume that all subjects had extensive overlearning and therefore judged that the minimum exposure time required to identify a dot pattern would serve as a valid index of its legibility.

Nolan and Kederis used a specially designed instrument, called the *tachistotactometer*, for their studies of legibility. This instrument is shown in Figure 5.3. The tachistotactometer controls the time during which dot patterns are available for tactual observation. Up to a full line

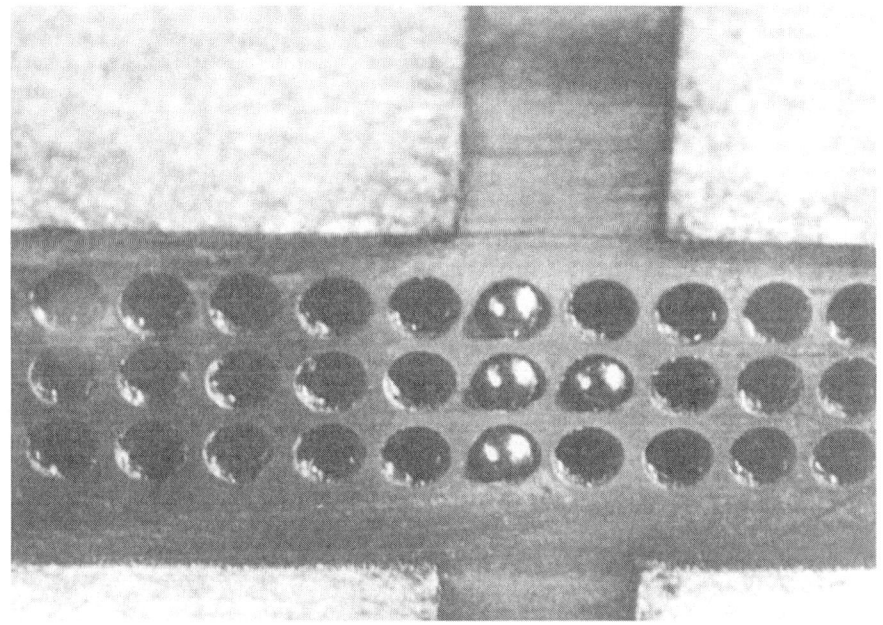

Figure 5.4. A close-up view of the display surface of the tachistotactometer.

of dot patterns may be presented at one time. The patterns to be presented are embossed on a sheet of suitable material. This sheet is placed on a platform elevated by solenoids. A tightly stretched metal membrane with holes in it corresponding to the dot positions in all of the cells in a line of braille writing is held just above the platform. When the platform is elevated, the dots on the sheet mounted on it protrude through the holes in the membrane to the height of the standard braille dot. They remain available for observation during a predetermined interval, and then, as the platform falls to its resting position, recede beneath the surface of the membrane again. Figure 5.4 is a close-up view of the display surface of the tachistotactometer with its platform elevated and a dot pattern on display.

The tachistotactometer made it possible for Nolan and Kederis to determine thresholds of legibility for most of the characters in the braille code, but like most instruments, it had problems. Because they were asking their subjects to report not just the detection but also the identification of stimuli, Nolan and Kederis were not free to use a standard psychophysical method in which the threshold value for a stimulus is determined by presenting several values of that stimulus that span the region in which the threshold is believed to lie. If such a method had been used, after the first exposure that was long enough to allow a subject to identify the test character, knowledge that the test character had been presented would permit a correct inference concerning its identity on subsequent exposures. This knowledge would be provided by the operating noise of the instrument alone.

One solution to this problem would be to present random permutations of all of the characters under test. However, this would have meant changing the sheet on which characters are embossed after each presentation of a stimulus, and the time needed to change sheets made this procedure impractical. The solution adopted by Nolan and Kederis was to emboss eight characters on a single sheet and to determine their thresholds before replacing the sheet with another one containing eight new characters. With only eight characters under test at any given time, subjects could easily remember those they had already identified, and as testing proceeded, they would soon be able to guess the identities of characters with an unacceptably high probability of success. Nolan and Kederis solved this problem by dispensing with the descending series of stimulus values called for by the method of limits, but in so doing, they increased the likelihood of systematic errors, such as errors of habituation.

Another problem with the tachistotactometer was the time required for one cycle of its operation. Because of the mass of its platform and the distance through which the platform must travel as it is elevated to the display position and then dropped to the resting position, it was not possible to adjust the instrument for exposure times that were brief enough to determine thresholds for a few of the characters. The minimum exposure time of which the instrument was capable was used as the threshold value for these characters.

In spite of these difficulties, the experiments made possible by the tachistotactometer have produced the best measures of the legibility of braille characters to date. Examples of these measures are shown in the third column of Table 5.1. The entries in the fourth and fifth columns will be explained later. The characters in column 3 are ranked according to their thresholds of legibility. As the threshold value increases, legibility decreases. Having determined the relative legibilities of the braille characters, Nolan and Kederis could search for those characteristics of a dot pattern that make it more or less legible than other dot patterns. They found that patterns with large numbers of dots and patterns with dots in the lowest third of the cell were relatively illegible.

A theory that accounts adequately for the performance of braille readers must be stated in quantitative terms, and to the extent that such a theory considers the legibility of braille characters, legibility must be

Table 5.1 *Legibility thresholds and identification times for characters in the braille code*

Print symbol	Dot pattern[a]	Legibility thresholds (sec) Nolan and Kederis (1969)	Kilpatrick (1974)	Identification times (sec) Challman (1978)
E	⠑	0.02	0.04	1.20
A	⠁	0.02	0.04	0.93
I	⠊	0.02	0.04	1.15
C	⠉	0.02	0.04	1.23
K	⠅	0.02	0.04	1.19
St	⠌	0.03	0.05	1.11
B	⠃	0.03	0.04	1.18
com	⠤	0.04	–	1.45
ch	⠡	0.04	0.04	1.22
in	⠔	0.04	0.05	1.22
Sh	⠩	0.04	–	1.18
ea	⠂	0.04	–	1.61
D	⠙	0.04	–	1.15
M	⠍	0.04	0.04	1.02
U	⠥	0.04	0.05	1.09
O	⠕	0.04	0.05	1.02
con	⠒	0.04	–	1.64
bb	⠆	0.05	0.05	1.25
ing	⠬	0.05	0.05	1.14
wh	⠱	0.05	–	1.26
en	⠢	0.05	0.06	1.28
J	⠚	0.05	–	1.20
G	⠛	0.05	0.04	1.25
H	⠓	0.06	0.04	1.14
his	⠦	0.06	–	1.14
ar	⠜	0.06	0.05	1.29
gh	⠣	0.06	–	1.29
X	⠭	0.06	–	1.09
L	⠇	0.06	0.04	0.97
S	⠎	0.06	0.04	0.99
N	⠝	0.06	0.05	1.13
V	⠧	0.06	0.05	1.22
ow	⠪	0.07	0.05	1.16
th	⠹	0.07	0.05	1.22
F	⠋	0.07	0.04	1.10

Table 5.1 (*cont.*)

Print symbol	Dot pattern[a]	Legibility thresholds (sec)		Identification times (sec)
		Nolan and Kederis (1969)	Kilpatrick (1974)	Challman (1978)
the	⠮	0.08	0.05	1.28
ff	⠖	0.08	–	1.27
ble	⠼	0.08	–	1.42
gg	⠶	0.08	0.06	1.28
was	⠴	0.08	–	1.45
and	⠯	0.09	–	1.14
Z	⠵	0.09	–	1.15
dis	⠲	0.09	–	1.41
Y	⠽	0.09	0.06	0.87
P	⠏	0.10	0.04	1.07
with	⠾	0.10	–	1.43
W	⠺	0.11	0.05	1.22
ed	⠫	0.12	0.05	1.35
T	⠞	0.12	0.05	1.38
ou	⠳	0.14	0.05	1.56
R	⠗	0.14	0.06	1.10
er	⠻	0.15	–	1.39
of	⠷	0.16	–	1.34
Q	⠟	0.18	–	1.42
for	⠿	0.19	–	1.38

[a] • = Used location in braille cell; o = Unused location in braille cell; – = no entries.

measured with accuracy and precision. An attempt to realize this objective was made in the Perceptual Alternatives Laboratory at the University of Louisville by building an improved tachistotactometer. Unlike the instrument used by Nolan and Kederis (1969), this instrument is limited by the ability to display only one dot pattern at a time, and hence it cannot be used in studies of the time required for word identification. Dot patterns are formed by metal pins that rise above its display surface to the height of a standard braille dot. Each pin is controlled by its own solenoid. Figure 5.5 is an overall view of the instrument with a subject observing its display. The small box with switches mounted on it is used by the experimenter to set up the dot pattern to be presented. The presence of the microphone and the timer will be accounted for later. Figure

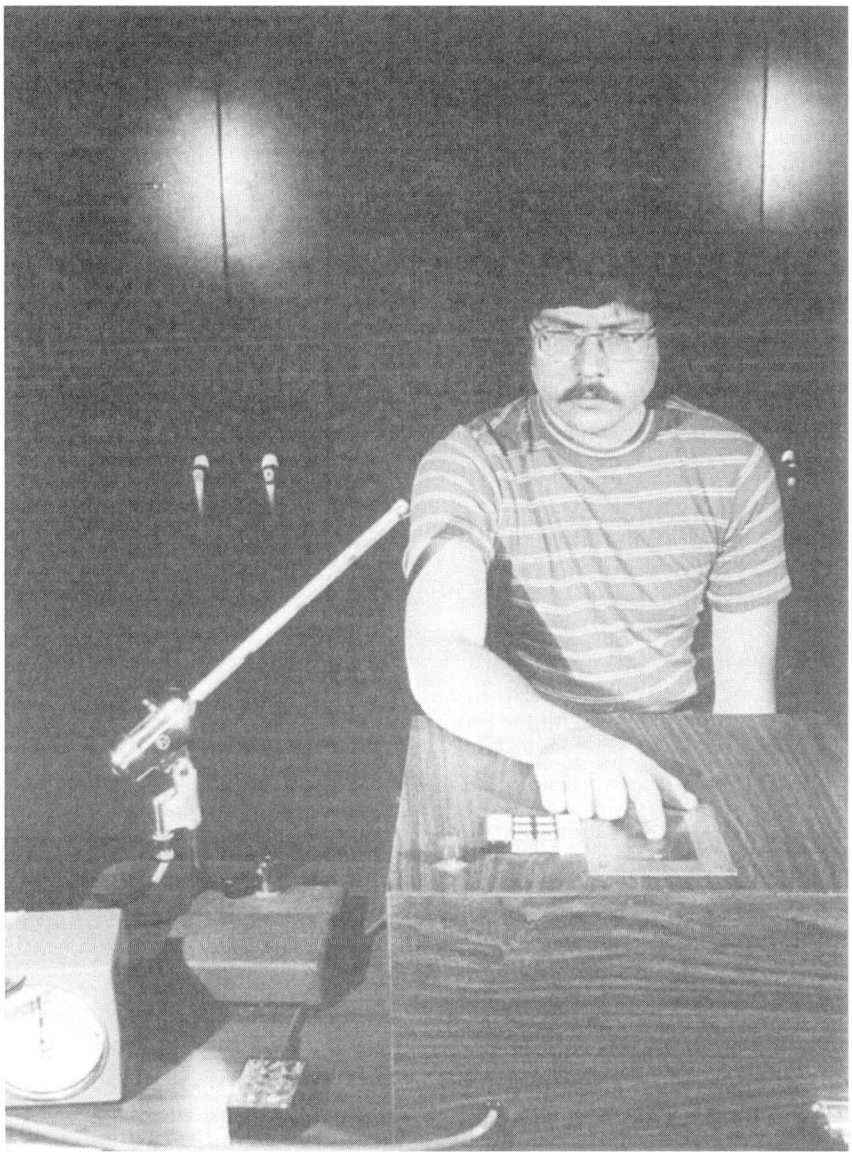

Figure 5.5. The redesigned tachistotactometer.

5.6 is a close-up view of the display surface with a braille character on display. This instrument can be used for the same purpose as the one employed by Nolan and Kederis. However, because any of the 63 characters in the braille code can be presented immediately simply by ener-

181

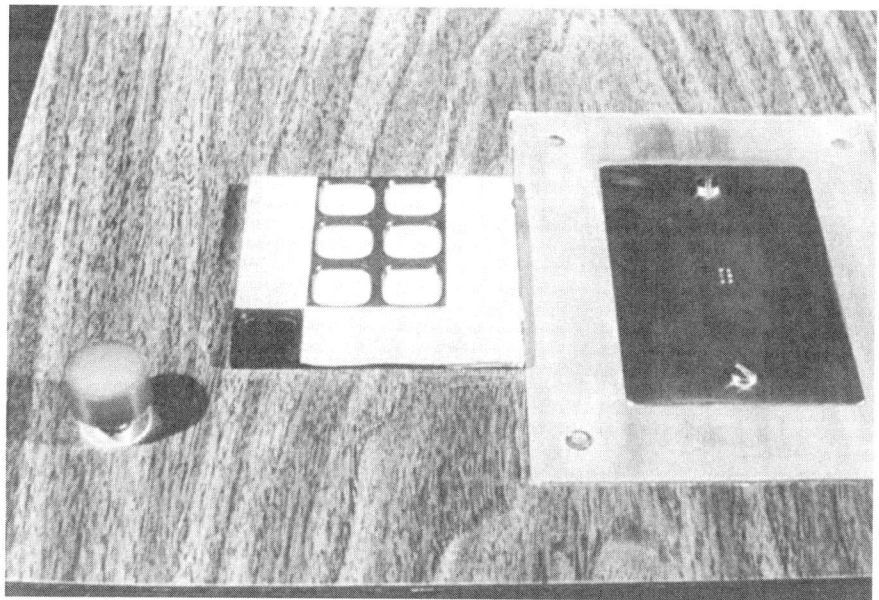

Figure 5.6. A close-up view of display surface of the redesigned tachistotactometer.

gizing the appropriate solenoids, it is not necessary to determine thresholds for only a few characters at a time; an unrestricted psychophysical method can therefore be used for the estimation of thresholds. Because there is a significant reduction in both the mass that must be moved and the distance through which it must be moved in order to present a character, briefer exposures can be provided, and it should be possible to determine threshold values for all of the characters in the braille code.

In addition to the use just described, the instrument can also be used to determine the amount of time needed to identify braille characters. In this mode of operation, the switch closure that presents a character also starts an electric stopclock. This is the timer shown in Figure 5.5. The subject identifies the character by pronouncing its name, and the signal generated by the microphone shown in Figure 5.5 stops the clock and removes the character from the display surface. Thus, the subject cannot stop the clock by making an inadequate vocal response and still retain the character for further observation.

This mode of operation was provided to test a hypothesis concerning the identification of braille characters. The process that culminates in the identification of a braille character is undoubtedly a complex one in which both perceptual and cognitive operations are involved. The initial perceptual operation is, in theory, to register an image of the stimulus pattern in short-term memory. Although this image probably decays, it is available for further cognitive processing during a brief interval. By comparing the image with information stored in long-term memory, the ensuing cognitive operations assign the image to an appropriate category of functionally equivalent stimulus patterns and abstract those inherent features common to all members of the category to which it belongs.

According to this reasoning, when Nolan and Kederis determined the minimum exposure time required to identify a character, they were accounting for that fraction of the total time that was spent in registering an image of the stimulus pattern in short-term memory. However, they did not measure response latencies, so they could not account for the time required for the remaining cognitive operations.

In an experiment conducted by Challman (1978), the tachistotactometer built in the Perceptual Alternatives Laboratory was used to determine the times needed to identify those characters for which Nolan and Kederis (1969) had determined thresholds of legibility. Challman reasoned that if the correlation between the identification times for characters and their legibility thresholds were low, the reading rate of a braille reader might be determined more by the time spent in identifying characters than by the time spent in registering stimulus patterns, because a registered pattern is not useful until it has been identified. Averages of the times needed by 10 subjects to identify the characters in the braille code are recorded in column 5 of Table 5.1. It is obvious that the correlation between identification times and thresholds of legibility is not high, and using the Spearman formula for rank order correlation, Challman found a correlation of 0.30.

This low correlation makes it plausible that the time spent in identifying characters is more predictive of reading rate than the time spent in registering stimulus patterns in short-term memory. However, neither Challman's data nor the data gathered by Nolan and Kederis can be used to evaluate this hypothesis. In both studies, raw data were reduced to averaged values for subsequent analysis, and thus individual differences were obscured. To test the hypothesis, a study is needed in which individual differences are preserved and a comparison is made between identification times and legibility thresholds as predictors of braille reading rate.

As already mentioned, the studies conducted by Nolan and Kederis were designed to discover differences in legibility among the characters in the braille code. Of course, such information is valuable, as is information concerning factors that affect legibility. However, if the performance of an individual braille reader is determined by the legibility of characters, what matters is how legible those characters are for that reader, not in the abstract. Studies designed to reveal differences among individual readers regarding the legibility and identifiability of braille characters would add useful data to what we already know in general terms. These studies of performance, together with behavioral studies of the sort conducted by Eatman (1942), should reveal some of the critical differences between good and poor braille readers, and this knowledge should contribute greatly to instructional design.

Both the tachistotactometer used by Nolan and Kederis (1969) and the one constructed in the Perceptual Alternatives Laboratory are subject to another criticism. The movement of cutaneous tissue is necessary for tactile stimulation. When dot patterns are briefly pressed into a stationary fingertip, as they are when an instrument like the tachistotactometer is employed, there is relatively little movement of cutaneous tissue compared to that produced by reading braille in the conventional manner. It could be argued that the stimulation provided by the tachistotactometer is not adequate and not enough like the stimulation that is produced when the fingertip is moved across a line of braille characters to warrant the generalization of tachistotactometric results to the braille reading situation. If this argument has force, an adequate method for measuring the legibility of braille characters would have to provide stimulation that more closely approximates stimulation during normal braille reading. The apparatus shown in Figure 5.7 was constructed in an effort to satisfy this requirement. It is a tape transport similar in operation to that of a conventional tape recorder. Paper tape, 2.5 cm (1 in) in width and of a weight suitable for embossing braille characters, is transferred from a supply reel across a display surface and onto a takeup reel. Tape speed is controlled by a capstan, driven by a well-regulated DC motor, the speed of which can be varied continuously through a wide range. Figure 5.8 is a close-up view of the top of the machine. Notice the word written in braille that is about to pass beneath the subject's reading finger.

Kilpatrick (cited in Foulke, 1974) used this machine to conduct a preliminary study of the legibility of certain braille characters. In his study, each subject experienced random permutations of the characters under test. Initially, the transport was adjusted for a tape speed too fast to permit identification of any of the characters. As testing proceeded, the tape speed was gradually reduced. When a subject had made three consecutive correct identifications of a character, the tape speed during the first three presentations was taken as the index of the character's legibil-

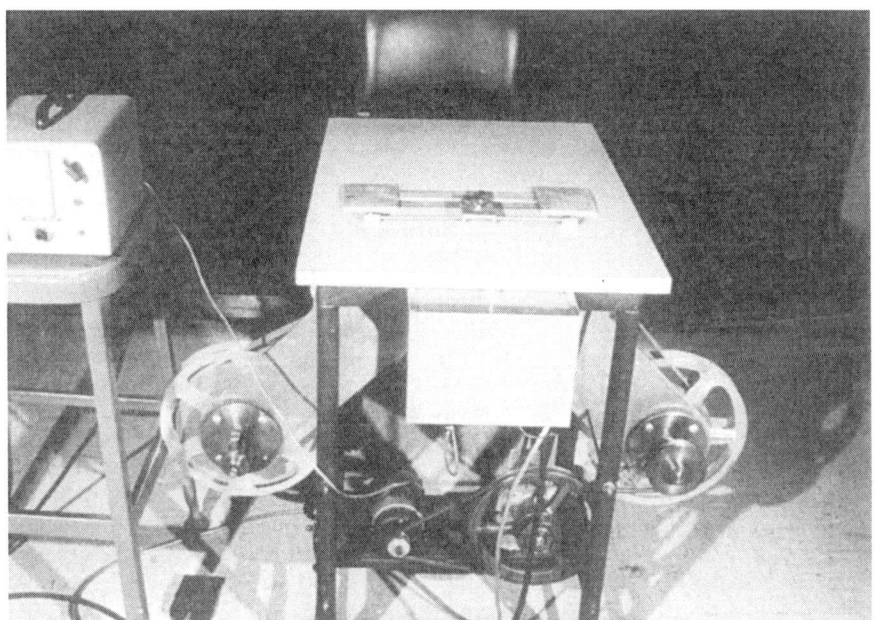

Figure 5.7. The PAL tape transport.

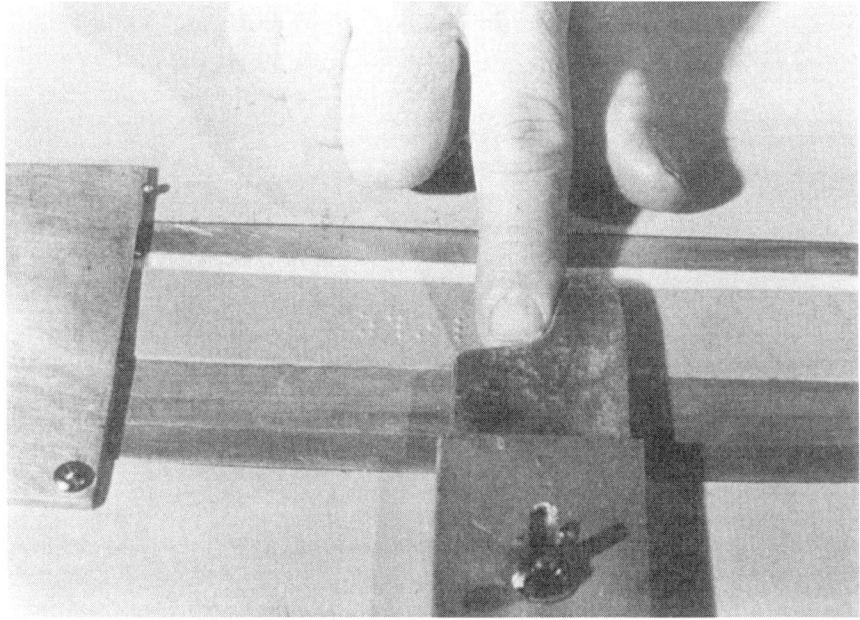

Figure 5.8. Close-up view of the PAL tape transport.

ity. Tape speeds were translated into exposure times by computing, at each of the tape speeds, the time required for 0.64 cm (0.25 in) of tape, the width of a letter space in a line of braille writing, to pass any point on the surface of the fingertip that was in contact with the moving tape. The averaged results for 10 subjects are shown in Table 5.1, column 4, along with the thresholds of legibility measured by Nolan and Kederis (1969) and the identification times measured by Challman (1978) for the same characters.

The thresholds of legibility measured by Kilpatrick appear to be lower than those measured by Nolan and Kederis. This may, in fact, be the case. Nolan and Kederis's subjects were children, whereas Kilpatrick's were experienced adult braille readers. On the other hand, Kilpatrick's lower threshold values may simply be a consequence of the way in which tape speeds were translated into exposure times. If exposure time had been defined as the total time a character was in contact with the portion of the fingertip used for sensing braille characters, Kilpatrick would probably have computed higher threshold values. In spite of these problems, Table 5.1 affords a comparison of relative legibilities as determined by the three methods. The rank order correlation between the entries in columns 3 and 4, columns 3 and 5, and columns 4 and 5 are 0.54, 0.30, and 0.73, respectively. The distributions of values produced by the three methods have some variance in common, but there are many disagreements in rank, and the choice among these measures will depend on their ability to predict significant aspects of braille reading performance.

Discrimination of dot patterns. If the methods just discussed are to be used to assess the legibility of braille characters, subjects must have had enough prior experience with those characters to learn both the dot patterns and the meanings associated with them. However, it may sometimes be worthwhile to gather information about dot patterns with which subjects have had no prior experience. For example, the overlearning of characters that are examined in studies of legibility may mask differences in their discriminability and ease of learning that could be taken into account in arranging the initial learning experiences of new braille readers. If the existing braille code were to be expanded, or if a new code of the same type were to be constructed, the selection of new dot patterns and the new meanings could not be guided by the learned performance of subjects who already knew the code. Of course, subjects could be required to prepare themselves for service in a legibility experiment by first learning the code, but it would not be practical to provide the overlearning characteristic of a typical legibility experiment. In the absence of such overlearning, the interpretations of legibility experiments of the type conducted by Nolan and Kederis would be ambiguous. Slow and/or incorrect identification of stimulus patterns might be due to incomplete learning of those patterns or of the names assigned to them, or to incomplete learning of the associations between names and dot patterns, or to some unspecifiable mixture of all three, and there would be no way to decide among these alternatives.

One solution to this problem is to change the task to one in which only discrimination is required. The discrimination task, in its simplest form, requires subjects to decide whether two dot patterns observed at the same time are alike or different. The difficulty of this task may be increased by requiring subjects to compare a present pattern with the memorial representation of a previously experienced pattern. The difficulty may be increased again by increasing the number of present patterns that must be compared with a remembered pattern or by increasing the number of remembered patterns that must be compared with a present pattern.

Such a task was employed in a series of experiments conducted by Foulke and Warm (1967, 1968), Warm and Foulke (1968, 1970), and Warm, Clark, and Foulke (1970). The purpose of these experiments was to determine the effects of variables such as complexity and redundancy on the speed and accuracy with which dot patterns resembling histograms can be discriminated.

The apparatus used to present the experimental task is shown in Figure 5.9. The subjects' side of the apparatus has a curtained opening through which subjects put their hands in order to examine dot patterns. There is a response keyboard to the left of the opening and another one to the right. Thus subjects are free to use either hand for observing dot patterns and the other for operating the keyboard.

Figure 5.10 shows the experimenter's side of the apparatus. There is an electric stopclock that measures response latency and a display with three light bulbs that informs the experimenter of the responses made. Figure 5.11 shows the hand of a subject attempting the discrimination task by examining dot patterns of the sort that might be presented during a trial. These patterns were formed in a cell with more positions for dots than the braille cell, and they were used to investigate the feasibility of expanding the braille code by adding characters formed in cells with more than six dot positions. An elevated runway on the floor of the compartment in which dot patterns are displayed guides the subjects' fingers to the dot pattern that serves as the standard stimulus. Touching the dot

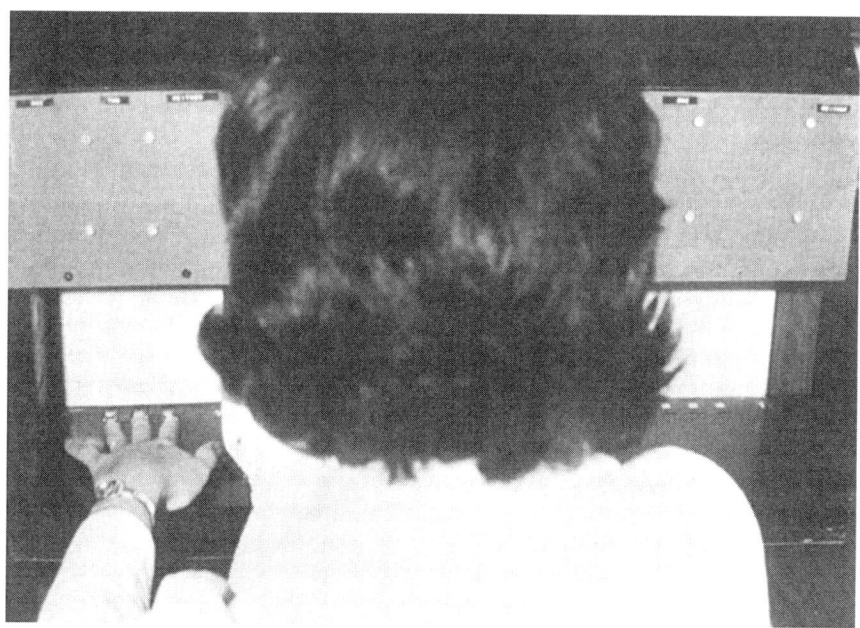

Figure 5.9. Subject's side of a discrimination apparatus.

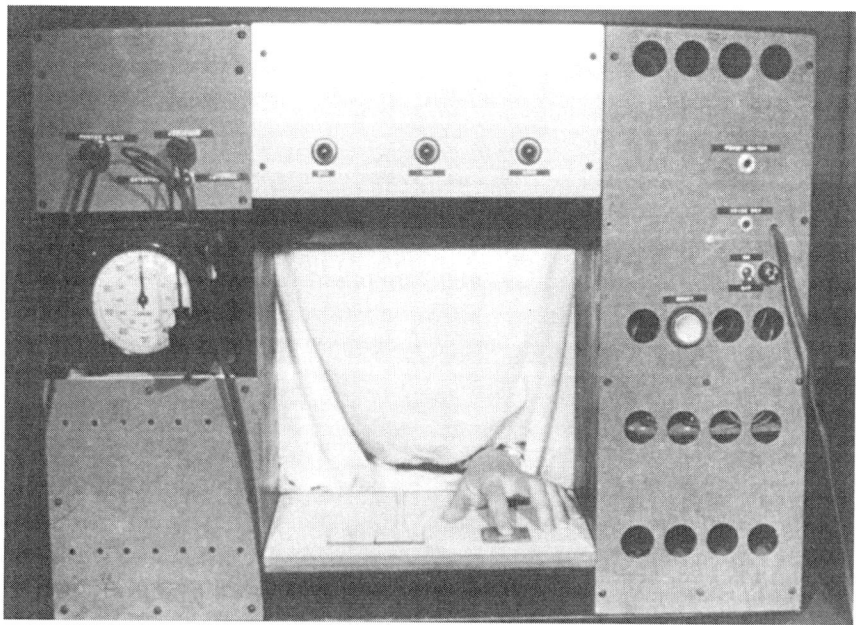

Figure 5.10. Experimenter's side of a discrimination apparatus.

188

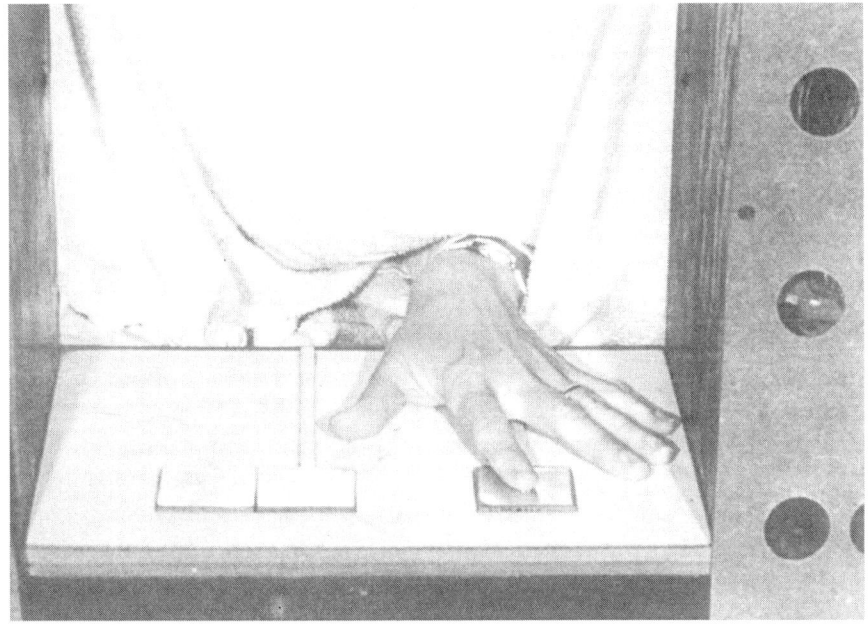

Figure 5.11. Subject's hand in a discrimination task.

pattern interrupts a beam of light focused on a photocell, and this event initiates a timed interval. At the end of this interval, subjects are informed by the sound of a buzzer that the time allowed for observation is over. Another elevated runway guides the subjects' fingers to the two dot patterns that serve as comparison stimuli. Touching either of these patterns interrupts the beam of light, which starts the stopclock. The subjects' task is to decide which if either of the two dot patterns being observed is like the dot pattern observed earlier. The choice is made by pressing one of three keys labeled "left," "right," and "neither." This response stops the clock and turns on the light that informs the experimenter of the response.

Though the results of discrimination experiments may guide the selection of dot patterns for such uses as expanding the present braille code or constructing a new code, in designing these experiments one must exclude alternative explanations of the performance. If a character is to serve in a touch reading code, it must be identifiable, and the two criteria relevant to identifiability are the speed and accuracy of identification after training. However, there are several factors that, if not controlled, can threaten the predictive significance of the discrimination experiment.

When the task is to determine whether two dot patterns are alike or

189

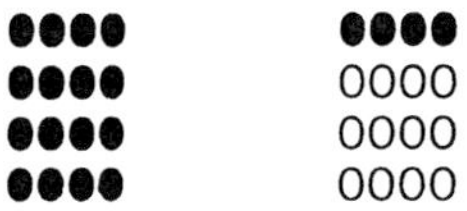

```
●●●●      ●●●●
●●●●      0000
●●●●      0000
●●●●      0000
```

Figure 5.12. Discrimination on the basis of pattern extension.

different, a subject might adopt the strategy of comparing the patterns systematically, element by element. If this sequence of comparisons did not disclose a lack of correspondence, the subject would report that the patterns are alike. Of course, response latency would be long, but the result would be accurate, and if prediction of identifiability after training were based on accuracy of discrimination alone, it would often fail. If at some point in the sequence of comparisons a discrepancy were discovered, the subject would report that the patterns being compared were not alike, and if this were discovered early, the subject's response would be both accurate and fast. Because the experimenter has little control over the subjects' observing strategies, the best way to minimize the effects of these strategies is to have the subject compare the test pattern with a variety of patterns that are the same, and a variety of patterns that are different, and to randomize the order. This would minimize the likelihood that a subject will expect a match or a mismatch on any given comparison.

Another threat to the predictive significance of the discrimination experiment arises when a subject can base judgments on the discriminability of compared patterns on gross differences between them of extension, the number of pattern elements, or the indentation of perimeters. For example, consider the patterns shown in Figure 5.12. These patterns can be discriminated easily by noticing only the difference in extension. In general, the greater the dissimilarity between patterns, the less a subject will need to know about them in order to discriminate between them. By proper selection of a set of dot patterns and of the comparisons to be made among members of that set, it would be possible to gather data indicating that the dot patterns under test were highly discriminable, and yet the results of subsequent training might indicate that many of them were relatively difficult to identify. A solution to this problem is to limit the size of differences between the dot patterns to be compared.

The following experiment by Foulke (1973, Chaps. 12 and 13) was designed to eliminate ambiguities of the sort just discussed so that data pertaining to discriminability could be used to predict identifiability after training. The purpose of the experiment was to forecast the legibility of a set of novel dot patterns proposed for use in an expanded braille

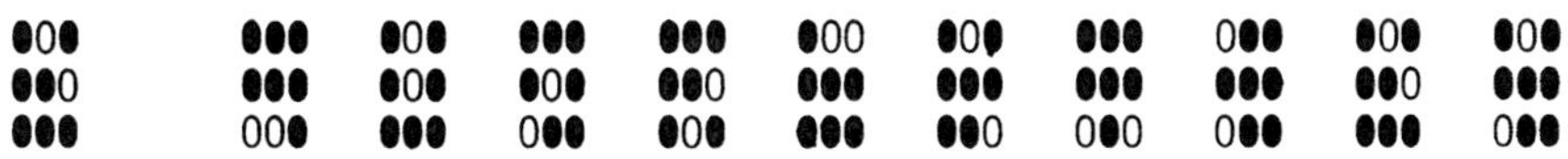

⬤○⬤ ⬤⬤⬤ ⬤○⬤ ⬤⬤⬤ ⬤⬤⬤ ⬤○○ ⬤○⬤ ⬤⬤⬤ ○⬤⬤ ⬤○⬤ ⬤○⬤
⬤⬤○ ⬤⬤⬤ ⬤○⬤ ⬤○⬤ ⬤⬤○ ⬤⬤⬤ ⬤⬤⬤ ⬤⬤⬤ ⬤⬤⬤ ⬤⬤○ ⬤⬤⬤
⬤⬤⬤ ○○⬤ ⬤⬤⬤ ○⬤⬤ ⬤○⬤ ⬤⬤⬤ ⬤⬤○ ○⬤○ ○⬤⬤ ⬤⬤⬤ ○⬤⬤

Figure 5.13. A match to sample with the standard and 10 comparisons.

code. Subjects examined a group of present dot patterns in order to find one that matched a memorial representation of a previously experienced pattern. If in such a task the number of present dot patterns is large enough to exclude chance as a significant factor in making correct matches, and if the present patterns are fairly similar to the remembered pattern, subjects should have to know as much about the remembered pattern in order to match it as they would in order to identify it in absolute terms.

Dot patterns were embossed on sheets of plastic 28 by 29 cm (11 by 11.5 in) in size. This is the size of the standard braille page. Plastic was used because dots embossed on plastic are more durable than dots embossed in paper. One trial pattern was presented on each line. A trial is shown in Figure 5.13. The dot pattern at the beginning of the line is the standard with which the remaining 10 patterns are to be compared. The experimenter placed the subject's preferred index finger on the standard, and the subject examined this dot pattern until informed by a signal that the time was up. The standard was then covered, and the subject searched among the remaining 10 dot patterns for one that matched it.

The position of the matching pattern was varied from trial to trial. In order to ensure a fair degree of similarity among the 11 dot patterns in a trial, each of the 10 patterns to be compared with the standard had to have the same number of dots as the standard, and at least one column in each comparison pattern had to match a column in the standard.

The measures of performance were the latency and accuracy of responses. If a response was incorrect, the pattern proposed by the subject as a match for the standard was noted, so that confusions could be analyzed.

In this experiment, 182 dot patterns were evaluated, and the 40 patterns for which matches were found with the greatest speed and accuracy were paired with familiar words to form an experimental code. This code was easily mastered by a group of subjects. Thus, when code characters were formed for assigning meanings to dot patterns that had been shown to be highly discriminable, the characters proved, after a few training trials, to be readily identifiable as well.

The reproduction experiment. The remaining type of experiment that can be used to predict the legibility of characters not yet learned is the reproduction experiment. The experimenter presents a dot pattern for observation and then requires the subject to reproduce it from memory. Like the discrimination experiment, the reproduction experiment avoids the ambiguities of an identification experiment in which dot patterns, their meanings, or the associations between dot patterns and meanings are not completely learned.

The reproduction experiment requires an apparatus that allows the experimenter to produce, on a display surface, the dot patterns to be observed and the subject reproduces observed dot patterns by placing dots at any of the positions in the cell in which dot patterns are formed. The subject must be able to remove and add dots until the pattern appears to be a faithful reproduction of the one observed. This apparatus must be simple enough to be learned quickly and easily, so that skill in operating it will not be a significant factor in determining the subject's ability to reproduce dot patterns. Furthermore, it is probably important for the reproduced pattern to be of the same type as the original pattern, and not just an analog. For instance, if the original pattern is formed with tangible dots, the reproduced pattern should not be formed by placing pencil marks in the appropriate squares in a printed grid. This problem is avoided if the same apparatus is used to form both the original and the reproduced pattern.

Figure 5.6 is the top view of the apparatus shown in Figure 5.5. In addition to the display area, there is a small grid of squares arranged in three rows and two columns, like the dot positions in a braille cell, and a seventh square just beyond the grid. This grid is the keyboard used by a subject to reproduce patterns. When the subject places a fingertip in a square and presses, a dot appears in the corresponding position in the braille cell on the display surface. If the same square is pressed again, the dot disappears. Thus, a dot can be added to a pattern, its effect on the pattern can be observed, and if the subject wishes, it can be removed again. If, at some point in the reproduction of the pattern, the subject wishes to clear the display and start over, this can be accomplished by pressing in the seventh square.

To form a pattern, the experimenter sets the appropriate toggle switches on a remote keyboard. The pattern is presented to the subject when the circuit is completed by an interval timer connected in the common return of the toggle switches. When the observation time is up, the interval timer opens the circuit again and the pattern disappears from the display. This disappearance starts an electric stopclock and signals

192

the subject to start reproducing the pattern. When a reproduction has been achieved that the subject is willing to submit for inspection, a vocal signal generates a microphone signal that is used to stop the clock. The subject is scored for speed and accuracy of reproduction, and if desired, incorrect reproductions can be examined for errors of various kinds.

An experiment requiring reproduction should directly reveal what a subject knows about the original pattern at the time of its reproduction. However, its outcome will be ambiguous in one respect. It will not always be possible to decide whether an error is due to misperception of the original pattern or to forgetting. Nevertheless, such experiments may provide useful information for the evaluation of novel dot patterns.

Manipulation of display variables

The third approach in investigating the factors in braille reading is the manipulation of variables relating to the manner in which braille characters are displayed. Similar research on the display of print characters has also been conducted, and the comparisons have facilitated our understanding of the reading of braille. Print readers can observe more of their display at one time than braille readers, and in general, print readers can read much faster. An obvious hypothesis is that the difference in favor of print readers is a consequence of the difference in the amount that can be observed at one time. A number of experiments varying the display of print and braille characters have produced results relevant to this hypothesis.

In 1886, Cattell reported an experiment in which the exposure time needed by his subjects to identify several characters displayed at the same time was no greater than the exposure time needed for only a single character. Since then, there has been considerable improvement in the instruments used to control and vary the exposure of visual stimuli, but Cattell's findings have generally been confirmed by experiments employing modern tachistoscopes.

Foulke and Wirth (Foulke, 1973, Chap. 8) used a tachistoscope that varies the exposure time in steps of approximately 1 msec. The minimum exposure time is approximately 5 msec. With this instrument, they determined the minimum exposure time required to identify single letters and words with two, three, four, and five, letters using the staircase method of limits (Cornsweet, 1962). They determined the median times needed by each subject to identify the stimulus items in each category and computed the means of these medians as follows: single letters, 35 msec; words with 2 letters, 35 msec; words with 3 letters, 36 msec; words with four letters, 37 msec; words with five letters, 39 msec. The differences among these means are quite small and not signficantly different.

The frequency of occurrence of a word may influence the time required for its identification. To control for this factor, Foulke and Wirth used only frequently occurring words as stimulus items on the assumption that such words were probably stored in the lexical memories of their subjects. The interaction of word length and frequency of occurrence was examined in an experiment by Doggett and Richards (1975). They found that the time required to identify an infrequently occurring word is increased by increasing its length. Whereas the time required to identify a familiar word is not. Furthermore, their results suggested the possibility that the length of a frequently occurring word may even serve as a cue that decreases the time required for its identification.

An interaction between word length and word frequency was also observed in an experiment by Newbigging and Hay (1962), who found that the effect of the length of a word on the time required for its identification was greater for freshmen and sophomores than for older students. Presumably the latter had more reading experience, and were therefore more likely to have stored in their lexical memories the longer and less familiar words employed by Newbigging and Hay.

The experiments just reviewed suggest that the time needed by visual readers to identify most words is not a function of the number of characters in those words. If this is true, the information available to visual readers at any given instant is much greater than that provided by a single character.

This is clearly not the case for braille readers. Nolan and Kederis (1969, Study 2) found that the time needed by braille readers to identify a word is a function of its length. This is true for both familiar and unfamiliar words and for both slow and fast readers. Furthermore, in many instances, the subject spent more time identifying a word than identifying all the characters in the word. Of course, the subjects tested by Nolan and Kederis occasionally used their knowledge of orthography and identified words without having to identify all of the characters in them, but their results strongly imply that at any given time, the braille reader is acquiring only the information that can be provided by a single character. If this is true, the braille reader must have to identify and remember all the letters in a word, and then integrate them in order to identify that word. The inevitable consequence of such a process would be a braille reading rate that is much slower than the visual reading rate.

If the visual reading rate is largely a consequence of the number of characters that can be observed at one time, then it should be increased by reducing the number of characters that can be observed at one time. In an experiment by Foulke and Smith (Foulke, 1973, Chap. 9), visual readers were required to read text a letter at a time, with freedom to manage their access to the display. They looked at the printed page with one eye, through a tube mounted on a pair of goggles. The lens in front of the other eye was painted to make it opaque. The material to be read was typed on vellum with a bulletin typewriter and backlighted. An aperture at the end of the tube was adjusted so that when one character was completely in view, the edges of adjacent characters could also be seen. Subjects were prevented from varying the distance between their eyes and the printed page by an aluminum tube 1.2 m (4 ft) in length attached at one end by a ball-and-socket joint to the wall behind the chair in which subjects sat, and at the other end by a ball-and-socket joint attached to a headband worn by the subjects. Thus, they could explore the page they were reading by moving their heads up and down, and from side to side, but they could not vary the amount seen at one time by moving their heads closer to or farther from the page. Under this condition, visual readers were forced to read the printed page just as tactual readers read a braille page. The college students who served as subjects found the task quite irritating, and only a few could be persuaded to endure enough training to reach a stable reading rate. However, those who persisted achieved reading rates ranging from 65 to 75 wpm. These rates approximate those reported for braille readers in junior high school (Nolan & Kederis, 1969). These results suggest that when visual readers of print are required to read under conditions that limit the number of characters that can be observed at one time to the number observed by tactual readers of braille, the two reading rates become equivalent.

In an experiment by Troxell (1967), visual readers read text displayed on an oscilloscope under two conditions. Under one condition, text was displayed a character at a time. Under the other condition, it was displayed a word at a time. Under both conditions, Troxell varied the rate at which items were presented and determined the maximum reading rate of each subject in words per minute. When text was displayed a letter at a time, the mean reading rate was 19.5 wpm; when it was displayed a word at a time, the rate was 108.5 wpm.

In another condition of Troxell's experiment, experienced braille readers read text presented a character at a time by sensing patterns of pins pressed against the tips of the fingers used to operate the keys on a braillewriter. Each of the six keys on a braillewriter produces one of the dots in the braille cell, and the dot patterns in the braille code are formed by pressing the appropriate combinations of keys. For example, pressing Keys 2 and 3 with the middle and ring fingers of the left hand, and Keys 4 and 5 with the index and middle fingers of the right hand, would produce Dots 2, 3, 4, and 5, the dot pattern to which the meaning *t* is assigned in the braille code. To present *t*, Troxell would stimulate simultaneously the fingertips just mentioned. Thus, his subjects were reading not braille characters but their analogs. Nevertheless, after only brief practice, they achieved a mean reading rate of 18 wpm, the maximum rate at which Troxell's instrument could be operated. It can be argued that if characters had been presented at a faster rate, his subjects might have learned to identify them at a faster rate; also, they might have been able to identify braille characters faster than the analogs they experienced. However, their rate closely matched that of Troxell's visual readers, and in the absence of evidence to the contrary, there is no reason to suppose that tactual readers of braille can identify characters presented one at a time faster than can visual readers of print.

In spite of its limitations, Troxell's experiment has important implications for the reading of braille. First, when the conditions of observation for the visual reader of print and the tactual reader of braille are equated by displaying only one character at a time, it appears that sequences of characters can be identified as rapidly by touch as by vision. The finding that visual readers were able to increase their reading rate from 19.5 to 108.5 wpm when allowed to experience all of the characters in a word at the same time suggests that they could treat whole words as single patterns. They read faster not because they identified the same units at a faster rate but because they identified larger units that provided more information at approximately the same rate.

It is unfortunate that Troxell's experiment did not include a condition in which braille readers were presented text in braille, a word at a time. Braille readers cannot observe as much at a time as visual readers. If they must read words a character at a time, they should not be able to use the additional information that visual readers of print gain when text is displayed a word at a time. Also, their reading rates should not be affected much by changing the display of text from a character at a time to a word at a time.

Troxell's experiment is interesting because of the comparisons it suggests, but the reading rates he found under all experimental conditions seem atypically low. They may have been a consequence of the novel text display and the reduced ability of his readers, visual or tactual, to deal with it. Under normal reading conditions the entire page is available, and the reader is free to vary the acquisition strategy with the continuously changing requirements imposed by the text. As already stated, when text was presented a character at a time, Troxell's subjects read it visually at a rate of 19.5 wpm. When it was presented so that they could observe several characters at a time, their reading rate increased to 108.5 wpm. When text is displayed on the printed page in the conventional manner, and when access to it is managed by the reader, there is another dramatic increase in reading rate. The average silent visual reading rate for high school students is about 250 wpm (Harris, 1947; Taylor, 1966), and if the average silent reading rate had been determined for Troxell's subjects, who were students at the Massachusetts Institute of Technology, it probably would have been still higher.

When text was displayed to Troxell's braille reading subjects a character at a time, they read 18 wpm. When text is displayed in braille on a page and read normally, the rate improves, but it is more modest than the improvement that occurs when text is displayed in print on a page and read normally. Though the reading rate of adult braille readers has not been adequately measured, the average is probably about 104 wpm (Foulke, 1964), and in the absence of better information, this figure will serve as the estimated average reading rate of Troxell's braille-reading subjects. Because of the way in which characters were presented, these subjects could not read a word at a time. However, if they could, they doubtless would have read faster than when text was displayed a character at a time. Their familiarity with orthographic and linguistic conventions, and their awareness of the context of meanings in which the text was embedded, would occasionally enable them to predict words and parts of words successfully without having to identify all the characters in them. However, because their perceptual limitations would not allow them to take advantage of the increased number of characters on display, they should receive less benefit than visual readers.

The experimental evidence reviewed in this section points to the conclusion that the difference in reading rate between visual readers of print and tactual readers of braille is a consequence of the difference in the number of characters that can be observed at one time by touch and by vision. However, in order to reach this conclusion, it has been necessary to make a number of assumptions, particularly in regard to the performance of braille readers. If, in a single experiment, visual readers of print and tactual readers of braille read text displayed a character at a time, a word at a time, and on a page in their normal manner, the resulting comparisons should permit an adequate evaluation of the hypothesis we have presented: that the difference in reading rate between visual readers of print and tactual readers of braille is accounted for by the difference in the number of characters that can be observed at one time.

The inclusion of another condition, in which text is displayed as a continuous line of characters embossed on a tape that moves from right to left beneath the finger(s) normally used for reading, might provide some indication of the ability of braille readers to identify temporally extended patterns consisting of several characters. If tactual readers of braille have this ability, they should be able to read text displayed on a moving tape faster than text displayed as a succession of discrete characters presented one at a time. Of course, because readers would not be able to manage their access to the information contained in such a display, they would not be able to increase their reading rate by skipping predictable words and parts of words. Therefore, their reading rate for text displayed in this manner should be slower than their rate when text is displayed on a page and read normally.

Obviously, there is a great deal of research to be done. Our current understanding of the braille reading process does not warrant final conclusions regarding the manner in which braille is read or how it might be read if it were properly displayed to adequately trained readers. However, the picture of the braille reading process that can be supported by current data is rather disappointing. Because of the limited sensing area on the fingertips, only about one braille character can be read at a time. Even if this were not the case, the mass of the finger, hand, and arm prevents the extremely rapid movement from one fixation to the next corresponding to the saccadic movements of the eyes. Furthermore, tactual perception requires movement of cutaneous tissue, and little movement takes place while the fingertip is at rest, as it would be during periods of fixation. The efficient perception of braille requires continuous lateral movement of the fingertip that is actively engaged in reading, and as a result of this movement, braille characters are encountered and perceived serially. This serial perception has been demonstrated by Nolan and Kederis (1969, Study 2), who have shown that the time required to identify a word written in braille is frequently greater than the sum of the times required to identify its characters. This is not always the case, because readers can predict some words and syllables, and the use of contractions sometimes reduces identification time, but there is a strong suggestion that braille readers must first register and accumulate percepts of single characters and then integrate them to perceive whole words.

There are many who dispute this model of the braille reading process. They maintain that although the patterns identified by braille readers are discovered temporally, there is no reason to believe that readers are necessarily limited to the serial perception of single characters. They believe that the patterns identified by braille readers can encompass entire words, and they point to a few exceptionally fast braille readers as proof of their contention. This point of view has merit, and it deserves to be investigated. However, there has been very little systematic observation of the behavior of unusually fast braille readers, and as yet, we have no data that could support a detailed description of the perceptual processes they employ.

Increasing the braille reading rate

Some investigators have attempted to increase the braille reading rate. This might be done by changing the reading behavior and perceptual ability of braille readers through training, by changing the braille display, or by changing the braille code itself. All of these approaches have been considered, but none has been thoroughly explored.

Changing the reading behavior and perceptual ability of braille readers

As an example of the first approach, braille-reading subjects were given tests that revealed the characters they identified slowly and/or inaccurately, and were then given practice in identifying these characters (Henderson, 1967; Umstead, 1970). The result of this training was an increase in the braille reading rate that, though modest, was worthwhile.

Eatman (1942) studied motion pictures of the hands of braille readers and found that fast readers engage in different reading behavior than slow ones. They usually read with the index fingers of both hands, but it appears that they do not use both index fingers for the perception of each character in the line. Instead, the left index finger reads the beginning of each line. As it passes the middle of the line, the reading task is transferred to the right index finger, which finishes reading that line. While this is happening, the left index finger finds the beginning of the next line. When braille is read in this manner, it is possible to make more efficient use of time. The index fingers of fast braille readers cover each line at a relatively fast and fairly constant speed and, as shown by several investigators (Bürklen, 1932; Holland, 1934; Kusajima, 1974), with relatively light pressure.

Slow braille readers, on the other hand, often read with only one index finger, and when two index fingers are used, there is no division of the reading task. The two index fingers read the same line together, make the return sweep together, and together find the beginning of the next line. Thus, the total reading time of the slow reader includes a large interval during which no reading takes place. Slow readers often stray from the line being read (Bürklen, 1932) and must take time to regain that line so that reading can proceed. Slow readers retrace more often than good readers, and sometimes, in an effort to identify characters, they scrub them with the reading fingers (Eatman, 1942). Consequently, the speed at which they cover a line is slow and variable (Kusajima, 1974).

Because these two behavior patterns can be observed and distinguished without difficulty, many educators (Kurzhals & Caton, 1973; Lowenfeld, Abel, & Hatlen, 1969) have hypothesized that reading speed might be increased by teaching slow readers to engage in the behaviors of fast readers. (Such a suggestion parallels the disputed view of training the eye movements of visual readers.) Unfortunately, although teaching practices have been based on this hypothesis, it has not received systematic evaluation.

Grunwald (1966), Flanigan (1964), Nolan (1964), and Ashcroft (1959) trained braille readers to read characters that moved from right to left beneath their stationary reading fingers. Although a display of this sort can be produced in several ways, the simplest is to emboss a continuous line of braille characters on paper tape that moves from a supply reel, across a display surface and beneath the reading finger(s) of the braille reader, and onto a takeup reel. As they read, the rate at which braille passed beneath their fingertips was gradually increased. By such pacing, it was hoped that they would learn to read at faster and faster rates, and that the effects of this perceptual training would transfer to the reading of braille displayed on a page. The results of these experiments were mixed, but more often negative than positive. As Nolan (1964) has pointed out, the increased reading rates occasionally associated with such training do not survive long, and they can be explained more reasonably by the increased motivation of experimental subjects than by a change in perceptual ability.

It may be, as Grunwald (1966) argues, that most braille readers read slowly because they were taught to identify characters one at a time, or at least were not taught to do otherwise. They can, he maintains, learn to identify temporally extended dot patterns that include several characters and specify syllables or words. According to him, those who have acquired this ability come to read at about 250 wpm, the rate he has observed.

The temporally extended patterns in question are not static. Before readers can learn to identify them, they must first learn the reading behavior that creates them. The fingertip(s) used for reading must be moved over the line at a fast and constant speed. If the speed is too slow, only individual characters will be perceived. If the speed is allowed to vary, the necessary conditions for the emergence of temporally extended patterns will not occur, and the patterns will not be available for perception. An analogy will help to make this point clear. Initially, students of Morse code learn to identify single characters, but as they gain experience, they begin to identify entire words. A given sequence of dots and dashes no longer sounds like the letters *a* and *n* and *d* but like the word *and*. The relative temporal values of dots and dashes, and of the intervals between characters, are critical to the perception of the code. If these temporal values were allowed to vary at random, the legibility of the code would be destroyed. Likewise, if braille readers moved their fingers across the line at a variable rate, the temporally extended dynamic patterns that could specify syllables, words, and even phrases would not emerge, and those readers would have no recourse but to identify individual characters, store them in memory, and then integrate them to perceive whole words.

This is a plausible hypothesis. It has been shown that fast braille readers do exhibit the reading behavior required for the emergence of temporally extended, dynamic patterns (Bürklen, 1932; Eatman, 1942; Kusajima, 1974). However, if some braille readers do have the perceptual ability to identify temporally extended dynamic patterns, the results of the research mentioned earlier, in which subjects were trained to read braille on a moving tape, suggest that this ability is not easily learned. It may be that subjects in these experiments did not receive enough training, or that they should have been trained to perceive individual words presented at a fast and constant speed before they were allowed to attempt continuous prose. It may be that they did acquire some perceptual ability to identify temporally extended dynamic patterns, but that this ability did not transfer to the reading of a braille page. The two reading situations are, after all, quite different. When braille characters are displayed on a moving tape, the fast, constant speed necessary for the emergence of patterns is assured by the tape mechanism. When braille embossed on a page is read in the ordinary way, readers must produce the behavior that will establish the necessary conditions; if they do not know how to do this, there is no reason to expect that transfer will occur. Whatever the case may be, it is clear that the results of the research to date will not permit evaluation of a hypothesis concerning the perceptual ability to identify temporally extended dynamic patterns of braille characters.

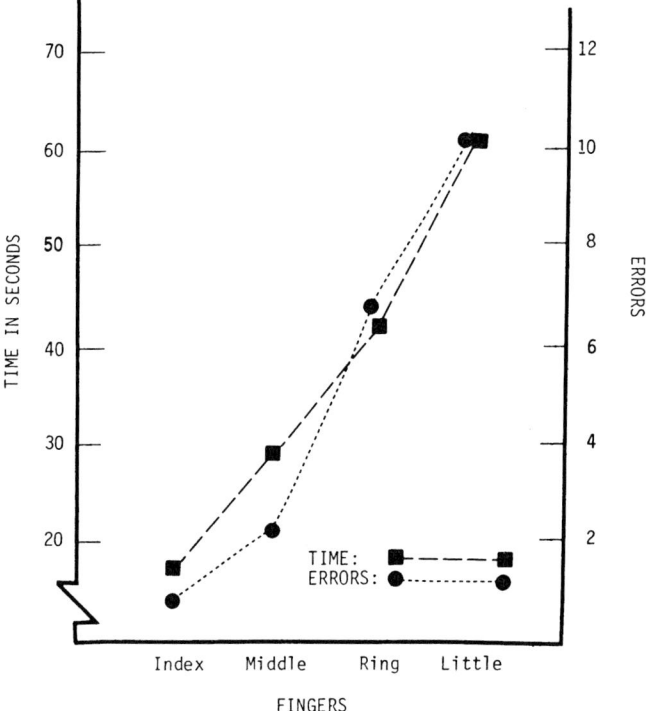

Figure 5.14. Time and errors as functions of fingers used in reading.

Changing the display of braille characters

Only the two index fingers are ordinarily used for reading braille. How-ever, other fingers may have useful sensory capacity, and if braille could be displayed so as to employ them, this sensory capacity might be ex-ploited. The sensory capacity of normally unused fingers was determined in an experiment by Foulke (1964). Subjects read random sequences of braille characters with each of the four fingers on both hands. Characters were arranged in groups of five, with five groups per line. A record was kept of the number of identification errors and the reading time for each line. The results are shown in Figure 5.14. For both hands, reading ability diminishes rapidly with progression from the index finger to the little finger. This loss in ability is indicated by both error scores and time scores. Though error scores were high and reading times were long when reading was done with the little fingers, these fingers clearly exhibited some sensory capacity.

202

The observed differences in sensory capacity might be a consequence of differences in the density of nerve endings in the cutaneous surfaces that were stimulated in this experiment, or of differences in the representation of those cutaneous surfaces in the cortex. On the other hand, the results might be explained by differences in perceptual learning. When braille characters are displayed in a straight horizontal line, and when a deliberate effort is made to scan the line with the index fingers, as in normal braille reading, the other fingers do not make systematic, reliable contact with the characters, and there is little opportunity for perceptual learning. It would be informative and useful to conduct an experiment in which braille readers were trained to employ normally unused fingers. It would also be useful to locate readers who, because of accidents involving their index fingers, have had to learn to read braille with other fingers, and to determine their reading rates.

Attempts have been made to display braille characters in columns instead of rows. Such a display would make it possible to present different characters to different fingertips at the same time, and there are two experiments in which this has been done (Funchess, 1934; Lappin & Foulke, 1973). The results are inconclusive. However, the braille-reading subjects had not been trained to employ normally unused fingers. Further exploration of the possibility of reading braille by columns instead of rows may be worthwhile.

Changing the code

The braille code includes the 63 combinations of dots that can be formed from the six possible dots in the braille cell. With only 63 dot patterns, the braille code is severely limited in comparison to the print code. Its symbology is adequate for literary purposes, but it cannot provide most of the symbols needed to represent meanings conveniently in scientific and technical reading matter.

Though the evidence is not yet conclusive, the results of the research to date suggest that for most braille readers, reading is necessarily slow because they must read a character at a time. If this is an inescapable requirement, the braille reading rate might possibly be increased by the use of symbols that contain more information than that provided by a single letter. The braille code takes limited advantage of this possibility. The dot patterns not used for letters or punctuation marks are used, as noted earlier, for contractions. If contractions reduce the number of characters that must be identified in order to perceive words, the result should be a faster reading rate. Although the relationship between read-

```
00
00
00
00


000
000
000
```

Figure 5.15. Expanded braille cells.

ing rate and the use of contractions is not a simple one (Ashcroft, 1959; Nolan & Kederis, 1969), this is generally true.

The braille reading rate might be further increased if more dot patterns were available for use as contractions, and scientific and technical matter might be written in braille with greater clarity and convenience if there were more dot patterns to which meanings could be assigned. There is no a priori reason to suppose that the braille reader can perceive only the 63 dot patterns in the standard braille cell. It is easy to augment the supply of dot patterns by adding dot positions to the cell. Each new dot position doubles the number of patterns that can be formed. Figure 5.15 shows a cell with four rows and two columns of dot positions in which 255 patterns can be formed, and a cell with three rows and three columns of dot positions in which 511 dot patterns can be formed. However, although new dot patterns can easily be generated, before these patterns can serve as characters in an expanded braille code, braille readers must be able to identify them with sufficient speed and accuracy.

This problem was investigated in a series of experiments by Foulke and Warm (1967, 1968); Warm and Foulke (1968); and Warm, Clark, and Foulke (1970). Subjects were required to discriminate between dot patterns formed in cells with three rows and three columns, four rows and four columns, five rows and five columns, and six rows and six columns. A record was kept of discrimination errors and response latencies. Although subjects performed beyond chance in discriminating between dot patterns formed in cells with five rows and five columns, and six rows and six columns, their error scores were high, their response latencies were long, and it was concluded that dot patterns formed in these cells could not be used in an expanded reading code. However, they discriminated between dot patterns formed in cells with three rows and three columns, and four rows and four columns, with enough speed and accuracy to suggest the feasibility of using such patterns in an expanded braille code.

In subsequent research (Foulke, 1973, Chap. 13), braille readers were taught two experimental codes: one with characters formed in cells with three rows and three columns and the other using cells with three rows and four columns. They learned these codes without difficulty, and although it was not possible to provide much practice, they were able to read simple text written in the codes. Encouraged by these results, Foulke took the next step toward practical application by proposing an expanded braille code.

In braille's short history, we have had more than enough experience with the problems caused by lack of standardization for those who produce, store, and read braille (Irwin, 1955). The present standardization is only a recent achievement, and those who defend it are understandably alarmed by proposals that threaten it. Accordingly, if expansion of the present braille code is to be considered, its advantages must be demonstrated beyond question.

The expanded code proposed by Foulke retains the characters in the present code. The cell in which these characters are formed provides three rows of dot positions, like the cell of the new code. The cell of the present code provides two columns of dot positions. In the cell of the expanded code, the number of columns is variable, depending upon the character to be formed. The separation between characters is indicated by a blank column. Thus, if only one or two columns of dot positions are required to form a character, as in the present code, only one or two columns are used. Because the number of rows in the cell is fixed whereas the number of columns is variable, Foulke has called it the *3-by-n code*. When standard braille is written in standard cells with three rows and three columns, the same amount of space is allotted to each letter, regardless of its size, as when print is typed on a standard typewriter. When standard braille is written in 3-by-*n* cells, the space allotted to each letter depends upon its size, as when print is typed upon a typewriter with proportional spacing. The first two rows of characters in Figure 5.16 provide a comparison of standard braille characters formed in standard cells and standard braille characters formed in 3-by-*n* cells. The third row contains samples of dot patterns formed in 3-by-*n* cells that might be included in an expanded braille code.

No code including new characters formed in the 3-by-*n* cells has yet been tested for legibility. In fact, no attempt has been made to expand the present code by assigning meanings to new dot patterns formed in 3-by-*n* cells. Obviously there is much research to be done before an expanded braille code can be given serious consideration. However, if a 3-by-*n* code with useful symbols not included in the standard braille

```
●0 ●0 ●0 0● ●0 ●0 ●0
●0 ●● 00 ●0 ●0 ●0 0●
00 ●0 00 00 ●0 ●0 00
```

Standard Braille Code

```
●0●0●0●●0●●0
●0●●0●0●0●0●
00●0000●0●00
```

Standard Braille in 3-by-n Cells

```
●●●    ●●●    ●000
●0●    0●0    ●●●●
●●●    ●●●    0●●0
```

Samples of Dot Patterns
Formed in 3-by-n Cells

Figure 5.16. A comparison of standard braille and 3-by-n cells.

code is ultimately shown to be at least as readable as the present code, it may have an advantage over the other expanded braille codes that might be proposed and tested. Because all of the characters in the standard braille code can be formed in 3-by-*n* cells, it would be possible to introduce new characters without rendering obsolete the reading skills of those who now read braille. New symbols in disciplines such as mathematics, chemistry, and physics would be learned by students of those disciplines and would not be encountered by the general reader. New contractions could be introduced slowly, giving the general reader the opportunity to learn them gradually.

Summary

Though there are notable exceptions, braille is generally read at a much slower rate than print. There is evidence to suggest that this slower reading rate is a consequence of the perceptual limitations of the braille reader. However, there is also some reason to believe that the fast braille reading occasionally observed may be achieved by using a perceptual strategy different from the one typically employed by the slow braille reader. If the perceptual strategy employed by fast readers can be described accurately and in detail, it may be possible to teach it to slow readers. It may also be possible to improve braille reading by changing the way in which braille characters are displayed or by changing the braille code itself.

References

American Association of Workers for the Blind/Uniform Type Committee. *Fourth biennial report.* (Reprinted in *New Outlook for the Blind,* 1913, *7,* 1–48.)

Ashcroft, S. C. *The IBM braille reader field test.* Unpublished progress report. Nashville, Tenn.: George Peabody College for Teachers, 1959.

Bürklen, K. *Touch reading of the blind.* (Translated by F. K. Merry) (Originally published 1917.) New York: American Foundation for the Blind, 1932.

Cattell, J. M. The time it takes to see and name objects. *Mind,* 1886, *11,* 63–65.

Challman, B. E. *Variables influencing the identification of single braille characters.* Unpublished master's thesis, University of Louisville, 1978.

Cornsweet, T. N. The staircase method in psychophysics. *American Journal of Psychology,* 1962, *75,* 485–491.

Doggett, D., & Richards, L. G. A reexamination of the effect of word length on recognition thresholds. *American Journal of Psychology,* 1975, *88,* 583–594.

Eatman, P. F. An analytic study of braille reading. Unpublished doctoral thesis, University of Texas, 1942.

Ethington, D. The readability of braille as a function of three spacing variables. Unpublished master's thesis, University of Kentucky, 1956.

Fertsch, P. An analysis of braille reading. *Outlook for the Blind,* 1946, *40,* 128–131.

Flanigan, P. J. Programmed learning and braille instruction for functional braille readers. *Proceedings of the 47th Meeting of the American Association of Instructors of the Blind,* Watertown, Mass. 1964, 10–16.

Foulke, E. Transfer of a complex perceptual skill. *Perceptual & Motor Skills,* 1964, *18,* 733–740.

The development of an expanded reading code for the blind, Part 2. (Final Progress Report. Project 7-1185, Grant OEG-O-8-0771185-1811(032). Washington, D.C.: U.S. Dept. of Health, Education and Welfare, Bureau of Education for the Handicapped, 1973.

The Perceptual Alternatives Laboratory: annual report to the dean of the graduate school, 1973–1974. Louisville, Ky.: Perceptual Alternatives Laboratory, University of Louisville, 1974.

Foulke, E., & Warm, J. Effects of complexity and redundancy on the tactual recognition of metric figures. *Perceptual & Motor Skills,* 1967, *25,* 177–187.

The development of an expanded reading code for the blind (Final Progress Report, Project 3104, Grant OE-6-10-035). Washington, D.C.: U.S. Department of Health, Education and Welfare, Office of Education, 1968.

Funchess. L. V. The psychology of reading braille with eight fingers. Unpublished Master's Thesis, Louisiana State University, 1934.

Gallo, D. R. *National assessment of educational progress: reading rate and comprehension, 1970–71 assessment* (Education Commission of the States, No. 02-R-09). Washington, D.C.: U.S. Government Printing Office, 1972.

Grunwald, A. P. A braille-reading machine. *Science,* 1966, *154,* 144–146.

Harris, A. J. *How to increase reading ability.* New York: Longmans, Green, 1947.

Henderson, F. M. The effect of character recognition training on braille reading. Unpublished specialist in education thesis, George Peabody College for Teachers, 1967.

Holland, B. F. Speed and pressure factors in braille reading. *Teachers Forum*, 1934, *7*, 13–17.

Irwin, R. B. *War of the dots*. Reprinted from *As I saw it*. New York: American Foundation for the Blind, 1955, pp. 3–55.

Kurzhals, I., & Caton, H. R. *A tactual road to reading*. Louisville, Ky.: American Printing House for the Blind, 1973.

Kusajima, T. *Visual reading and braille reading: an experimental investigation of the physiology and psychology of visual and tactual reading*. New York: American Foundation for the Blind, 1974.

Lappin, J., & Foulke, E. Expanding the tactual field of view. *Perception & Psychophysics*, 1973, *14*, 237–241.

Lowenfeld, B., Abel, G. L., & Hatlen, P. H. *Blind children learn to read*. Springfield, Ill.: Charles C. Thomas, 1969.

Meyers, E., Ethington, D., & Ashcroft, S. C. Readability of braille as a function of three spacing variables. *Journal of Applied Psychology*, 1958, *42*, 163–165.

Newbigging, P. L., & Hay, J. The practice effect in recognition thresholds as a function of word frequency and length. *Canadian Journal of Psychology*, 1962, *16*, 177–184.

Nolan, C. Y. Cues in the tactual perception of patterns (Progress Report, NIH Grant NB-3124-09). Louisville, Ky.: American Printing House for the Blind, 1964.

Nolan, C. Y., & Kederis, C. J. *Perceptual factors in braille word recognition*. American Foundation for the Blind Research Series, no. 20. New York: American Foundation for the Blind, 1969.

Shaw, R., & Pittenger, J. Perceiving change. In H. L. Pick, Jr., & E. Saltzman (Eds.), *Modes of perceiving and processing information*. Hillsdale, N.J.: Erlbaum, 1978, pp. 187–204.

Taylor, E. A. *The fundamental reading skill, as related to eye movement photography and visual anomalies*. Springfield, Ill.: Charles C. Thomas, 1966.

Troxell, D. E. Experiments in tactile and visual reading. *IEEE Transactions on Human Factors in Electronics*, HFE-8, 1967, 261–263.

Umstead, R. G. *Improvement of braille reading through training*. Unpublished Doctoral Thesis, George Peabody College for Teachers, 1970.

Wait, W. B. Alphabets and books for the blind. In *Thirty-third annual report of the managers of the New York Institution for the Blind, to the legislature of the state, for the year 1868*. New York: George F. Nesbitt, 1869.

Warm, J., Clark, J. L., & Foulke E. Effects of differential spatial orientation on tactual pattern recognition. *Perceptual & Motor Skills*, 1970, *31*, 87–94.

Warm, J., & Foulke, E. Effects of orientation and redundancy on the tactual perception of form. *Perceptual & Motor Skills*, 1968, *27*, 83–89.

Effects of rate of signal rise and decay on reaction time to the onset and offset of acoustic stimuli. *Perception & Psychophysics*, 1970, *7*, 159–160.

6. Dynamic tactile displays

JAMES C. CRAIG & CARL E. SHERRICK

In Chapter 6, James Craig and Carl Sherrick review much of what is known about dynamic tactile displays, which present changing patterns of stimulation to passive skin surfaces. Most displays of this type are electrical, electronic, or electromechanical, and most are designed to present coded information (e.g., speech, printed language, or other graphic patterns) to perceivers.

The authors neatly summarize a large body of work with the Optacon and related devices. This class of devices was designed for and is widely used by blind persons. Much Optacon use is related to reading ink-print via tactile transformations of scanned print (rather than braille). Problems related to reading rate, letter processing, and letter-group processing are explored. Research and practical applications of the related TVSS are also examined, with special reference to using the system as a mobility aid.

The authors then review some considerations many consider to be basic in tactile perception and communication – our ability to deal with stimulus dimensions such as frequency, amplitude, duration, and the locus of stimulus application. The import of masking phenomena for tactile displays is also explored. The authors concur with others in this volume that temporal masking of tactile stimuli is a basic and major problem in using the skin as a system for rapid processing of information. They also note, however, that Kirman holds an alternative position that may circumvent the problem. The chapter also examines perceived movement and ways of displaying movement in tactile displays. This chapter is a must for psychologists and engineers involved with the presentation of dynamic information to the skin and exploration of the potentials of the skin for mediating temporally extended inputs, or passively perceived *events*.

WILLIAM SCHIFF

Introduction

Dynamic tactile displays differ from most of the other types of displays discussed in this volume in a number of ways, most obviously in that dynamic displays usually generate tactile patterns on a stationary skin surface rather than having the skin surface move across the display. On the active–passive touch dimension, then, dynamic displays compared with tangible graphic displays should be placed near the passive end of the dimension (Kirman, 1978; but cf. Chapter 2).

The purpose of this chapter is to introduce the reader to what is known about dynamic displays or what can reasonably be inferred about them from the available data. It will be obvious that what we know with certainty about dynamic displays is not extensive. Moreover, the studies involving these displays were not designed, understandably, with this chapter in mind. In comparing one study with another, one finds a variety of approaches to the problem. Two studies may employ different types of displays on wholly disparate body surfaces with widely separated frequencies of vibration to present dissimilar types of information. It is not always possible, therefore, to state with assurance that one particular variable produced the major difference between the two studies. However, short of replicating the entire history of research on these displays, we are forced to make comparisons across studies. The reader is forewarned that some of the conclusions may ultimately prove inaccurate.

The first half of this chapter describes some of the displays that have been developed. The second half examines some of the stimulus considerations that have emerged from the development of dynamic displays and influenced their design. The chapter will not deal with displays whose primary purpose is the communication of speech information; that topic is covered in Chapter 7. The present chapter will confine its discussion to mechanical stimulation of the skin, which is the mode of stimulation most often favored in dynamic tactile displays.

Displays

The Optacon

A general rule has been that dynamic displays have been developed solely for experimental purposes, but a notable exception is the tactile display that is part of the Optacon. The Optacon (the word stands for *op*tical-to-*ta*ctile *con*version) is a commercially available direct ink-print reading aid for the blind consisting of a small hand-held camera that is moved across the material to be read. Within the camera is an array of photosensitive elements, 6 columns wide by 24 rows high. The photosensitive array registers the pattern of light and dark produced by a letter passing beneath the camera. The pattern is transferred to a 6-by-24 array of pins measuring 1.1 by 2.7 cm (0.43 in by 1.06 in) on which the user places a fingertip. The pins vibrate to reproduce the pattern that the

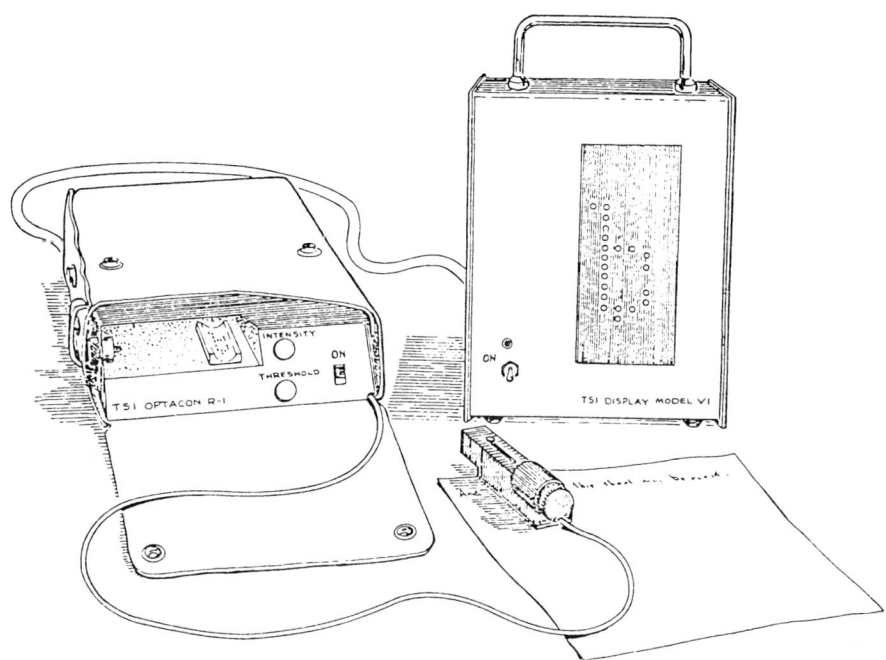

Figure 6.1. Drawing of an Optacon showing camera and visual display.

camera "sees"; for example, the letter O produces a circular pattern of vibration on the user's fingertip. Moving the camera causes the vibrotactile pattern to move across the fingertip after the fashion of moving electric signs such as the Times Square display (Bliss, 1974; Bliss, Katcher, Rogers, & Shepard, 1970). Whether or not this movement of the camera by a user activates some of the mechanisms involved in active touch is not clear; nevertheless, attaching the camera to a device that moves it automatically across the material to be read does not seem to interfere with reading and may, in fact, lead to higher reading rates (Telesensory, 1973). Clearly, the user's operation of the camera is not a necessary component of reading.

In order to make use of this reading aid, people must receive fairly intensive training. After the 9-day training program conducted by the manufacturer, Telesensory Systems, Inc., the average reading rate is about 10 to 12 wpm. (Bliss, 1978). With further training and experience, reading rates of 30 to 50 wpm are obtained (Goldish & Taylor, 1974), and for certain individuals rates of up to 100 wpm may be achieved(Craig, 1977; Moore & Bliss, 1975). If reading rates are calculated on the basis of 5.5 letters per word, then 50 wpm means that users are able to perceive

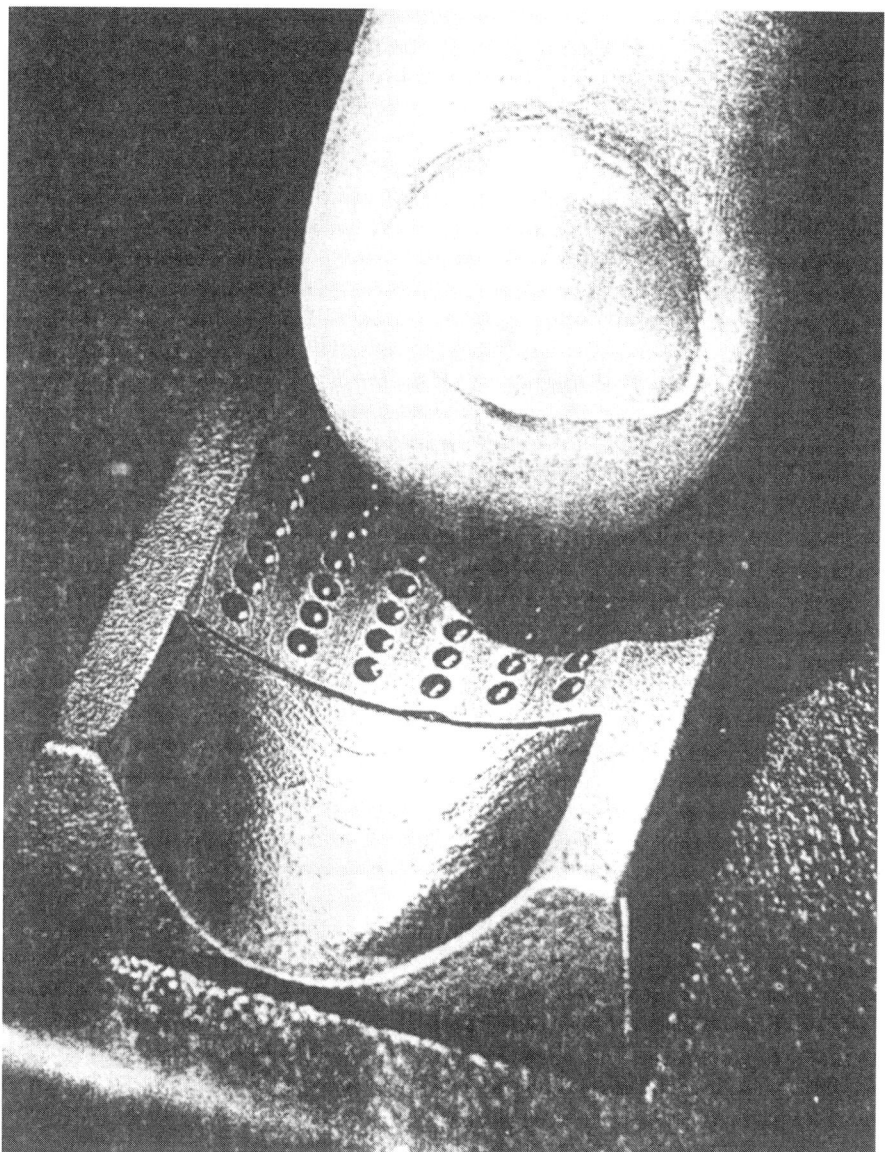

Figure 6.2. Close-up of an Optacon display.

letters coming at a rate of 4.5 per second, or 220 msec per letter plus interletter space. There may be ways to achieve good pattern recognition in far less time than 220 msec, a possibility that will be discussed later in this chapter, but no method has gone beyond this rate in presenting meaningful, continuous information to users.

212

The Optacon display was the result of considerable previous work. Some of this work involved a display that employed jets of air as the stimuli. The display was created by a matrix of outlet ports 12 columns wide by 8 rows high. Letters were generated using half of the display, a 6 by 8 matrix, which was placed beneath the subject's pronated hand and extended across the four fingers. The patterns were produced by air pulses repeated at a rate of 200 Hz. Pairs of letterlike patterns were presented to subjects while both the duration and time between patterns were varied. Subjects were able to identify both members of a pair of patterns more accurately as the duration of presentation and the time between pairs of stimuli were increased. The latter result suggests that reducing the mutual interference or masking that the two patterns produce leads to improved pattern recognition (Bliss, Crane, Link, & Townsend, 1966). The effects of pattern duration and masking will be considered later in this chapter.

In addition to the air-jet display, several other tactile displays were constructed by Bliss, Linvill, and their co-workers. One early display utilized both tactile and kinesthetic stimulation. The device, which could move the subject's fingers in any one of six directions, received some preliminary investigation as a possible way to encode letters (Bliss, 1963), as did another display in which the letters of the alphabet were coded to a particular place on the fingers being stimulated (Hill, 1971). However, more significant to the development of reading aids for the blind and the study of dynamic displays in general is a study by Hill (1974) on the effect of using a larger Optacon display on reading rates. Early studies had shown that increasing the width of the tactile display from one to four columns (Bliss & Linvill, 1966) or from one to six columns (Bliss, Katcher, Rogers, & Shepard, 1970) led to more accurate word recognition and higher reading rates. Such a result is to be expected, particularly in light of the fact that a single letter will, when centered on the tactile display, extend across six columns and that the six columns could fit against one finger. Hill enlarged upon these earlier studies by extending the width of the Optacon display to include the presentation of more than one letter at a time. The analogy with visual reading is direct. With the increase in the number of letters viewed visually at a single time, the reading rate increases (Gibson & Levin, 1975; White, 1974). Such was not the case with tactile reading, however: The reading rate did not increase as the display was doubled in width to include two letters. In one experiment the tactile display extended over two fingers; in another, the width was doubled, with the display remaining in contact with a single finger (Hill, 1974). The fact that reading rate did not improve as the size of the display increased is important not only for what it indicates about limitations in reading through the skin but also for what it might indicate about the skin's ability to integrate information coming from spatially separated points on the skin. Whether the skin's ability to integrate information from two fingers at the same time or from a larger array in contact with one finger is a result of some basic sensory limitation of the skin, or whether the inability is more the result of the high-level processing task of reading through the skin, is not clear. Some work with larger arrays, described later, indicates that in some tasks subjects are able to use information coming from widely separated points on the body.

TVSS

Both the Optacon and the next display to be considered, the Tactile-Vision Substitution System (TVSS), share a common purpose, to overcome visual handicaps, as well as a common approach of converting visual information to patterns for the skin. The TVSS, developed at the Smith-Kettlewell Institute in San Francisco, is a device that utilizes a TV camera and an array of vibrators built into the back of a chair to generate tactile patterns from optical patterns. The purpose of the TVSS was, as its name indicates, fairly ambitious. Indeed, the title of one of the articles written by the group that developed the TVSS is "Seeing with the skin" (White, Saunders, Scadden, Bach-y-Rita, & Collins, 1970). The idea was that the TV camera would replace the lens of the eye and the skin of the back would replace the retina. The possibility of such a replacement was subsumed under the general heading of "sensory plasticity" (Bach-y-Rita, 1972).

The TV camera was connected through an electronic processing network to a 20-by-20 array of vibrators that formed a square 25 by 25 cm (9.84 in). The vibrators were either on or off in the presence of light or dark stimuli, hence showed no gradation in intensity of light. In using the TVSS, subjects scanned the TV camera across an object to be identified, thereby generating a corresponding pattern of vibration on their backs. Blind subjects who had received some practice with the device were able to discriminate horizontal from vertical lines, and even to judge the slant of a checkerboard. They were also able to identify which one of a group of 25 objects, such as a stuffed animal, a telephone, or a cup, had been placed in front of the TV camera. It was also reported that subjects with additional experience began to localize the objects

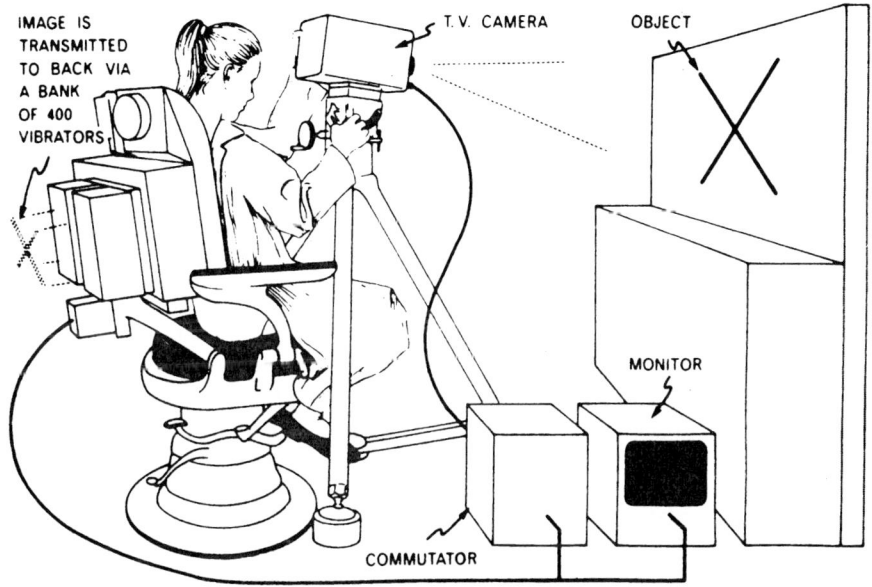

Figure 6.3. Drawing of the TVSS system. (From White et al. 1970)

out in front of them in space rather than on their backs. The subjects reported considerable difficulty in identifying the internal details of a pattern, such as facial features in a photograph (White et al., 1970). Working with a similar display, Craig (1974) observed that subjects also had difficulty recognizing internal details, such as the diagonal line in the letter *N*.

To what extent does the TVSS permit the skin to substitute for the eye? It would appear that there is considerable doubt about this possibility. The failure "to find solid evidence for three-dimensional organization in cutaneous stimulation" (White, 1974, p. 16) has led one of the investigators working with the TVSS to express doubts about using the skin to gain visual space information. Another investigator working with the TVSS concluded that more basic research on tactile stimulation would be required before any kind of mobility aid might emerge (Jansson, 1978). White also expressed doubts about the skin's ability to identify complex visual patterns, although as Kirman (1978) points out, White (1974) is somewhat more hopeful about presenting language information through the skin.

215

Pictorial versus coded approaches

The development of the TVSS and the initial findings obtained with it raised a number of issues for consideration in creating dynamic displays. One of the most important issues has been referred to as the *pictorial versus coded approach* by Geldard (1974) or the *analogic versus synthetic systems approach* by Sherrick (1975). The issue is a complicated one. It concerns the extent to which one deliberately sets out to create a set of patterns for the skin or instead imposes the information intended for another modality, in this case vision, almost directly on the skin. Clearly, devices like the Optacon and the TVSS are representative of pictorial displays. In fact, White and his co-workers (1970) clearly believed that the success they reported with the TVSS is largely the result of this pictorial approach. To the extent that the initial optimism about the TVSS has been reduced, as noted above, the advantages of the pictorial approach may be questioned.

It has been shown that pictorial information is not entirely necessary for recognizing some cutaneous patterns, such as letters of the alphabet. Craig (1974) used a device similar to the TVSS that converted visual patterns to patterns of vibration on a display that could be brought in contact with a subject's back or abdomen. The tactile array was made up of 100 vibrators arranged in a square, 10 columns by 10 rows. These were connected to an array of 100 photocells also arranged in a 10 by 10 matrix. By moving a letter across the photocell array, the subject generated a pattern of vibration on the skin. In the pictorial arrangement, the spatial relations among the various parts of the letter were preserved as much as possible when presented to the skin. The left panel of Figure 6.4 shows the letter Z presented pictorially. In a second method of presentation, the scrambled arrangement, the connections between the columns of the photocell array and the columns of the vibrating array were rerouted to produce a pattern that no longer looked like the letter generating it. The right panel of Figure 6.4 shows the letter Z as it appeared when presented in this scrambled fashion. A comparison of subjects' performances in recognizing letters presented with the two arrangements showed that subjects did no better in recognizing letters presented pictorially than when scrambled. These results indicated that pictorial information does not have to be preserved in tactile displays for such tasks as letter recognition.

The question that arises is, what information are subjects using to recognize cutaneous patterns with spatially extended displays such as the TVSS? By observing how subjects scanned the TV camera across the

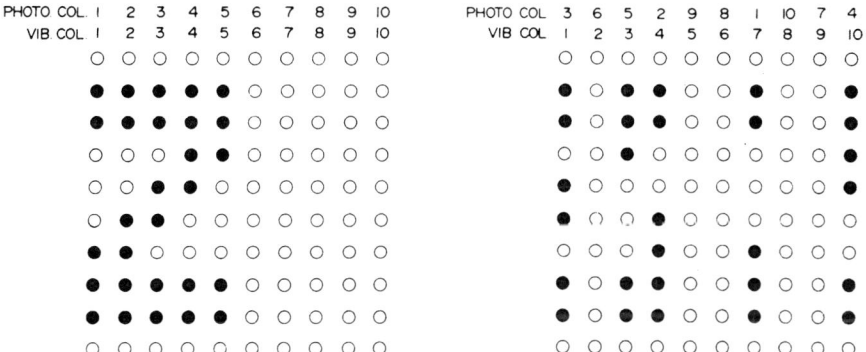

Figure 6.4. Representations of the vibrators energized in the tactile display when the letter Z was presented. The figure on the left shows Z in the pictorial mode. The figure on the right shows Z in the scrambled mode. (From Craig, 1974)

forms to be identified, White et al. (1970) concluded "that the discrimination is largely based upon contour changes in the leading edge of the figure" (White et al., 1970, p. 24). Craig (1974) reached a similar conclusion, based in part on his observations of the way subjects moved the letters to be identified across the 10 by 10 array he used.

The issue of pictorial versus coded approaches to pattern recognition may be important to the designer of tangible graphic displays for the blind. Designers of such displays attempt to incorporate symbols that suggest the object they are meant to represent (see Chapter 10). If pictorial approaches are not necessarily superior to coded approaches, then the search for the haptic equivalents of visual objects needs to be broadened. It should not be assumed that some direct, albeit reduced, representation of a visual object makes the best representation for the skin.

Experimental displays

As previously noted, the majority of the tactile displays developed have been designed for experimental use. One of the earliest of these was developed by Geldard and his co-workers. The approach taken by Geldard exemplifies the coded approach in constructing tactile displays. In a series of studies summarized by Geldard (1957, 1960, 1961), subjects were tested for their ability to discriminate between vibrotactile stimuli that were varied along a single stimulus dimension. Subjects were tested to see how well they could discriminate various amplitudes of vibration from one another, various durations of vibration, and places of stimulation on the skin. As a result of this work, a vibratory code called Vibratese was devised, which involved placing five vibrators in an X pattern against the subject's chest. In Vibratese only one vibrator was energized at a time for one of three durations, 100, 300, or 500 msec, and at one of three amplitudes, weak, medium, or strong. From the combination of five vibrators at five different loci on the skin times three durations times three amplitudes, 45 usable signals were created (see Figure 6.5). The signals were then individually assigned to the 26 letters of the alphabet, the numerals 0 through 9, and short words such as *of* and *the*. There is obviously no a priori connection between the letter *e* and a brief, strong buzz in the upper right quadrant of the chest. Subjects had to learn the code, and after several training sessions, one subject was able to receive messages at a rate of about 35 wpm (Geldard, 1957, 1961).

Vibratese had only one vibrator energized at a time in order to prevent interaction among the signals generated at the various loci. The next display examined by Geldard and his co-worker, Sherrick (1965), also attempted to minimize interaction among loci even though in this case up to 10 vibrators could be turned on at the same time. Interaction was minimized by strapping 10 specially designed vibrators (Bice, 1961) to widely separated loci on the skin. The locations of the vibrators are shown in Figure 6.5.

In an examination of some of the possibilities of cutaneous spatial discrimination, subjects were presented pairs of patterns in which pair members comprised equal numbers of vibrators. The subjects were required to say whether the two patterns were the same as or different from one another. The results showed, not too surprisingly, that as the number of vibrators in a pair increased, the percentage of errors also increased. A detailed analysis of the data revealed that a more important cause of errors was not the number of vibrators per se but rather the number of elements shared by the pair members, that is, the amount of communality. Thus, if the second member of a pair of patterns, made up of four vibrators each, differed from the first by the location of a single vibrator ($3 \div 4 \times 100 = 75$ percent communality), the error rate in discriminating this pair would be approximately the same as that resulting from a pair of patterns composed of eight vibrators in which the second pattern differed from the first by two vibrators (again, $6 \div 8 \times 100 = 75$ percent communality). The importance of the principle of communality in predicting errors has also been reported in a study using a 64-element array placed against the ventral surface of a subject's thigh (Gottheil, Cholewiak, & Sherrick, 1978). As in the above study, subjects were required to discriminate between pairs of patterns varying in percent of communality. Again, communality appeared to be the important

218

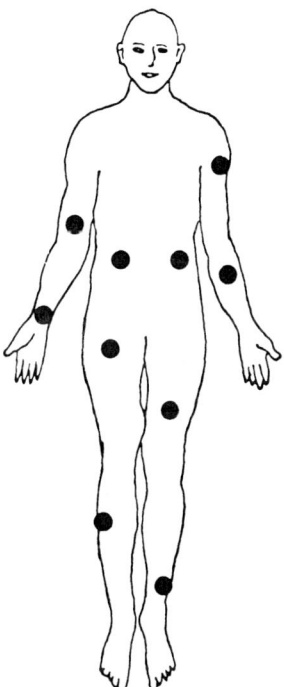

Figure 6.5. Locations of vibrators. (From Geldard & Sherrick, 1965)

factor in determining errors. There was the interesting finding that from levels of 0 percent communality (the first pattern shared no elements in common with the second pattern) to 60 percent communality, there was a gradual increase in errors. As the percent of communality increased beyond 60, the error rate rose sharply. In addition, comparing the results from this 64-element array with the 10-element array used by Geldard and Sherrick (1965) showed that for the same percent of communality fewer errors were produced with the more widely spaced 10-element array.

The work with a 10-element simultaneous display was extended to the fingertips by Gilson (1968), who found that replacing widely separated body loci with the 10 fingers led to a greater error rate than that produced on the body unless interaction among the sites of stimulation was reduced. The nature of this interaction appeared to be both neural and physical. Better discrimination was achieved when the vibrators produced relatively confined stimulation (reduced physical propagation), and the fingers were stimulated at noncorresponding points, presumably reducing neural interaction.

219

All elements in both of the 10-vibrator displays and the 64-element display just described were turned on and off simultaneously, a mode of presentation that is called *static*. This mode of generating patterns does not take advantage of the skin's ability to make fine temporal discriminations, nor does it produce the perception of movement that might be used to enhance the vividness of patterns. In part to remedy this situation, Geldard (1966) changed the input to his 10-vibrator array, reduced to nine for this experiment, to accommodate a nine-element photocell array arranged in a column in an optical pickup. When letters were passed beneath the pickup, the pattern of light and dark was registered by the photocells, much as it is in the Optacon, and transferred to the vibrators. The result was a pattern of vibration that appeared to sweep across the body as a symbol passed beneath the photocells. Geldard found that with this device, called the *optohapt*, the letters of the alphabet did not produce the most highly discriminable patterns. Simpler patterns produced by punctuation marks turned out to be better candidates for a cutaneous code. In fact, in the assignment of characters for alphabetic coding, only the letters *I*, *J*, and *V* were used.

An additional group of experimental displays should be considered together inasmuch as they have been designed to accomplish the same task, namely, tracking a target. The elements making up these displays have been configured to produce circular displays, cross displays (a vertical line of vibrators crossing a horizontal line of vibrators) (Triggs, Levison, & Sanneman, 1974), two-vibrator displays, and linear displays (Hill, 1970), among others. Using these displays on different body sites, investigators have measured how well subjects were able to track a target. In a 1970 study Hill placed his two-vibrator display on several locations on the skin, such as on the same finger or the same forearm, or one vibrator on one forearm and the second on the other forearm, and found no significant difference in tracking accuracy. Using a linear air-jet display, however, Hill did find some differences in performance between placing the display on the back of the hand versus the forearm, with the former producing lower error scores than the latter. Increasing the spacing between sites of stimulation on the forearm improved performance such that it was now comparable to that produced by placing the display on the hand. Of particular interest to designers and users of tactile displays is the fact that comparisons can be made between targets tracked visually and tactually. It is not surprising that under most conditions visual tracking is superior, but sometimes tactile tracking approaches and equals it (Geldard, 1960; Hill, 1970; Triggs et al., 1974).

Another experimental display with possible usefulness in tracking involves a unique method of stimulation: water. Using a device resembling an oral hygiene appliance, Loomis and Collins (1978) measured the ability of subjects to detect the direction of movement of a stream of water directed against a thin rubber dam placed between the water stream and the skin. With this display, subjects were able to identify the direction of very small movements.

Stimulus considerations

Frequency, amplitude, duration, locus

In the course of designing and testing dynamic displays and also as a result of basic measurements of vibrotactile sensitivity, investigators have reached a number of conclusions concerning stimulus parameters that should be employed in displays. Typically these conclusions are in the form of recommendations about what stimulus values should be selected for enhancing cutaneous pattern recognition or discrimination. We shall first consider the recommendations concerning the four primary dimensions of vibratory stimulation – frequency, amplitude, duration, and locus.

Using the air-jet display, Rogers (1970) found that a stimulus rate of 160 pulses per second produced better letter recognition than a rate of 20 pulses per second. Gilson (1968), in the study referred to earlier using the 10 fingers as sites of stimulation, found a slight decrease in errors as frequency was increased from 60 to 500 Hz. Based on the above results, it seems best to use a higher frequency in a display, perhaps one close to 250 Hz, a frequency that not only permits finer spatial discrimination than lower frequencies (Bliss, 1974) but is also in the region of maximal absolute sensitivity (cf. Verrillo, 1962). Indeed, the frequency of vibration of the Optacon display is 230 Hz.

The boundaries for amplitude variation can be easily stated. One would not want the intensity of vibration set so weak that subjects had difficulty detecting it or so strong as to be painful. Within this rather broad range, however, there is a question of whether intensity has much effect on pattern perception. Gilson (1968) found no effect on the ability of subjects to discriminate pairs of patterns when the amplitude of vibration was varied from 3 to 28 dB above threshold. Similarly, there seems to be little correlation between reading performance with the Optacon and the amplitude of the vibration generating the letters. Optacon users are simply encouraged to find a comfortable level of stimulation (Telesensory, 1973). However, a definite effect of amplitude was found using the Optacon display, not in reading but in a letter recognition task. With increasing display amplitude, recognition of single letters improved, an effect dependent upon the pattern presentation mode (Craig, 1980). There are a number of reasons why the improvement in single letter recognition with amplitude of vibration would not improve reading performance, among which is that increasing the intensity of a single pattern would also increase its effectiveness as a masking stimulus for adjacent letters.

Limits similar to those proposed for amplitude can be specified for duration of presentation. One would not select durations so brief as not to be detectable or so long as to result in a ponderous rate of information transmission. There may be certain types of displays in which one would want to avoid durations so brief that the vibratory signals would be reduced to pokes and jabs (Geldard, 1957). The general effect of increasing the presentation time is, as noted before, to improve pattern recognition and discriminability. Studies with the air-jet and Optacon displays have shown that as the display time was increased, letter recognition and word recognition improved (Bliss et al., 1966; Craig, 1980; Rogers, 1970; Taenzer, 1970). In one experiment with the air-jet display mentioned previously, the pairs of letters were presented to subjects for durations varying from 50 to 400 msec. Increases in duration of the briefer stimuli produced more improvement in letter recognition than comparable changes at longer durations (Bliss et al., 1966). A similar result was found by Craig (1980) with the Optacon display. However, Craig also found that the increase in correct percentage accompanying increasing duration was apparently the result of increasing the sensory magnitude of the pattern rather than increasing the duration per se. A briefer display duration that ordinarily produced a lower percentage of correct letter recognition than a longer duration would yield exactly the same correct percentage if the display amplitude at the shorter duration was increased until letters presented at the two durations were perceived as equally intense. This result was limited to a static presentation of the patterns.

Many problems associated with dynamic displays can be subsumed under the general heading of "locus." In keeping with the discussions of frequency, amplitude, and duration, the first problem is, what area of the skin should the array contact? The most common choice appears to be the fingers, mainly because they possess the obvious advantages of high sensitivity to small amplitudes of vibration and excellent spatial acuity. Both of these advantages permit a tactile display designed for the fingertips to be small and portable. However, the fingers and hand are often called upon to perform tasks that might make it impossible to stay in contact with the display. For example, in a recent demonstration of the potential usefulness of keeping the hands free, a blind technician was trained in an assembly task involving the use of both hands and, ordinarily, visual inspection. The visual inspection part of the task was accomplished by a modified TVSS-type display in contact with the technician's abdomen (Bach-y-Rita, Scadden, & Collins, 1975). There have been very few direct comparisons of performance, on a similar task with a similar array, between the fingers and body loci. As noted above, Gilson (1968) did find that repeating a set of measurements made with body loci on the fingers initially led to poorer performance by the fingers, but that some stimulus manipulations improved performance with the fingers until it was made comparable to that of the body loci.

One additional point should be made about the selection of locus. In a study using the TVSS, Scadden (1973) found that subjects trained to recognize patterns presented to their backs showed almost immediate transfer when the patterns were presented to the thigh or abdomen. In fact, the abdomen produced the highest percentage of correct letter recognition even when the subjects had received all their training with the array against their backs. Results with the Optacon indicate that there is transfer from one finger to another, although it is apparently not immediate (Hill, 1974; Telesensory, 1973).

Masking

A commonly investigated problem with dynamic displays, and one of great potential importance to users, is masking. *Masking* is usually defined as a condition in which one stimulus interferes with the detection of another stimulus. The definition has been broadened to include interference not only in detection but also in pattern recognition. In nearly every display so far described, investigators have studied masking directly or noted its effects. An early display, a kind of vibrotactile braille, consisted of six vibrators, three strapped to each arm (Geldard & Hahn, 1961). One of the most striking observations with this display was that subjects were usually unable to detect the presence of the middle vibrators on each arm when both of the outside vibrators were energized, that is, the middle vibrator was masked and therefore certain patterns would be indistinguishable from one another. A more systematic examination of detection masking on body loci was carried out by Gilson (1969a, b), who measured the detectability of a test vibrator on the upper thigh in the presence of masking vibrators located at other sites on the body. It is probably not surprising that as the longitudinal distance between the test site and the masking site increases, the amount of masking decreases. However, the decrease in masking with increased distance could be offset by changing the time interval between the test vibrator and the masker to compensate for neural conduction time. Thus, a vibrator on the upper arm that had its onset delayed 10 msec relative to the onset of a test vibrator on the upper thigh produced nearly as much masking as a vibrator located next to the test vibrator (Gilson, 1969a). It follows and is the case that, for stimuli close together on the skin, increasing the time interval between the test and masking stimuli will reduce masking (Craig, 1978; Gilson, 1969a; Sherrick, 1964). Gilson (1969b) found, in addition, that as the number of vibrators in a pattern increases, so does the masking effect on a single test vibrator.

Measurements of the effect of masking stimuli on pattern recognition parallel those of detection. The presence of extraneous vibration on the TVSS display, for example, interfered with the subjects' recognition of letters. The closer the masking stimulus was to the letter and the more intense the masker, the greater was the interference effect (Loomis & Apkarian-Stielau, 1976). As with detection, varying the time interval between the pattern to be identified and the masking stimulus changes the amount of recognition masking. If the time interval exceeds approximately 150 to 200 msec, the masker produces little interference (Bliss et al., 1966; Craig, 1976, 1978, 1980). For both the air-jet display and the Optacon, presenting the masking stimulus immediately after the pattern (a condition referred to as *backward masking*) produces more interference than presenting the masking stimulus immediately before the target (i.e., *forward masking*). This result, in which the relative efficiency of the backward masker is greater than that of the forward masker, is not entirely paralleled by results in detection masking. Craig (1978) found that in detecting a brief vibrotactile signal on the fingertip, forward masking was more potent than backward masking, whereas for recognizing a letter on the Optacon, the reverse was true. The fact that detection and recognition masking effects in cutaneous displays are not entirely comparable is not surprising; different processes undoubtedly underlie the two tasks of detection and recognition, in agreement with a hypothesis currently favored for auditory and visual stimuli as well (Massaro, 1975; Turvey, 1973).

A moment's reflection on the masking data will reveal why masking can be so troublesome for the designer of cutaneous displays. A high rate of information transmission, which most designers would like to achieve, demands that patterns arrive rapidly one after another. Compact, portable displays require that patterns be generated on the skin at the same or closely adjacent areas. Thus, two conditions usually sought by display designers are just those that tend to maximize masking.

A rather different view of masking and the need to avoid it has been advanced by Kirman (1973). He has pointed out that masking is an indication of interaction among stimuli and that for certain types of displays such interaction should not be avoided but encouraged. Interactions of this kind, particularly in the presentation of speech information through the skin, might produce new spatiotemporal patterns through mechanisms of integration and perhaps lead to better information transmission (Kirman, 1973).

Movement

The title of the present chapter, "Dynamic Tactile Displays," highlights what for many investigators is the importance of movement in tactile perception. Indeed, the importance of movement has been pointed out a number of times in this volume, particularly in Krueger's discussion of Katz's contributions to tactile sensitivity (Chapter 1). Such movement is usually generated when the skin is passed over some surface, as in active touch. Although the present discussion of dynamic displays is concerned with movement generated across skin surfaces that are stationary, here too the importance of movement is evident. With both the air-jet display (Bliss et al., 1966), and an Optacon-like display (Bliss and Linvill, 1966), moving the pattern to be identified across the display yielded better recognition than did a static presentation of the pattern. The term *static* needs clarification in the present context. The mode is actually dynamic when viewed as a spatiotemporal phenomenon. The term, as noted before, is commonly applied to those displays in which all the matrix elements that make up the pattern are turned on and off together. There is, therefore, not the same spatial elaboration of contour over the matrix as there is in dynamic displays. Nonetheless, the static display does produce a spatiotemporal elaboration of contours, inasmuch as the growth and decline of vibratory intensity over time and across the matrix represent a changing pattern of disturbance throughout the sensory sheet. As the disturbance continues, the observer's perceptual report may shift from that of a compact, sharply localized feature set to a less dense, somewhat fuzzy grouping of tactile sensations (see von Békésy, 1967). In the static mode, many of the natural elaborative processes of the skin and the somatosensory system are called into play, including magnitude growth, the time constants of funneling, and adaptation. The dynamic modes include the same processes, but in addition, they provide for their systematic distribution through the tactile space–time domain, thereby augmenting or attenuating their effective interrelations.

A dynamic mode was generated in one study with the TVSS by subjects panning the camera. This movement produced by the camera allowed subjects to identify patterns that they could not recognize when the camera was stationary (Bach-y-Rita, 1972). Subjects also recognized letters more readily when they were moved across the tactile display than when presented in a stationary mode (Loomis, 1974). Geldard (1966), working with the optohapt, commented on the "vividness" of patterns produced when they contained movement. The general recommendation would obviously be to include movement in both large and small tactile displays. One or two exceptions to this recommendation will, however, be noted below.

Simply recommending the use of movement in dynamic displays ignores the fact that there are certain movement effects one might wish to incorporate or avoid. These include apparent motion, sensory saltation, and the phantom of lateralization. *Apparent motion* on the skin or, as it is sometimes called, *cutaneous phi,* is a striking phenomenon resulting from successive stimulation at several loci on the skin. Under the proper conditions, the result is "a powerful 'gouging' that moved from one stimulus site to the other at a rate depending on the distance between sites and the time between onsets" (Sherrick & Rogers, 1966, p. 177). In general, as the duration of the tactile signals increases, the time between the onsets of the two signals must be increased to produce the best apparent motion. For two vibrotactile stimuli of 50-msec duration, optimal movement is obtained when the onsets differ by 80 msec, whereas for two stimuli of 400-msec duration, optimal movement is obtained when the onsets differ by 250 msec. Apparent motion is not only a vivid phenomenon, it is also a fairly robust one. For example, it may be obtained bilaterally, with one vibrator on one forearm and the second on the other forearm. The movement is perceived in space between the two arms (Sherrick, 1968).

Another striking effect involving movement on the skin is *cutaneous saltation,* better known to its friends as the *rabbit.* When several tactile stimulators are energized to produce a series of taps and their number and timing are adjusted properly, the result is a clear perception of taps "hopping" from one stimulator to the next and on to the next, very much as though a small rabbit were moving across the skin (Geldard, 1975; Geldard & Sherrick, 1972). In one demonstration, 15 taps were presented through three vibrators placed on the forearm. Five taps were generated by the first vibrator, followed by five taps at the second vibrator and five at the third. The taps were presented at intervals of 50 msec. The result was a vivid perception of taps more or less evenly spaced along the arm from the first to the third vibrator. The rabbit can be generated with electrical and thermal stimuli, and with auditory and visual stimuli as well (Geldard, 1975).

The third phenomenon that can produce a perception of movement, the *phantom of lateralization*, is perhaps less vivid and stable than cutaneous phi or the rabbit but nevertheless has received considerable attention for its potential usefulness in tactile displays. The phenomenon is generated by presenting tactile stimuli to two separate loci on the skin within 1 or 2 msec. The result is often a single tactile sensation, a phantom, located between the two sites of stimulation (von Békésy, 1967), that may be moved to various positions between the two sites by changing the relative onset times or intensities of the stimuli at the veridical sites. The phantom will shift toward the site of the more intense stimulus or the stimulus presented first. A change of a few milliseconds is sufficient to move the phantom along its full range from one site to the other. The phantom has been investigated for its possible use in signaling elbow position in a prosthetic device and as a way to represent space in a mobility aid for the blind (Mann, 1974).

The three phenomena can be ordered in terms of the temporal conditions required for their appearance from the phantom to the rabbit to apparent motion, with the briefest times between stimuli required for the phantom and the longest times required for apparent motion. It is likely, however, that in a complex display such as the TVSS or the Optacon or optohapt, all three phenomena and additional ones might emerge as the displays are used (Kirman, 1978). All three phenomena not only produce perceptions of movement from stationary arrays but also allow the display designer to "fill in" between adjacent stimulating points on the skin. Thus, one could imagine an array composed of a few elements that might, by taking advantage of movement phenomena, produce effects similar to those obtained in a much denser array. The blessing is not unmixed, because there is also the potential problem of creating "sensations" where one wishes to avoid them.

Modes of presentation

The topics of movement and specific movement effects lead to the consideration of various modes of presenting cutaneous patterns. Once a particular display has been chosen, what is the best way to use it to present information? The answers here, as nearly everywhere in the cutaneous realm, are sketchy. Moreover, these answers are likely to be derived from only a few types of information-processing tasks such as recognition of letters, position in space, or orientation of a line.

Loomis (1974) compared five different modes of letter generation on the TVSS, including a full-field static presentation of the letter (all elements turned on and off simultaneously), a full-field moving letter (scan condition), and three modes in which the letter was exposed through a narrow slit. In one mode, a vertical slit two columns wide was passed over a static letter. In the second mode, a moving letter was passed behind the vertical slit. In the third mode, a diagonal slit was passed across a static letter. The poorest letter recognition was obtained with the full-field static mode, bettered slightly by the full-field moving letter. The slit modes, in which only a portion of the letter is presented at a time, proved to be superior to the full-field modes, a finding that is at odds with some results mentioned above, particularly those obtained with the Optacon in a reading task. One- or two-column displays proved to be poorer than displays in which all six columns of the array were employed (Bliss, et al., 1970). Following a suggestion by Taenzer, Loomis (1974) indicated that the difference in results may have been due to the amount of practice subjects had with the display. Apparently it is only with practice that Optacon users perform better with the full six-column display than with the one- or two-column displays. In a second study with the TVSS, two additional modes of presentation were examined. Subjects attempted to identify geometric forms and letters of the alphabet when they could pan the camera across the form or letter, as is the usual mode of presentation with the TVSS, or have the pattern "drawn" across the array as though someone were writing the letter on the subject's back. The results showed that drawing the pattern proved to be the superior mode as measured by both the latency and accuracy of performance (Beauchamp, Matheson, & Scadden, 1971).

A second study involving an array on body loci was reported by Sherrick (1979). The vibratory array, 7 by 7, was placed against the ventral thigh of the subjects, who were required to identify in which of four orientations, vertical, horizontal, left or right diagonal, a line had been presented. Five modes of presentation were used to generate the lines to be identified, namely, a static mode, a scan mode, a slit-scan mode with a slit three columns wide and a second seven columns wide, and finally, a mode involving the rabbit. In the last mode, several pulses were presented at each locus along a line, thereby defining the line by creating a cutaneous rabbit. The most salient result was that the scan mode was clearly inferior to the other four modes, surpassed surprisingly even by the static mode. The other four modes did not differ from one another.

228

Because of the overwhelming weight of evidence favoring movement in cutaneous pattern recognition, it was conjectured that the superiority of the static mode to the scan mode would disappear if more complex patterns were used (Kirman, 1978). However, a similar result was obtained in a study using the Optacon in a letter-recognition task. In this study, the static mode was again found to be superior to the scan mode, particularly at the shorter durations. For example, at a display time of 26 msec, the percent of correct letter recognition in the static mode was approximately 65, whereas in the scan mode it was approximately 25. The difference in performance decreased as display time increased, until at longer durations the two modes produced approximately equal levels of performance (Craig, 1980).

Both of the latter studies carried the examination of presentation modes beyond recognition of patterns presented alone to pattern recognition in the presence of a masking stimulus. In the study by Sherrick (1979), the masking stimulus was generated by a group of 10 vibrators pulsed on and off at the same time as the line to be identified. When the static, scan, and slit-scan modes were tested, it was found that once again the scan mode led to the poorest performance, with the other two modes producing better and similar results. In the Craig (1980) study, the masking stimulus was generated by turning on the stimulators in the Optacon array either before or after the letter had been generated, that is, subjecting the letters to forward or backward masking. The two modes examined, static and scan, showed similar masking functions.

The concern with modes of masking clearly shows the presentation of a single pattern will probably be only a minor use of a dynamic display. In addition, Sherrick (1979) points out that "the decision concerning the effectiveness of a mode cannot be made exclusively on the basis of single character performances; it is well-known in the analysis of lip-reading and signing skills, to give only two examples, that single-element scores are not predictive of those obtained in continuous discourse" (p. 50).

The last point needs to be expanded. This chapter has described some displays that have been tried and made some suggestions for stimulus parameters and perceptual phenomena that might be used. However, it should also be clear that these suggestions have limitations. One of the most serious is the information being presented by the particular display. Some suggestions may work out well when the information to be transmitted is a letter of the alphabet but may fail to communicate position in space. The caveat for the designer of displays is clear: The display employed and the stimulus parameters selected need to be tested with the actual material to be transmitted and with the final users (Elliott &

229

Sherrick, 1976). For the experimentalist in information processing there are equally clear route markers, established more than a decade ago by Bliss and his co-workers, who used the digital computer to generate tactile displays (Bliss, et al., 1966). Current usage by Craig (1980) and Sherrick (1979) has been limited to programmatic display sequences, but the next milestones are in sight: the pickup by sensing systems of optic or acoustic information, its conversion to digital form, and its display via tactile arrays to the skin. In a similar manner, the subject's movements can be transduced and converted to the digital code to modify the output of the same or another tactile (or auditory) array. In addition, the information coming to the computer from the environment or from the subject's behavior can be reconstituted by computer operations to add to, subtract from, or otherwise modify the events to enhance or attenuate various aspects of the ultimate tactile patterns being presented (Mann, 1974). The computer thus becomes the instrument of an enterprise that might be labeled *Psychophysical surgery.*

Acknowledgments

Portions of this chapter were prepared under DHEW grant NS 09783 to Indiana University and under Grant NS 04755 to Princeton University from the National Institutes of Health.

References

Bach-y-Rita, P. *Brain mechanisms in sensory substitution.* New York: Academic Press, 1972.

Bach-y-Rita, P., Scadden, L. A., & Collins, C. C. Tactile television system. SRS Final Report (Research Grant No. N-P-55282). San Francisco: Smith-Kettlewell Institute of Visual Sciences, Division of Research and Demonstration Grants, Social and Rehabilitation Service, 1975.

Beauchamp, K. L., Matheson, D. W., & Scadden, L. A. Effects of stimulus-change method on tactile-image recognition. *Perceptual & Motor Skills,* 1971, 33, 1067–1070.

Békésy, G. von. *Sensory inhibition.* Princeton, N.J.: Princeton University Press, 1967.

Bice, R. C. Electromechanical transducer for vibrotactile stimulation. *Review of Scientific Instruments,* 1961, 32, 856–857.

Bliss, J. C. Tactual–kinesthetic perception of information. *Proceedings of the International Congress on Technology and Blindness.* New York: American Foundation for the Blind, 1963, pp. 309–323.

Summary of Optacon-related cutaneous experiments. In F. A. Geldard (Ed.), *Cutaneous communication systems and devices.* Austin, Tex.: Psychonomic Society, 1974, pp. 84–94.

Reading machines for the blind. In G. Gordon (Ed.), *Active touch. The mechanism of recognition of objects by manipulation: a multidisciplinary approach.* Oxford: Pergamon Press, 1978, pp. 243–248.

Bliss, J. C., Crane, H. D., & Link, S. W. Effect of display movement on tactile pattern perception. *Perception & Psychophysics,* 1966, 1, 195–202.

Bliss, J. C., Crane, H. D., Link, S. W., & Townsend, J. T. Tactile perception of sequentially presented spatial patterns. *Perception & Psychophysics*, 1966, *1*, 125–130.

Bliss, J. C., Katcher, M. H., Rogers, C. H., & Shepard, R. P. Optical-to-tactile image conversion for the blind. *IEEE Transactions on Man–Machine Systems*, MMS-11, 1970, 58–64.

Bliss, J. C., & Linvill, J. G. A direct translation reading aid: reading alphabetic shapes tactually. In R. Dufton (Ed.), *Proceedings of the international conference on sensory devices for the blind*. London: Arrowsmith, 1966, pp. 389–407.

Craig, J. C. Pictorial and abstract cutaneous displays. In F. A. Geldard (Ed.), *Cutaneous communication systems and devices*. Austin, Tex.: Psychonomic Society, 1974, pp. 78–83.

Vibrotactile letter recognition: the effects of a masking stimulus. *Perception & Psychophysics*, 1976, *20*, 317–326.

Vibrotactile pattern perception: extraordinary observers. *Science*, 1977, *196*, 450–452.

Vibrotactile pattern recognition and masking. In G. Gordon (Ed.), *Active touch. The mechanism of recognition of objects by manipulation: a multidisciplinary approach*. Oxford: Pergamon Press, 1978, pp. 229–242.

Modes of vibrotactile pattern generation. *Journal of Experimental Psychology: Human Perception and Performance*, 1980, *6*, 151–166.

Elliott, L. L., & Sherrick, C. E. NINCDS workshop on tactile aids for the deaf. *Journal of the Acoustical Society of America*, 1976, *59*, 486–489.

Geldard, F. A. Adventures in tactile literacy. *American Psychologist*, 1957, *12*, 115–124.

Some neglected possibilities of communication. *Science*, 1960, *131*, 1583–1588.

Cutaneous channels of communication. In W. A. Rosenblith (Ed.), *Sensory communication*. Cambridge, Mass: MIT Press, 1961, pp. 73–87.

Cutaneous coding of optical signals: the optohapt. *Perception & Psychophysics*, 1966, *1*, 377–381.

Preface. In F. A. Geldard (Ed.), *Cutaneous communication systems and devices*. Austin, Tex.: Psychonomic Society, 1974, pp. ii–v.

Sensory saltation: metastability in the perceptual world. Hillsdale, N.J.: Erlbaum, 1975.

Geldard, F. A., & Hahn, J. F. *Virginia cutaneous project*. Progress Report, No. 45, 1961. Charlottesville, Va.: Psychological Laboratory, University of Virginia.

Geldard, F. A., & Sherrick, C. E. Multiple cutaneous stimulation: the discrimination of vibratory patterns. *Journal of the Acoustical Society of America*, 1965, *37*, 797–801.

The cutaneous "rabbit": a perceptual illusion. *Science*, 1972, *178*, 178–179.

Gibson, E. J., & Levin, H. *The psychology of reading*. Cambridge, Mass.: MIT Press, 1975.

Gilson, R. D. Some factors affecting the spatial discrimination of vibrotactile patterns. *Perception & Psychophysics*, 1968, *3*, 131–136.

Vibrotactile masking: some spatial and temporal aspects. *Perception & Psychophysics*, 1969, *5*, 176–180. (a)

Vibrotactile masking: effects of multiple maskers. *Perception & Psychophysics*, 1969, *5*, 181–182. (b)

Goldish, L. H., & Taylor, H. E. The Optacon: a valuable device for blind persons. *New Outlook for the Blind*, 1974, *68*, 49–56.

Gottheil, E. F., Cholewiak, R. W., & Sherrick, C. E. The discrimination of vibratory patterns on a tactile matrix. *Bulletin of the Psychonomic Society*, 1978, *11*, 21–24.

Hill, J. W. A describing function analysis of tracking performance using two tactile displays. *IEEE Transactions on Man–Machine Systems*, MMS-11, 1970, 92–101.

Processing of tactual and visual point stimuli sequentially presented at high rates. *Journal of Experimental Psychology*, 1971, *88*, 340–348.

Limited field of view in reading letter shapes with the fingers. In F. A. Geldard (Ed.), *Cutaneous communication systems and devices*. Austin, Tex.: Psychonomic Society, 1974, pp. 95–105.

Jansson, G. Human locomotion guided by a matrix of tactile point stimuli. In G. Gordon (Ed.), *Active touch. The mechanism of recognition of objects by manipulation: a multidisciplinary approach*. Oxford: Pergamon Press, 1978, pp. 229–242.

Kirman, J. H. Tactile communication of speech: a review and an analysis. *Psychological Bulletin*, 1973, *80*, 54–74.

Tactile pattern perception and tactile displays. Paper presented at the Conference on Interrelations of the Communicative Senses, Asilomar, Calif., September 1978.

Loomis, J. M. Tactile letter recognition under different modes of stimulus presentation. *Perception & Psychophysics*, 1974, *16*, 401–408.

Loomis, J. M., & Apkarian-Stielau, P. A lateral masking effect in tactile and blurred visual letter recognition. *Perception & Psychophysics*, 1976, *20*, 221–226.

Loomis, J. M., & Collins, C. C. Sensitivity to shifts of a point stimulus: an instance of tactile hyperacuity. *Perception & Psychophysics*, 1978, *24*, 487–492.

Mann, R. W. Technology and human rehabilitation: prostheses for sensory rehabilitation and/or sensory substitution. *Advances in Biomedical Engineering*, 1974, *4*, 209–353.

Massaro, D. W. *Experimental psychology and information processing*. Chicago: Rand McNally, 1975.

Moore, M. W., & Bliss, J. C. The Optacon reading system. *Education of the Visually Handicapped*, 1975, *7*, 15–21.

Rogers, C. H. The importance of vibration frequency in tactile pattern perception. Unpublished doctoral thesis, Stanford University, 1970. Cited by J. C. Bliss, Summary of Optacon-related cutaneous experiments. In F. A. Geldard (Ed.), *Cutaneous communications systems and devices*. Austin, Tex.: Psychonomic Society, 1974, pp. 84–94.

Scadden, L. A. Tactile pattern recognition and body loci. *Perception*, 1973, *2*, 333–336.

Sherrick, C. E. Effects of multiple simultaneous stimulation of the skin. *American Journal of Psychology*, 1964, *77*, 42–53.

Bilateral apparent haptic movement. *Perception & Psychophysics*, 1968, *4*, 159–162.

The art of tactile communication. *American Psychologist*, 1975, *30*, 353–360.

Cutaneous communication. In W. D. Neff (Ed.), *Contributions to sensory physiology*. New York: Academic Press, 1979.

Sherrick, C. E., & Rogers, R. Apparent haptic movement. *Perception & Psychophysics*, 1966, *1*, 175–180.

Taenzer, J. C. Visual word reading. *IEEE Transactions on Man–Machine Systems*, MMS-11, 1970, 44–53.

Telesensory Systems, Inc. *Optacon training*. Palo Alto, Calif.: TSI, 1973.

Triggs, T. J., Levison, W. H., & Sanneman, R. Some experience with flight-related electrocutaneous and vibrotactile displays. In F. A. Geldard (Ed.), *Cuta-*

neous communications systems and devices. Austin, Tex.: Psychonomic Society, 1974, pp. 57–64.

Turvey, M. T. On peripheral and central processes in vision: inferences from an information-processing analysis of masking with patterned stimuli. *Psychological Review*, 1973, *80*, 1–52.

Verrillo, R. T. Investigation of some parameters of the cutaneous threshold for vibration. *Journal of the Acoustical Society of America*, 1962, *34*, 1768–1773.

White, B. W. What other senses can tell us about cutaneous communication. In F. A. Geldard (Ed.), *Cutaneous communications systems and devices.* Austin, Tex.: Psychonomic Society, 1974, pp. 15–19.

White, B. W., Saunders, F. A., Scadden, L., Bach-y-Rita, P., & Collins, C. C. Seeing with the skin. *Perception & Psychophysics*, 1970, *7*, 23–27.

7. Current developments in tactile communication of speech

JACOB H. KIRMAN

In Chapter 7, Jacob Kirman discusses a set of problems pertinent to deaf and deaf–blind people's apprehension of speech, as well as the receptive-communicative capacities and potential of the skin senses. Kirman traces the historical failures to develop a tactile display of speech information, noting that many such efforts were abandoned before sufficient training had taken place to evaluate fully their possibilities, and without a full consideration of the capabilities of the skin as an information-processing system. He elaborates on the necessity to consider separately and evaluate the roles of speech signals, their transformation, and their mode of presentation in working with speech perception devices.

Examining systems as diverse as the Tadoma method (in which training in speech comprehension involves placing the auditor's hand(s) on the speaker's face) and microprocessors analyzing acoustical patterns and driving electrocutaneous stimulators, Kirman reviews and evaluates the import of recent research, both basic and applied. He discusses problems associated with several forms of sensory interaction as they pertain to tactile displays of speech patterns. He then raises the intriguing possibility that such problems may be circumvented by treating the skin like a slower-acting basilar membrane, which extracts meaningful information from such sensory interactions, rather than the interactions masking clearer and more punctate information. He then introduces the possibility that the skin's apparent capacity for making sense out of coherent, two-dimensional spatiotemporal patterns unfolding over time may have been neglected in work focusing on unidimensional spatial displays. The general import of J. J. Gibson's ideas concerning temporally extended stimulation effective for visual and tactual perception again looms large (Gibson, 1966, 1979).

After examining a number of machine-oriented techniques for presenting speech to the skin, Kirman examines the stimulation patterns of the more successful Tadoma method, attempting to develop templates for a better haptic speech perception device. For those interested in the applications of problems of speech comprehension, in prosthetic devices for deaf or deaf–blind persons, this chapter provides a wealth of material to consider, digest, and utilize in future work.

WILLIAM SCHIFF

Introduction

There are estimated to be over 13 million hearing-impaired people in the United States, of whom some 300,000 to 600,000 may be classified as having a profound hearing loss (Elliott, 1978). In addition, it is estimated there are about 10,000 to 15,000 deaf–blind Americans (Freiberger, Sherrick, & Scadden, 1977). Among them, those with a severe sensorineural hearing loss have no medical remedy available. Although there is currently considerable interest in the development of surgically implantable cochlear prostheses, it is not yet clear that such prostheses will have applicability to a wide range of deaf persons or be superior to less invasive tactile aids. Research is also aimed at improving and tailoring auditory hearing aids to the individual needs of the deaf, but there is evidence that whatever benefit the profoundly deaf obtain from auditory amplification is derived via a vibrotactile channel, even though such aids are not designed to engage effectively the tactile sense (Erber, 1978). These observations provide a powerful motive for the development of tactile aids for the communication and production of speech. This motive has been joined in recent years to a renewed optimism concerning the feasibility of using the skin for such purposes. More than a dozen laboratories are currently working on some aspect of this problem.

Modern interest in using the skin to transmit speech was sparked by the work of Gault in the 1920s (1924, 1926a,b, 1927; Gault & Crane, 1928), and several projects were begun during the following decades (Guelke & Huyssen, 1959; Keidel, 1958, 1968; Kringlebotn, 1968; Lovgren & Nykvist, 1959; Lucas, Steward, & Kreul, 1964; Nelson, 1959; Newman, 1960; Pickett, 1963; Pickett & Pickett, 1963; Wiener & Wiesner, 1949–1951). None of these efforts was rewarded by unequivocal success, leading to a widespread sense that the skin was not capable of transmitting a signal as complex as the speech stream. Such pessimism was reinforced by an influential theory that speech was a special code that could in principle be comprehended only by an intact auditory system (Liberman, Cooper, Shankweiler, & Studdert-Kennedy, 1967). From that perspective, there seemed little point in attempting to substitute another sense for defective hearing. The efforts at tactile communication of speech during this period as well as the theoretical issues involved were reviewed in earlier papers (Kirman, 1973; Levitt and Nye, 1971; Nickerson, 1975; Pickett, 1968).

Current workers in the area seem undeterred by earlier failures. It is now widely believed that the early work was often abandoned before a reasonable amount of training had permitted valid evaluations, and furthermore, due to a lack of sufficient information concerning both the limitations and capabilities of the skin, speech information was not applied so as to engage optimally a tactile perceptual capacity. Although the same problems of adequate training and effective matching of speech information to tactile perception continue to bedevil current workers, they tend to regard such difficulties as challenges to research ingenuity and patience rather than as indications of inherent limitations in the tactile sense. The argument that speech is a special code, and that any attempt to utilize substitute modalities is doomed to failure, is less compelling today. Some aspects of this argument can be questioned (Kirman, 1973), and recent dramatic demonstrations that subjects can learn to read speech spectrograms in a relatively short time (Cole, 1978) suggest that the acoustic speech signal may be decipherable by senses other than the auditory. The demonstrated usefulness of the Tadoma method (Norton, Schultz, Reed, Braida, Durlach, Rabinowitz, & Chomsky, 1977) is proof that tactile perception of connected speech is possible and encourages all current work. This successful method of tactile speech reading, which enabled the famous Helen Keller to communicate at normal speaking rates by placing her hand on the face of a speaker, will be discussed later in the chapter. It is true that this display gives a direct indication of articulation and is therefore, from the point of view of the speech code theory, less encoded. Should future research indicate that a direct reference to articulation is essential for any nonauditory display of speech, current developments in computer processing of speech permit the abstraction of many articulatory parameters from the acoustic stream with reasonable accuracy. Microprocessor technology promises to make such transforms available in real time even to portable tactile displays.

Tactile speech aids may be designed to assist the deaf or deaf–blind to achieve correct articulation or production of speech (production aids) or to improve the comprehension of spoken language (reception aids), either in conjunction with lipreading or as self-sufficient speech reception channels. They may be intended for use by adventitiously deafened, linguistically competent adults, congenitally deaf adults with linguistic skills, or prelingual deaf children or infants. A researcher may be concerned either with the portability and comfort of such aids or with the effectiveness of the system without regard for immediate wearable application. Current work is primarily concerned with the development of reception aids, and these seem to be about evenly divided between intended applications in conjunction with lipreading and as self-sufficient channels. The choice of combining an aid with lipreading or not seems to depend more on the beliefs and aspirations of the researcher than on the demonstrated capacity or limitation of any given device. Although several workers have expressed an awareness that early application of such devices to young prelingual children should have the greatest impact, almost all research is done with linguistically competent adults or older children, and the most common research subjects are normally hearing adults who have been artificially deafened by masking noise during testing. This choice is apparently dictated by both convenience and the belief that these subjects are likely to permit a first-level evaluation of various transformation and display schemes, and that only such aids with proven value with adult subjects should be tried on very young children. Very few devices have thus far been designed to be totally portable, again reflecting the opinion that further development and evaluation are likely to be necessary before the extensive engineering efforts required to produce portable aids are justified.

Tactile speech: its source, transform, and mode of display

Any attempt to communicate speech through the tactile sense must consider several interrelated questions: (1) Which of the physical manifestations of speech shall be selected for presentation? (2) How shall these events be transformed, if at all? (3) How shall the resulting signals be applied to activate the tactile sense? In the history of research on tactile speech communication, these questions have rarely been separately considered or independently evaluated. Almost all workers have investigated a single device that incorporated one specific method of displaying a particular version of speech information. Although efforts have often gone into improving a given device after initial testing, such efforts have consisted of refinements rather than comparative examinations of various possible transforms or display modes. The style of work has been more characteristic of the individual inventor than of the systematic researcher. Any effort to review published results for the purposes of comparative evaluation of different devices is impeded by the use of different training methods and subject populations, and even if one could conclude, however tentatively, that one device is superior to another, it would not be clear whether the superiority is due to differences in the signals applied to the skin or to differences in the mode of presentation. It has therefore not yet been possible to disentangle the respective contributions of the information source, the transform, and the mode of display to the overall performance of each system. This has contributed to a situation, often noted, in which workers find it difficult to build upon previous efforts in developing more effective designs. Only very recently

237

have workers in this area been interested in investigating the relative effectiveness of various modes of presentation of the same information. Perhaps the applied nature of this many-faceted problem and a sense of urgency concerning its solution have led to impatience with its systematic and analytic exploration. However, even if one or more of the current efforts at tactile speech communication should prove highly useful, future attempts to optimize such devices will require firm knowledge about how different modes of tactile display can cope with various aspects of speech.

Articulatory displays

Given various sources of information about speech events the major distinction is between those derived more or less directly from monitoring the articulatory gestures of a speaker and those derived from the acoustic speech signal. In addition to posing entirely different problems for the design of appropriate tactile displays, these two categories would have very different areas of application. The acoustic displays have more uses in situations in which the distance between the speaker and the listener is too great for direct tactile contact, or when the speaker cannot readily be encumbered by monitoring devices.

Direct tactile perception of articulatory gestures has long been used by teachers of the deaf. In the 1920s, Alcorn (1932) brought to the United States a systematic method of teaching speech reception and production to the deaf–blind based on this approach: the Tadoma method. In this method, which has been described by Vivian (1966), the deaf–blind student places a hand on the speaker's face and learns to distinguish a sufficient number of speech events to be able successfully to comprehend ordinary connected speech. Given that this is the only method that has been proved effective, it is remarkable that systematic study of the basis for its success has begun only in the past 2 years. Preliminary reports of this work currently underway at MIT (Norton et al., 1977) have substantiated, at least for one subject, that successful communication at normal speaking rates is possible with this method. This research is clarifying which aspects of speech are best transmitted. For example, this subject has been shown to detect consonants better than vowels and manner cues better than place cues. As might be expected, consonant confusions were most common in a manner class in which lip movements or rounding provided minimal distinctive information (e.g., /l/ vs. /n/ and /t/ vs. /k/). He did well in detecting voicing and in judging the syllabic length of sentences, but he did not detect nasality or utilize intonation and stress

238

cues even though he could detect them. Interestingly, this subject performed better on identification than on discrimination tasks, and he showed a much greater use of context in identifying sequences of words than do normal listeners. Whether these last two observations are peculiar to this subject or reflect a general adaptation to the requirements of this speech display must await further investigation, but they may suggest that Tadoma users deal with speech in larger perceptual units than do normal listeners.

In the Tadoma method, the articulatory source of speech information is not subject to experimental transformation, nor is the mode of tactile display capable of being seriously altered, with the exception of variations in hand placement on the speaker's face. The MIT group, however, plans to build an artificial Tadoma display that will be controlled by sensing devices placed on the speaker's face. This intriguing project will not only make it possible to analyze precisely the contribution of all the articulatory cues, as begun by Hansen (1964) but should also allow the introduction of different transforms of the source signals as well as different modes of tactile display of this information. It may well be that a better match can be achieved between articulatory information and tactile capacity than that naturally obtained with a hand on a face. It is quite remarkable that Tadoma users do so well, considering that facial speech movements and tactile perceptual capacity did not develop together in the course of human evolution with the kind of mutual interdependence that occurred between speaking and hearing. There is no guarantee that the tactile salience of cues is proportional to their information contribution. In addition, it is clear that some important articulatory cues, which are derivable by the normal listener from the acoustic signal, are not available on the speaker's face – as preliminary research has already demonstrated. This synthetic Tadoma display, in addition to permitting transformations and remapping of articulatory signals to tactile display features, will allow the introduction of signals derived from the acoustic signal. Such linguistic cues, not available from sensors on the speaker's face, should make a valuable contribution to a hybrid display based on both acoustic and articulatory sources of information about speech events.

Acoustic displays

The most straightforward tactile display of the acoustic speech signal consists of feeling it directly with the skin; that is precisely how modern research on this topic began. Gault's first attempts at tactile speech communication (1924) consisted of speaking through a hollow tube, 4.3 m (14 ft) long, which was held against the palm of a subject whose hearing had been masked. Even with this simple arrangement, several dozen words could be distinguished. In the interest of improving on this display, Gault then proceeded to the next simplest display of the speech signal – a single vibrator display of the electronically amplified signal. Gault's further efforts (1924, 1926a, b, 1927; Gault & Crane, 1928) with such vibratory speech displays did show early promise in discriminating sentences, isolated words, and vowel sounds, but most segmental phonemic discriminations were not possible, and his early hope that he had "demonstrated the possibility of acquiring the art of interpreting speech by means of touch" (1926b, p. 132) ended in disappointment. It is now generally agreed that the skin does not have the temporal resolving power to deal with the high-frequency content of the speech signal.

The skin, though faster than the eye on several measures of temporal resolution, is clearly much slower than the ear. Von Békésy (1967) found that the time required for a vibratory stimulus to reach full sensation is about 1.2 sec compared with about 0.2 sec for the ear. Lechelt (1974) has shown that the skin is considerably better than the eye at estimating the number of pulses in a stimulus train at rates of presentation above 3 per second, but it deteriorates sharply at faster rates compared with the ear. Gescheider (1970) demonstrated that the time interval necessary to resolve two pulses at separate loci was about 10 msec for the skin and less than 2 msec for the ear. Efron (1973) reported that the skin was poorer than the ear in perceiving a "micropattern" consisting of two rapidly successive stimuli of different frequencies applied to the same locus. Tactile discrimination of vibratory frequency was found by Goff (1967) to fall off severely at rates approaching 200 Hz. Equally discouraging for vibratory frequency encoding in tactile displays is the observation (von Békésy, 1967) that perceived vibratory pitch is markedly influenced by stimulus amplitude. On the positive side, Franzen and Nordmark (1975), using a different psychophysical method and short (1.5 msec) rectangular pulses as inputs to their vibrator rather than sinusoids, found frequency discrimination to be much better than Goff had reported, with a Weber fraction of about 0.03 for all frequencies up to 256 pulses per second. Rothenberg, Verrillo, Zahorian, Brachman, and Bolanowski (1975) also observed frequency discrimination to be better with short pulses (though not as good as those reported by Franzen and Nordmark) and found that variations in pulse repetition rate do not produce changes in subjective magnitude. Furthermore, pulsed stimuli produce lower absolute thresholds and greater suprathreshold sensitivity than sinusoidal vibrations and offer an additional codable dimension – pulse rise and fall times –

that Rothenberg et al. report is "felt as a parameter clearly different from the pulse amplitude or frequency over a wide range of frequencies" (p. 9). In short, modulated pulse trains may offer a significant improvement over sinusoidal vibration for tactile displays.

Even though vibratory presentation of the amplified time waveform of speech is an inadequate display for speech reception, it has been shown to provide some important linguistic information that can supplement other limited presentations of speech, such as lipreading. Gault's original work, as well as the observations of others (Fraisse, 1963; Katz, in Krueger, 1970; Manning, Pasquali & Smith, 1975), indicate clearly that a single vibrator can transmit the syllabic structure of speech and that vibratory rhythms are very well perceived. Schulte (1977) has been using a single vibrator both in speech training and as an adjunct to lipreading. The recent work of Erber (1972, 1978) has demonstrated that vibratory displays can provide considerable information about the gross time–intensity envelope of speech and can serve as a useful aid to lipreading. Erber estimates that such vibratory displays can increase comprehension scores about 10 percent over lipreading alone.

Anyone interested in transmitting additional information about the segmental features of speech to the skin must clearly do more than amplify the acoustic signal. Once it is granted that some transformation is necessary, a limitless range of possibilities is open. Although we have considerable information on which aspects of the acoustic signal can serve as cues for the auditory perception of speech, the question of what information should be used in a tactile display of speech is still open. Pickett (1978) suggests that researchers on speech aids tend to fall into one of two camps: the "brain" workers, who hope that the brain will somehow manage to organize linguistically a rich, complex tactile speech display, and the "machine" workers, who prefer the use of machines to preprocess the speech signal into a form more compatible with the presumably limited information-processing abilities of the skin. Currently available transformations of the speech signal can differ widely in terms of how much of the original information in the acoustic signal is preserved in the tactile transformation. At one extreme would be those transformations that attempt to preserve all of the acoustic information, or at least as much as possible, while mapping this information onto some suitable set of dimensions of tactile stimulation. One example of such a display is a single-channel vibratory or pulsed device operating in the frequency domain that transposes the frequencies of the acoustic signal down to a range more compatible with the skin's vibratory sensitivity. Interestingly, although such transposition devices have been tested with auditory displays, no systematic evaluation of a comparable tactile display has been made. At the other extreme is a display that uses a microprocessor to analyze the speech signal and make linguistic decisions as to the phonemic categorization of segments of the speech stream. The output of such a device would be a string of phonemic elements or features, representing perhaps 60 bits per second of information compared with the thousands of bits in the original acoustic signal. Again, although such phonemic feature-extracting devices have been tested, more work has been done with the visual modality (Cornett, 1977; Upton, 1968) than with the tactile sense. The transformations of the acoustic signal that have been investigated for tactile displays have typically been intermediate between the above extremes and have usually relied on some form of spectral analysis based on sets of band-pass filters.

Although most such frequency domain transforms have attempted to use arrays of vibrators or electrocutaneous stimulators to represent frequency information spatially on the skin, a few have applied such outputs to a single locus. Traunmuller (1977) has reported on a sophisticated single vibratory display to be used in conjunction with lipreading. The signal that energizes his vibrator has its frequency determined by the ratio of energies in high-pass and low-pass bands of the acoustic signal, and its amplitude is a suitably compressed version of the amplitude envelope of the original signal. Traunmuller has found that this display transmits a significant amount of segmental phonemic information in addition to the prosodic information usually available from single vibratory displays of the untransformed speech signal. Scott, De Filippo, Sachs, and Miller (1977) have developed a combined vibratory-electrocutaneous display that aims at presenting to the same region of the hand an integratable stimulus that preserves the time–intensity envelope of speech and uses the differences in sensation quality contributed by mechanical and electrical stimulation to provide some spectral information. Interestingly, one of their electrocutaneous stimulators, recently added to the display, not only represents the output of a band-pass filter but is an amplitude-modulated train of square waves whose frequency is proportional to that of the first formant. Thus, in this sophisticated addition, they have used a form of parameter tracking and combined it with pulsed square waves whose frequency and amplitude convey information. Their display, when used as an adjunct to lipreading, has been shown to increase the rate of speech reception for two subjects from 36 and 54 wpm for lipreading alone to 54 and 71 wpm for the combined presentation.

One-dimensional spatial displays

The device developed by Scott et al. (1977) is unique in that it presents spectral information in the form of variations in the quality of tactile sensation experienced at essentially the same locus of stimulation. The other devices that transform the acoustic waveform into the frequency domain, usually with filter banks, attempt to utilize spatial locus as the tactile dimension onto which frequency is mapped. This approach, taking into account the limited temporal resolving power of the skin, and cognizant that the ear transforms a temporal pattern at the eardrum into a spatiotemporal pattern on the basilar membrane, attempts to accomplish tactile transmission of speech by supplying the skin with some form of external cochlea.

The most direct application of this idea is the work of Keidel (1974). He and his co-workers have been using the electromechanical model of the cochlea developed by von Békésy (1955), in which traveling waves presumably similar to those developed on the basilar membrane are applied directly to the skin of the forearm. Early reports of this work (1958, 1968) indicated considerable success with phoneme and word recognition, although the results were described in a somewhat sketchy fashion and the technique was hampered by the necessity of slowing the speech input by a factor of 1:4, thereby eliminating the possibility of real-time speech reception or correlation with lipreading or articulation. Keidel's recent report (1974) describes a computer approach to the solution of this problem in which the frequency components of speech are lowered by removing segments of the speech signal and joining the remaining segments with smooth transitions. Keidel reported that this system was under investigation and that "the preliminary results are very promising, because (a) it now works in real time, (b) tactile memory is not overloaded, and (c) vibrotactile information can be combined with that from other sensory modalities" (1974, p. 31). The results that might bear out this promise, however, have not yet been reported.

Several earlier projects had utilized some form of tactile vocoder to map speech frequencies into a spatial dimension. The vocoder, developed at Bell Telephone Laboratories in the late 1930s, divides the speech spectrum into a number of frequency channels by means of a set of band-pass filters. The output of each filter, after suitable rectification and low-pass filtering, constitutes a relatively slowly changing voltage that is proportional to the vicissitudes of energy in that pass-band of the spectrum. Such filter outputs can modulate the intensities of a set of audio oscillators (to reconstruct an acoustic version of the original speech signal), or a set of lights (as in experiments on visible speech), or a set of vibrators, as in the work discussed here. Again, Gault was the first to use this approach (Gault & Crane, 1928). He divided the speech spectrum by means of five band-pass filters, the outputs of which were used to activate vibrators on each of the five fingers. Wiener and Wiesner (1949–1951) explored a very similar five-channel device, which was then expanded to include seven pass-bands. A later version (Witcher, 1956) used six channels to control small vibrators arranged in the format of a braille cell. Guelke and Huyssen (1959) developed a more refined version of this kind of display utilizing eight filter channels, each of which was further subdivided by 20 tuned resonant reeds, resulting in a display that resolved the speech spectrum from 410 to 2,880 Hz into 160 tactile loci on one hand. Lovgren and Nykvist (1959) described a tactile vocoder that utilized 10 filter channels applied to the 10 fingertips. This device was more systematically evaluated in later reports by Pickett (1963; Pickett & Pickett, 1963). Kringlebotn (1968) reported on a five-channel device that used various divisions of speech zero-crossings to activate each vibrator. These devices have been considered in greater detail in an earlier paper (Kirman, 1973). All these efforts had two features in common. First, they all represented the frequency domain of the speech signal by a linear arrangement of vibrators (except that the Guelke and Huyssen device ran this linear arrangement up and down the length of all five fingers), and the amount of energy in each pass-band was represented by vibratory amplitude. Second, they were all abandoned after relatively brief evaluation, and none was used in a long-term systematic training program.

Recent projects aimed at mapping the frequency domain of the speech signal onto a tactile locus have attempted to improve on these earlier efforts either by implementing a more systematic and longer period of training or by trying a different mode of displaying spectral information, or both. Although most current researchers on this problem place more emphasis on the need for adequate training and testing procedures than did the early workers, Englemann and Rosov (1975) are perhaps the most emphatic. As they say:

> The present experiment was based on the idea that the vocoding devices used in the past were adequate to provide a suitable display of speech. However, adequate training was lacking . . . Previous . . . investigators seemed to assume that if the display provided the information needed for adequate speech perception, the subject would learn quickly, if not instantly. The assumption underlying the present study was that a great deal of practice would be needed. (p. 244)

Accordingly, they have used a straightforward tactile vocoder of 23 channels, activating a corresponding number of vibrators linearly arranged in sets of four or five and placed either on the fingers, forearms, or legs. Fifteen channels divided the frequency range from 200 to 4,000 Hz into equal logarithmic intervals, with four low-frequency channels extending the range to 85 Hz and four high-frequency channels extending the upper range to 10,000 Hz. Their initial report (1975) of results with normal and deaf subjects indicated that both groups were able to learn substantial vocabularies of tactually presented words, with one deaf child acquiring 152 words after 48 weeks of training. Interestingly, they observed that new words could be learned more quickly as training proceeded. Another noteworthy observation was that subjects did quite well at perceiving sentences composed of familiar words, even though relatively little training time had been devoted to working with connected speech. A more recent paper (Englemann & Skillman, 1977) is focused entirely on a systematic instructional procedure. These authors concluded that "even very fine speech discriminations were mastered with practice and . . . the prosthesis . . . was capable of providing the basis for normalizing the speech and language behavior of profoundly deaf children" (p. 2). These reports suggest that with sufficient practice, any speech feature can be successfully discriminated with this display, although no analytical data are presented to indicate the relative ease of learning various features of speech or, indeed, to certify that all features can be reliably perceived.

Saunders, Hill, and Simpson (1976) have also utilized a vocoder transform in a project that has paid considerable attention to training. They have implemented a computer-assisted instructional program that permits a sophisticated and flexible approach to training. Their 20-channel filter bank, which ranges from 190 to 6,200 Hz, activates an electrocutaneous display. The amount of energy in each pass-band determines the subjective intensity of each correlated stimulator by controlling the number of biphasic, constant-current pulses in successive bursts presented at a 100-Hz rate. The stimulating electrodes, designed by Saunders to be pain free, are arranged linearly on a belt worn around the waist. Early phonemic discrimination tests obtained accuracy scores ranging from 66 to 80 percent for pairs of vowels; 85 percent for the voicing contrast in /t–d/ and /s–z/; 82 percent for the nasality feature; 87 percent for fricative place of articulation; 58 percent for plosive place of articulation; and chance performance for discriminations between /l–r/ and /m–n/. In addition, scores between 72 and 85 percent were obtained on tests with sets of isolated words after very limited training, and good preliminary results were obtained as well with the perception of words combined into sentences. Systematic evaluation and training with this device are continuing, and future reports should indicate its potential and limitations.

All of the vocoder devices translating frequency into space thus far mentioned utilized a one-dimensional spatial array along which each locus was stimulated in varying amplitudes according to the energy in the corresponding pass-band. The number of such loci ranged from 5 to 160, and the unidimensional array was positioned along the fingertips, up and down the length of all the fingers of one hand, or on the arms, legs, or waist; but nonetheless they all used location along one spatial dimension to indicate frequency, and they all represented energy at each frequency by stimulator amplitude. A subject confronted with such a display must base perceptual judgments on the locus and relative intensity of several simultaneously active and shifting points of stimulation along a single spatial dimension. The early workers using this type of display commented on the interference produced by such simultaneous stimulation. Gault and Crane (1928) observed that several of the vibrators could not be perceived when all five were simultaneously active, and Guelke and Huyssen (1959) similarly noted the difficulty of "determination and localization of two or more simultaneous stimuli" (p. 804). Pickett and Pickett (1963) also found that "only one diffuse peak of a momentary pattern could be easily discerned" (p. 219). More recent workers have not described such effects, though it is doubtful that they have ceased to exist.

Tactile stimulus interactions

Interactions among simultaneous tactile stimuli have been discussed in a recent paper (Kirman, 1978).

> Multiple simultaneous stimulation of the skin is beset with gross interactions, such that few stimulated loci may be perceptually resolved, and even these are likely to be altered in subjective intensity and spatially displaced (Békésy, 1967; Gilson, 1969). As the number of simultaneously applied point stimuli is increased beyond two or three, their localization and detection accuracy decrease sharply even when the stimulators are widely separated on the body surface and regardless of whether the stimuli are electrocutaneous or vibratory pulses or single pressures (Allusi, Morgan, & Hawkes, 1965; Brown, Nibarber, Ollie, & Solomon, 1967; Geldard & Hahn, 1961; Posey & James, 1976). Masking effects with such multiple stimulators have been shown to be a nearly additive func-

tion of the number of simultaneous stimuli (Gilson, 1969). Even with only two equally "loud" stimulators, the subjective experience will be of one "phantom" sensation located midway between the stimulators, provided the distance between them is not too great. Békésy (1967) has named this effect "funneling" because the resulting unitary sensation shows amplitude summation from both sources. He reported an especially impressive demonstration of funncling with five vibrators, each activated with equal loudness at a different frequency and spaced 2 centimeters apart on the forearm. Only the center vibrator was felt at its frequency, but with the other four masked vibrators contributing to its loudness. There is evidence that such funneling is central in origin. (Gardner & Spencer, 1972; Kirman, 1978, p. 5)

To complicate matters further, tactile stimuli have been shown to interact grossly even when they are not simultaneous.

Previous investigations with two loci have demonstrated extensive spatiotemporal interaction. As has been discussed earlier . . . two points stimulated simultaneously can be experienced as only one point sensation situated midway between the two stimulators. If a time difference is introduced between the two stimulators, the subjectively experienced point begins to move toward the point first stimulated, becoming totally localized under that stimulator as the time interval is increased to between 2 msec. (Békésy, 1967) or 6 msec. (Gescheider, 1974). By the time the interval has exceeded about 20 msec., Geldard (1975) reports a third "phantom" pulse in the region between the two stimulators (though he says this phenomenon is more vivid if the first pulse is preceded by an additional "localizing" pulse at the first stimulator). As the interval is lengthened still further, the "phantom" pulse shifts closer to the first stimulator, until at about 300 msec., it is no longer differentiated from the first veridical pulse. Beyond this 300 msec. interval, such interactions are no longer found. In addition to such mislocalizations, interactions that affect apparent intensity – both enhancement and suppression – occur within this time period. If such interactions as the above occur between only two successive points, it is evident that a succession of many points . . . must produce a complex situation. (Kirman, 1978, pp. 11–12)

One may take the position that such simultaneous and successive stimulus interactions occur to some degree on all sensory surfaces, and that they are only a psychophysicist's bird's-eye view of perceptual organization. It is true that von Békésy's work on funneling effects on the skin was at least partly motivated by an interest in understanding similar processes occurring on the basilar membrane. One might hope that the stimulus interaction on the skin is sufficiently like that on the basilar membrane so that such interactions will facilitate rather than impede the extraction of linguistically meaningful percepts from the welter and flux of stimulation. Such a belief was reflected in Gault's early proposition that the skin is an evolutionary ancestor of the ear, and Keidel's work with the cochlear model also seems to suggest that the skin is a kind of slower basilar membrane. However, it is interesting that workers attempting to use the skin as a substitute for vision have suggested that the skin is much like a rudimentary retina (Apkarian-Stielau & Loomis, 1975; Daley & Singer, 1975; Loomis, 1974). Although it may be true that both the eye and the ear have evolved from a more basic sensory surface, it is likely that the skin – or better, the haptic sense (Gibson, 1966) – has followed its own evolutionary course, and it may be more appropriate to treat it as an independent perceptual system rather than as an ancient relative of the ear or the eye. In practical terms, this suggests that mapping auditory or visual stimuli onto the tactile sense would be optimized by a prior understanding of tactile perceptual organization in its own right. Although there are a few studies in the literature on this organization, the area is largely terra incognita at the present time.

Two-dimensional spatial displays

In an earlier paper, I suggested that whereas the ear is most effective with temporal patterns and the eye with static spatial patterns,* the skin is most effective with coherent spatiotemporal patterns (Kirman, 1973). That paper also argued that unidimensional spatial displays, such as those discussed above, cannot optimally engage the skin's capacity for organizing spatiotemporal patterns, and that it is unnatural to ask the skin to recognize which fingertip or which of several points on a line were being stimulated and to what degree. It was proposed instead to present patterns on a two-dimensional display in which successive points of stimulation would be integrated by tactile apparent movement into spatiotemporally coherent shapes unfolding over time.

Several such displays of speech have since been reported. It is difficult to judge the relative effectiveness of one- and two-dimensional displays because each project used different subjects and training methods, and

---

* Editor's note: Many perceptual psychologists would disagree with this conceptualization, holding instead that the visual system has also evolved to be especially responsive to spatiotemporal patterns. (W. S.)

comparisons are impeded by a lack of analytical data in some reports. However, one study that investigated both methods did find a two-dimensional display to be superior. This project first investigated a 16-channel vocoder whose outputs energized a 3 by 16 matrix of piezoelectric vibrators that was about 0.6 by 1.5 cm (0.24 by 0.59 in) in size (Ifukube & Yoshimoto, 1974). Although the design of this matrix would have permitted the use of two spatial dimensions, identical spectral information was displayed on the three columns, resulting effectively in a unidimensional spatial array. After a brief period of training (20 to 30 min), they found that five vowels were identified with an accuracy of 91 percent, and five consonants paired with the vowel /u/ were identified with an average of 66 percent accuracy. The second report on this project (Ifukube, Yoshimoto, & Shoji, 1977) described a modification of the display such that the three columns no longer represented the same speech information. Instead, the spectrum at any moment was displayed on the right column of 16 vibrators, with spectral values that occurred 5 msec previously displayed on the center column and values that occurred 10 msec previously displayed on the left column. The authors refer to this as a *scanned mode*. The display now utilized both spatial dimensions, one for frequency and one for time, and should have produced short, undulating, curved segments across the display. This modification improved consonant identification scores from 66 percent with all three columns carrying the same information (spatially unidimensional) to about 77 percent with the two-dimensional display. An additional modification of the scanned mode consisted of reducing the intensity of vowel portions of the speech signal; this increased consonant identification scores to about 83 percent. The authors also explored the effect of slowing the vocoder output presentation rate. They found that the unidimensional display was markedly affected, with the best results obtained by a reduction of 1:4. The scanned modes were less influenced by rate, and the scanned mode with reduced vowel intensities gave almost the same results at any rate.

Yeni-Komshian and Goldstein (1977) investigated a very similar piezoelectric matrix, a modified Optacon. They used 18 of the 24 available rows of the 24 by 6 Optacon array to display the outputs of an 18-channel vocoder in a manner analogous to that used by Ifukube and his associates. The second spatial dimension, in this case the six columns, was utilized in quite a different manner, however. Instead of presenting time-delayed versions of the vocoder outputs, as had Ifukube, they used the six columns to represent the intensity of each channel. From one to six of the vibrators in each row were activated according to the momentary intensity of the corresponding vocoder channel. The normal adult subjects were trained over a 6-week period in 30 half-hour sessions on three sets of speech sounds: four synthetic vowel durations, three vowels, and four spondee words. The results were surprisingly poor. After this relatively extensive training (compared with the 20 to 30 min used by Ifukube), subjects achieved identification scores of 94 percent on the six vowel durations, 75 percent on the three vowels, and 71 percent on the four spondee words. When these results on small sets of relatively simple stimuli are compared with those obtained by Ifukube, it would appear that a frequency versus intensity display is inferior to a frequency versus time display, but a study of the two presentation modes on the same subjects under the same conditions would be necessary to settle the matter.

One other frequency versus intensity display has been investigated by Sparks, Kuhl, Edmonds, and Gray (1978). This group used a belt of 36 by 8 electrocutaneous stimulations worn around the abdomen and driven by the output of a 36-channel cochlear filter. Frequency was represented by the 36 rows, and channel intensity was displayed on the eight columns. Unlike the Yeni-Komshian and Goldstein display, however, only one stimulator was active regardless of channel intensity, and only the position of that stimulator in the row of eight indicated intensity. Normal adult subjects were trained for a year in 35 sessions lasting about 90 min. This device, conceived as an aid to lipreading, was used in training and testing in conjunction with lipreading as well as by itself. Only results for the tactile-alone condition will be reported here. By the end of the training period, one subject was able to identify eight vowels in a /b–d/ context with an accuracy of 95 percent for tokens from a single talker and was then tested in a multiple-talker situation with a resulting identification score of 76 percent. Two other subjects were trained for a shorter period on consonant recognition in consonant–vowel (CV) syllables with both constant and varying vowel contexts. Identification scores for six stops and two nasal consonants were between 20 and 45 percent for one subject with a constant vowel context and about 50 percent with a varying vowel context after further training. The other subject, who was trained with a single vowel in CV, vowel–consonant–vowel (VCV), and vowel–consonant (VC) contexts, achieved identification scores that approached 50 percent with the consonant in final position and somewhat lower scores with the consonant in initial and medial positions. These data were also analyzed in terms of phonemic feature recognition. Voicing was distinguished among stop consonants with an accuracy approaching 100 percent, whereas place of articulation was correctly identified only 40 percent of the time. The manner distinction between stops and nasals was perceived with an accuracy of nearly 100 percent. A fourth subject was trained and tested with nine fricative consonants in a CV context with a single vowel over eight sessions. Identification of these fricatives asymptoted at about 70 percent correct. A phonemic feature analysis showed that voicing was correctly detected with an accuracy of over 90 percent, and the score for place of articulation approached 80 percent. These data indicate that a considerable amount of segmental information was transmitted by this device, but differences in the transform, region of skin used, and training procedure make it difficult to isolate the effects of the display mode for comparison with the two piezoelectric displays described above.[1]

Two additional reports described the use of two-dimensional displays in a frequency versus time mode. Kirman (1974) used a 15 by 15 matrix of solenoid vibrators spaced 0.2 in apart, which was felt by the palm. The speech samples were analyzed by a formant-tracking computer program to obtain the two lowest formants displayed on the vibrator array. These two frequency values, sampled at a 100-Hz rate, were entered vertically on the leftmost column of the array and were then shifted one column to the right every succeeding 10 msec as new formant values were entered on the left. The display thus presented current formant values along with the preceding 14 values, thereby simultaneously displaying a 150-msec time window of the speech sample. No information about speech or formant intensity was displayed. Normal adult subjects were trained for about 30 sessions on a list of 15 common words selected to contain only vowels and vowellike speech sounds (that is, no fricative, plosive, or nasal consonants were included). Subjects were first trained on a slowly spoken pronunciation of the list, then on a fast pronunciation by the same speaker. They were tested on both pronunciations and then were tested without further training on three additional pronunciations by this speaker and three by three different speakers. After training, subjects averaged 83 percent correct identifications on the first pronunciation, 70 percent on the second, and 54 percent on the three additional new pronunciations by the same speaker. When tested on three different speakers, the average identification score was 35 percent. The data were analyzed in confusion matrices, and the major phonemic contributors to erroneous performance were identified. It should be noted that, although these scores were not very high, they were achieved solely with the display of frequency information about the first two formants, with none of the indication of speech intensity that was included in all the other displays discussed.

251

Spens (1975) used a similar transform on an Optacon display. He sampled speech every 16 msec and used a computer to calculate the intensity and center of gravity of two frequency ranges, 50 to 800 Hz and 700 to 3,600 Hz, selected to cover the regions of the first and second formants, respectively. The two frequencies representing the centers of gravity of the formants were coded on the 24 rows of the Optacon, and their intensities were presented by energizing, in addition to the vibrator representing the center frequency, the one above it for moderate intensities and both the one above and the one below for high intensities. Normal adults were tested on recorded pronunciations of the 10 Swedish numerals, and after about 7,000 trials, one subject achieved an asymptotic accuracy of about 94 percent. When tested on a faster pronunciation by the same speaker, 81 percent accuracy was obtained, and with a normally spoken pronunciation by a different speaker, a score of 86 percent was obtained. Noting that Kirman's display had used 15 columns, each presenting previous formant values separated by 10 msec with a resulting total time window of 150 msec, Spens was interested in varying this window to determine its optimum value. He investigated this by extending Ifukube's technique of controlling the number of columns that displayed the same time sample of spectral values. For a minimum time window, all six columns of the Optacon received the same current spectral values; for a window of 32 msec, the previously sampled spectral values were displayed on three of the columns, along with a presentation of the current values on the remaining three columns. In this manner, additional time windows of 48 and 96 msec were tried as well. There was some indication in the data obtained that the 48-msec time window yielded the best results, but in a later report (Spens, 1977), the transmission of speech information was found to increase with increasing time windows out to 96 msec, which was the maximum that could be tested with the six column Optacon and a 16-msec sampling rate. Spens concluded that, although the optimum value for this window was not yet established, some such window did improve tactile reception of speech. This result is in accord with that of Ifukube (who tested two values of this time window with a faster sampling rate). Both of these studies represent all too rare examples of systematic exploration of display parameters in the tactile presentation of speech information.

With respect to my suggestion (Kirman, 1973) that two-dimensional spatial displays would present coherent spatiotemporal patterns more congenial to tactile perceptual organization than those available from linear displays, the evidence thus far is equivocal. Although frequency versus time displays have been shown to be superior to linear displays in both studies that compared the two, at least one report of a frequency versus intensity two-dimensional display described rather poor results. Even though projects differ on so many variables as to preclude valid comparisons on the effects of display mode, the data suggest that the manner in which the two spatial dimensions are utilized will influence the results. It is, however, not clear whether the apparent superiority of frequency versus time displays is due to the suitability for tactile organization of the stimulus patterning in space and time; to the transformation of rapid temporal patterns into more enduring shifting spatial patterns; to the relief provided tactile preperceptual memory by accumulating for simultaneous presentation the recent history of the spectral pattern of speech; or perhaps to some other unspecified factor.

Phonemic tactile displays

Several projects have presented one or more phonemic or articulatory features to the tactile sense. Some have derived these features from the acoustic speech signal, and others have directly monitored articulatory events (Edmondson, 1977; Ling and Sofin, 1975; Martony, 1974; Miller, Engebretson, & De Filippo, 1974; Spens, 1975; Stratton, 1974; Willemain & Lee, 1972). Such displays have been shown to be of value in improving speech articulation by the deaf as well as augmenting speech reception in conjunction with lipreading. No reports have yet appeared, however, on a device that attempts to take maximum advantage of current technology for the reduction of speech information, a tactile display of machine-categorized phonemic strings. There is no doubt that such machine recognition would produce erroneous categorizations. But although such errors are a major impediment for completely autonomous machine recognition of speech, the human perceiver of a tactile display of automatically categorized phonemes would be able to supply a knowledge of context and syntax not available in any computer system. The tolerable machine error rate for such a human–machine system is not yet known, but this information may soon be forthcoming from anticipated experiments on the question by H. Levitt and his colleagues (Levitt, pers. comm., 1978). The effectiveness of such a tactile display of machine-recognized phoneme strings should be increased if the tactile output is made to reflect the probability of correctness of each phonemic segment. That is, phonemic elements that are categorized with a high degree of confidence by the processer could be tactually displayed by a specific, definite, and salient tactile pattern, whereas those phonemic elements that are categorized with very low confidence could be displayed by tactile patterns that are themselves perceptually ambiguous. It may be possible to devise tactile patterns that are intermediate in their perceptual categorization between two or more contending phonemic elements. Such patterns should reflect the degree of ambiguity in the phonemic categorization. When, for example, the processer is fairly certain that a segment is a fricative, but is not confident of which specific fricative is indicated, the tactile display could also indicate a fricative but be ambiguous about its identity. This approach should reduce the most catastrophic effects of misidentifications by the machine processer while preserving as much information as possible in the tactile output.

Researchers considering this approach to tactile speech communication would have to face squarely problems of tactile perceptual organization that workers with other speech-transforming devices have dealt with only marginally. Given the freedom to devise any tactile output for a machine-recognized phonemic string, it would be necessary to consider how to compose a set of tactile patterns that are salient, distinctive, and capable of comprehension at rapid rates of presentation.

There should be little difficulty in obtaining some set of tactile patterns that could be mapped on to the set of phonemes. One could use the set of braille characters, alphabetic shapes, or a unique tactile set such as that designed by Geldard (1966). All of these are likely to work, but only at the relatively slow rates produced in their past applications to reading. Of these alphabets, braille is probably the fastest, but it is by no means clear that it is an optimal tactile code, especially because the output of a phoneme recognizer would present the equivalent of uncontracted braille. It is likely that the superimposition of prosodic patterns of stress and rhythm on the phonemic string would assist the tactile perceiver in segmenting and organizing the tactile stream in a manner that has not been possible with current embossed tactile displays. This addition in itself should improve the speed of comprehension, but other considerations may be relevant.

In particular, it may be necessary to devise the alphabet so that sequences of phonemes, especially those with high sequential dependencies, are displayed by tactile patterns that can be readily integrated over time into salient higher-order percepts. An exclusive focus on the perceptibility of individual phonemic segments is likely to lead to a display that can be comprehended only slowly. Many authors have commented on the apparent uniqueness of speech as a rapidly comprehensible code. Green (1978), for example, contrasts the wide range of perceptual alternatives and the rapid speed permitted by speech to the narrow range of alternatives and slow speed of all artificial codes devised in the laboratory. Liberman et al. (1967) have suggested that the remarkable speed of speech is attributable to the fact that the individual phonemes are not encoded in the speech stream as independent acoustic entities but are woven into units of at least syllabic size. The listener is thus presented with fewer perceptual segments per unit of time, and phonemes are processed in parallel. For this reason, among others, Liberman et al. claimed that speech is special. When, however, artificial codes based on sequences of physically simple stimulus patterns are considered in terms of the range and complexity of stimulus patterns that exist in nature and to which organisms typically respond, it appears, as Gibson (1966) has stressed, that the "special" codes are the artificial ones. Though apparently fundamental from the point of view of psychophysics, displays built up from concatenations of independent psychophysically defined stimulus energies do not exist in nature and do not optimally engage an organism's perceptual systems. Sequences of independent stimulus energies or patterns such as Morse code or braille are ideal for input to a computer, which would be befuddled indeed by a string of context-dependent, interactive elements such as is typically found in nature generally and in speech in particular. Natural stimulus streams, including speech, are characterized by an organic interdependency of elements that nevertheless preserve higher-order invariances to which the senses are attuned. It is clear that even when a stimulus stream consists of independent elements, as with sequences of pure tones, the human perceiver does not treat them as independent except at relatively slow rates of presentation. As Warren and Ackroff (1976) say about such auditory stimuli;

> Acoustically, the stimuli used in the present studies may be considered as a series of discrete sounds, but perceptually they appear to be treated as a succession of separate sounds only at item durations of 200 msec and above. At shorter item durations, complex acoustic sequences seem to be recognized and differentiated as overall or holistic patterns. These statements . . . seem to apply not only to sequences of unrelated sounds, but to speech and music as well. (p. 392)

The fact, therefore, that phonemes are interwoven and physically inextricable from syllables in the acoustic speech stream does not create a unique problem for rapid auditory comprehension because any such rapid sequence would be perceptually interwoven and inextricable in any case. That is, holistic (or parallel) processing occurs with any rapid auditory stream, over at least the typical duration of syllables (over 200 msec), and is not peculiar to speech. What is peculiar to speech is its suitability for such rapid processing.

255

The task facing designers of artificial codes, including the development of a tactile display for speech, is to imitate nature, and in particular, speech; to elucidate the organizational principles involved in the perception of natural events, including speech; and to exploit these principles in the design of novel artificial displays. One aspect of the speech signal that should be imitated in a tactile display is the integration of units of at least syllabic size. It is significant that such units have a typical duration of about 250 msec. As indicated above, the auditory system does not treat successive stimuli occurring within this interval as independent. There is considerable evidence that this is true of vision and touch as well (Kirman, 1973). Individual letters and other patterns presented to either sense more rapidly than three or four per second tend to obscure one another; therefore, in order to preserve their perceptual integrity to permit linguistic comprehension, the maximum rate of presentation is held to this limit. It is reasonable to suppose that this factor accounts for the relatively low upper limit on reading speed of the Optacon. It would be valuable to investigate Optacon readers over the first years of their training to determine whether experience permits them to organize perceptual units extending over several letters, or whether they are constantly held to the single-letter units found by Hill (1974). Craig (1977) has reported on Optacon readers with remarkably rapid reading speeds and found that these subjects differed from slower readers in their relative absence of successive masking effects. This observation certainly deserves closer investigation. Although braille can be read more rapidly than an Optacon display, the reasons for its superiority have not been elucidated. It is apparently not yet established whether experienced braille readers can perceptually integrate significantly more than one character at a time. It would be worthwhile to examine both experienced braille and Optacon readers to determine which sequences of characters and letters, if any, can be perceptually integrated into larger units. Such an investigation would provide clues to the designer of tactile speech displays who is interested in building the structure required for such integrated perceptual units into a display. It is clear that not just any sequence of tactile patterns can be assigned to the output of a phoneme-recognizing device and permit syllable-sized perceptual organization and therefore reasonably rapid comprehension. Some suggestions for facilitating such perceptual organization were made in an earlier paper (Kirman, 1973). In addition to such integration within syllables, it is clear that rapid speech perception is aided by the suprasegmental structures of intonation and stress. It would certainly be desirable to incorporate into any tactile display a clear presentation of these segmenting and organizing rhythms of speech, especially because it has been demonstrated that the skin is adept at perceiving and utilizing these rhythms (Erber, 1978; Gault, 1926a).

At the present time, none of the artificial tactile displays of speech has been demonstrated to rival the success of the Tadoma method in communicating connected speech. It may be useful to conclude this discussion with a brief review of the distinctive characteristics of this display. First, it is likely that successful Tadoma users have had far more practice than the subjects tested on other displays. Given the long time normally required to learn to perceive speech by ear in original language learning or in learning other languages, it has been argued that none of the other devices has had a comparable opportunity to demonstrate effectiveness over a sufficiently long period of training. Second, only the Tadoma method presents cues that directly relate to the articulatory movements of the speaker, whereas most other displays present either a spectral transform of the acoustic speech signal or some version of the time waveform itself. Considering the possibility that articulatory reference in a tactile display may be superior to a spectral transform of the acoustic signal, it would be reasonable to test tactile displays that present articulatory features derived by computer from the acoustic signal. Although such processing, at the present state of the art, would make mistakes, the error rate might not preclude useful speech comprehension. Third, the Tadoma method provides a display that is much richer in phenomenally distinctive tactile features than any of the artificial displays. The observer's hand feels a shaped object with characteristic transformations of jaw opening and lip protrusions and separations; this object and its movements probably engage both superficial and deeply embedded pressure receptors as well as receptors in the muscles and joints of the fingers, providing an impression of the dynamics of articulation, the temporal and spatial distribution of muscular effort by the speaker. In terms of the dimensions of sensation, surface touch, deep pressure, and muscular effort or strain, as well as kinesthesis or movement, all contribute in a coordinated manner. In addition, the Tadoma method presents to surface touch distinctive patterns of breath flow and vibratory patterns of the vocal cords and the resonant vibrations of the vocal cavity with and without the nasal cavity occluded. In contrast, all the other tactile displays being investigated are restricted to engaging surface touch, and the patterns they present, though sometimes highly complex in their own way, do not seem to constitute the kinds of stimulus configurations that result in salient, distinctive tactile features. Although it is possible that a trained observer may come to experience a comparable perceptual richness in a matrix of vibrators, all such displays that I have experienced have a relatively homogeneous perceptual quality of various portions of the stimulus stream that carry information about very different speech sounds. The major goal of a tactile display of language might be to engage not only the speech code but also the tactile code – that is, to generate a stimulus stream that presents linguistic information in a mode that optimally utilizes the object–perceptual capacity of the tactile sense.

Note

1 After this paper was prepared, an article of considerable interest appeared: Sparks, D. W., Ardell, L. A., Bourgeois, M., Wiedmer, B., & Kuhl, P. Investigating the MESA (Multipoint Electrotactile Speech Aid): the transmission of connected discourse. *Journal of the Acoustical Society of America*, 1979, *65*, 810–815. This article evaluates the performance of the MESA tactile speech aid with connected discourse. That device had been shown to permit reasonably high recognition accuracy of isolated syllables when used alone as well as in conjunction with lipreading. These promising results, described in an earlier paper by Sparks et al. (1978), demonstrated that the device was capable of transmitting much information about segmental features of speech–when tested with isolated syllables. This current article reports surprisingly poor performance when the device was used with connected discourse over a reasonably long training period. As the authors state: "After an initial period of learning, combined visual and electrotactile receptive performance exceeds lipreading-alone performance. After extensive learning, however, performance in lipreading alone or MESA plus lipreading is practically equivalent" (p. 810). The authors point out that in their earlier study of isolated speech tokens, "Observers often required several seconds . . . before coming to a decision about which token had been presented. Obviously, this processing time is not possible when phonemes are housed within the context of running speech" (p. 814). These observations underscore the relevance of the task discussed in the last section of the present chapter: the need to create distinctive, integratable tactual perceptual units, extending over relatively long segments of speech, that permit rapid tactile communication of speech in real time.

References

Alcorn, S. The Tadoma method. *Volta Review*, 1932, *34*, 195–198.

Allusi, E. A., Morgan, B., & Hawkes, G. Masking of cutaneous sensations in multiple stimulus presentations. *Perceptual & Motor Skills*, 1965, *20*, 39–45.

Apkarian-Stielau, P., & Loomis, J. M. A comparison of tactile and blurred visual form perception. *Perception & Psychophysics*, 1975, *18*, 362–368.

Békésy, G. von. Human skin perception of traveling waves similar to those of the cochlea. *Journal of the Acoustical Society of America*, 1955, *27*, 830–841.

Sensory inhibition. Princeton, N.J.: Princeton University Press, 1967.

Biber, K. W. Ein neues Verfahren zur Sprachkommunikation über die menschliche Haut. Thesis, University of Erlangen, Germany, 1961.

Brown, R. L., Nibarber, D., Ollie, G., & Solomon, A. A differential comparison of two types of electropulse alphabets based on locus of stimulation. *Perceptual & Motor Skills*, 1967, *24*, 1039–1044.

Cole, R. Reading visible speech: They said it couldn't be done. Talk presented at the City University of New York Graduate School and University Center, New York, 1978.

Cornett, O. R. Automatic cued speech. Talk presented at the Research Conference on Speech-Processing Aids for the Deaf. Washington, D.C.: Gallaudet College, May 1977.

Craig, J. C. Vibrotactile pattern perception: extraordinary observers. *Science,* 1977, *196*, 450–452.

Daley, M. L., & Singer, M. A spatial resolution measure of cutaneous vision. *IEEE Transactions on Systems, Man, and Cybernetics*, 1975, 124–125.

Edmondson, W. H. Experience in schools with a new vibrotactile speech training aid for the deaf. Talk presented at the Research Conference on Speech-Processing Aids for the Deaf, Washington, D.C.: Gallaudet College, May 1977.

Efron, R. Conservation of temporal information by perceptual systems. *Perception & Psychophysics,* 1973, *14*, 518–530.

Elliott, L. L. Development of communication aids for the deaf. *Human Factors,* 1978, *20*, 295–306.

Engelman, S., & Rosov, R. Tactual hearing experiment with deaf and hearing subjects. *Journal of Exceptional Children*, 1975, *41*, 243–253.

Englemann, S. & Skillman, L. D. Developing a tactual hearing program for deaf children. Talk presented at the Research Conference on Speech-Processing Aids for the Deaf. Washington, D.C.: Gallaudet College, May 1977.

Erber, N. P. Speech-envelope cues as an acoustic aid to lipreading for profoundly deaf children. *Journal of the Acoustical Society of America*, 1972, *51*, 1224–1227.

Erber, N. P. Vibratory perception by deaf children. *International Journal of Rehabilitation Research*, 1978, *1*, 27–37.

Fraisse, P. *The psychology of time.* New York: Harper & Row, 1963.

Franzen, O., & Nordmark, J. Vibrotactile frequency discrimination. *Perception & Psychophysics*, 1975, *17*, 480–484.

Freiberger, H., Sherrick, C. E., & Scadden, L. *Report of the workshop on sensory deficits and sensory aids.* San Francisco: Smith-Kettlewell Institute of Visual Sciences, March 1977.

Gardner, E. P., & Spencer, W. A. Sensory funneling, II. Cortical neuronal representation of patterned cutaneous stimuli. *Journal of Neurophysiology,* 1972, *35*, 954–977.

Gault, R. H. Progress in experiments on tactual interpretation of oral speech. *Journal of Abnormal and Social Psychology*, 1924, *14*, 155–159.

On the interpretation of speech sounds by means of their tactual correlates. *Annals of Otology, Rhinology, and Laryngology*, 1926 3.(a)

Touch as a substitute for hearing in the interpretation and control of speech. *Archives of Otolaryngology*, 1926, *3*, 121–135. (b)

Hearing through the sense organs of touch and vibration. *Franklin Institute Journal*, 1927, *204*, 329.

Gault, R. H., & Crane, G. W. Tactual patterns from certain vowel qualities instrumentally communicated from a speaker to a subject's fingers. *Journal of General Psychology*, 1928, *1*, 353–359.

Geldard, F. A. The Optohapt. *Perception & Psychophysics*, 1966, *1*, 377–381.

Sensory saltation: metastability in the perceptual world. Hillsdale, N.J.: Erlbaum, 1975.

Geldard, F. A., & Hahn, J. F. Virginia Cutaneous Project, Progress Report No. 45, 1961. Charlottesville, Va.: Psychological Laboratory, University of Virginia.

Gescheider, G. A. Some comparisons between touch and hearing, *IEEE Transactions on Man–Machine Systems*, MMS-11, 1970.

Temporal relations in cutaneous stimulation. In F. A. Geldard (Ed.), *Cutaneous communication systems and devices*. Austin, Tex: Psychonomic Society, 1974, pp. 33–37.

Gibson, J. J. *The senses considered as perceptual systems*. Boston: Houghton Mifflin, 1966.

The ecological approach to visual perception. Boston: Houghton Mifflin, 1979.

Gilson, R. D. Vibrotactile masking: effects of multiple maskers. *Perception & Psychophysics*, 1969, 5, 181–182.

Goff, G. D. Differential discrimination of frequency of cutaneous mechanical vibration. *Journal of Experimental Psychology*, 1967, 74, 294–299.

Green, D. M. Functional aspects of the auditory sense. Paper prepared for the Conference on the Interrelations of the Communicative Sciences, Asilomar, Calif., Sept. 29–Oct. 2, 1978.

Guelke, R. W., & Huyssen, R. M. J. Developement of apparatus for the analysis of sound by the sense of touch. *Journal of the Acoustical Society of America*, 1959, 31, 799–809.

Hansen, R. J. Characterization of speech by external articulatory cues as the basis for a speech-to-tactile communication system for use by the deaf–blind. Unpublished doctoral thesis, MIT, 1964.

Hill, J. W. Limited field of view in reading lettershapes with the fingers. In F. A. Geldard (Ed.), *Cutaneous communication systems and devices*. Austin, Tex: Psychonomic Society, 1974, pp. 95–105.

Ifukube, T., & Yoshimoto, C. A sonotactile deaf-aid made of piezoelectric vibrator array. *Journal of the Acoustical Society of Japan*, 1974, 30, 461–462.

Ifukube, T., Yoshimoto, C., & Shoji, H. A fingertip tactual vocoder with feature extracting system. Research Conference on Speech Processing Aids for the Deaf. Washington, D.C.: Gallaudet College, May 1977.

Katz, D. Cited by L. E. Krueger. David Katz's Der Aufbau der Tastwelt (The World of Touch): a synopsis. *Perception & Psychophysics*, 1970, 7, 337–341.

Keidel, W. D. Note on a new system for vibratory communication. *Perceptual & Motor Skills*, 1958, 8, 250.

Electrophysiology of vibratory perception. In W. D. Neff (Ed.), *Contributions to sensory physiology*, vol. 3. New York: Academic Press, 1968.

The cochlear model in skin stimulation. In F. A. Geldard (Ed.), *Cutaneous communication systems and devices*. Austin, Tex.: Psychonomic Society, 1974, pp. 27–32.

Kirman, J. H. Tactile communication of speech: a review and an analysis. *Psychological Bulletin*, 1973, 80, 54–74.

Tactile perception of computer-derived formant patterns from voiced speech. *Journal of the Acoustical Society of America*, 1974, 55, 163–169.

Tactile pattern perception and tactile displays. Paper prepared for the Conference on the Interrelations of the Communicative Sciences, Asilomar, Calif., Sept. 29–Oct. 2, 1978.

Kringlebotn, M. Experiments with some visual and vibrotactile aids for the deaf. *American Annals of the Deaf*, 1968, 113, 311–317.

Lechelt, E. C. Some stimulus parameters of tactile numerousness perception. In F. A. Geldard (Ed.), *Cutaneous communication systems and devices*. Austin, Tex.: Psychonomic Society, 1974, pp. 1–5.

Levitt, H., & Nye, P. Sensory training aids for the hearing impaired. Proceedings of a conference, 1970. Washington, D.C.: National Academy of Engineering, 1971.

Liberman, A. M., Cooper, F. S., Shankweiler, D. P., & Studdert-Kennedy, M. Perception of the speech code. *Psychological Review*, 1967, 74, 431–461.

Ling, D., & Sofin, B. Discrimination of fricatives by hearing impaired children using a vibrotactile cue. *British Journal of Audiology*, 1975, 9, 14–18.

Loomis, J. M. Tactile letter recognition under different modes of stimulus presentation. *Perception & Psychophysics*, 1974, 16, 401–408.

Lovgren, A., & Nykvist, O. Speech transmission and speech training for the deaf child by visual and tactual means using special devices. *Nordisk Tidskrift Dovundervvisn*, 1959, 122–143.

Lucas, R. L., Steward, J. L., & Kreul, E. J. Communication without (conventional electromechanical) acoustic transducers (Research Report AL-TDR-64-243). Wright-Patterson, Ohio: Air Force Base, Air Force Avionics Laboratory, Research and Technology Division, Air Force Systems Command, September 1964.

Manning, S. K., Pasquali, P. E., & Smith, C. A. Effects of visual and tactual stimulus presentation on learning two-choice patterned and semirandom sequences. *Journal of Experimental Psychology: Human Learning & Memory*, 1975, 104, 736–744.

Martony, J. On lipreading with visual and tactual lipreading aids. *Proceedings of the sixth Danavox Symposium*, Copenhagen, 1974.

Miller, J. D., Engebretson, A. M., & De Filippo, C. L. Tactile speech-reception aids for the hearing impaired. *Journal of the Acoustical Society of America*, 1974, 56, S47(A).

Nelson, M. Electrocutaneous perception of speech sounds. *Archives of Otolaryngology*, 1959, 69, 445–448.

Newman, R. The feasibility of speech transmission using the skin as a sensor. Paper presented at the Air Research and Development Command Seventh Annual Science and Engineering Symposium, Boston, November, 1960.

Nickerson, R. S. *Speech training and speech reception aids for the deaf* (Rep. No. 2980). Cambridge, Mass.: Bolt, Beranek and Newman, 1975.

Norton, S., Schultz, M., Reed, C., Braida, L., Durlach, N., Rabinowitz, W., & Chomsky, C. Analytic study of the Tadoma method: background and preliminary results. MIT pre-publication manuscript, 1977.

Pickett, J. M. Tactual communication of speech sounds to the deaf: comparisons with lip-reading. *Journal of Speech and Hearing Disorders*, 1963, 28, 315–330.

Recent research on speech-analyzing aids for the deaf. *IEEE Transactions of Audio and Electroacoustics*, 1968, AU-16, 227–234.

On somesthetic transforms of speech for deaf persons. Draft paper for the Workshop on Prosthetic and Sensory Aids for the Deaf. New York: National Technical Institute for the Deaf, Aug. 14–18, 1978.

Pickett, J. M., & Pickett, B. H. Communication of speech sounds by a tactual vocoder. *Journal of Speech and Hearing Research*, 1963, 6, 207–222.

Posey, T. B., & James, M. R. Numerosity discrimination of tactile stimuli. *Perceptual & Motor Skills*, 1976, 42, 671–674.

Rothenberg, M., Verrillo, R. T., Zahorian, S. A., Brachman, M. L., & Bolanowski, S. J. Vibrotactile frequency for encoding a speech parameter. Pre-publication copy, 1975.

Saunders, F. A., Hill, W. A., & Simpson, C. A. Hearing substitution: a wearable vocoder for the deaf. Talk given at the meeting of the American Association for the Advancement of Science, 1976.

Schulte, K. Acquisition of speech by means of definable tactual and visual-kinetic transforms. Talk given at the Research Conference of Speech-Processing Aids for the Deaf. Washington, D.C.: Gallaudet College, May 1977.

261

Scott, B. L., De Filippo, C., Sachs, R. M., & Miller, J. D. Evaluating with spoken text a hybrid vibrotactile–electrotactile aid to lipreading. Talk given at the Research Conference on Speech-Processing Aids for the Deaf. Washington, D.C.: Gallaudet College, May 1977.

Sparks, D. W., Kuhl, P. K., Edmonds, A. E., & Gray, G. P. Investigating the MESA (multipoint electrotactile speech aid): the transmission of segmental features of speech. *Journal of the Acoustical Society of America*, 1978, *63*, 246.

Spens, K. E. Pitch information displayed on a vibrator matrix as a speech reading aid: some preliminary results. *Speech Transmission Laboratory Quarterly Progress and Status Report*, 1975.

Is there an optimal time window for tactually conveyed spectral patterns derived from the speech signal? Talk given at the Research Conference on Speech-Processing Aids for the Deaf. Washington, D.C.: Gallaudet College, May 1977.

Stratton, W. D. Intonation feedback for the deaf through a tactile display. *Volta Review*, 1974, *76*, 26–35.

Traunmuller, H. The Sentiphone, a tactual speech communication aid. Talk given at the Research Conference on Speech-Processing Aids for the Deaf. Washington, D.C.: Gallaudet College, May 1977.

Upton, H. W. Wearable eyeglass speechreading aid. *American Annals of the Deaf*, 1968, *113*, 222–229.

Vivian, R. M. Tadoma method: a tactual approach to speech and speech reading. *Volta Review*, 1966, *68*, 733–737.

Warren, R. M., & Ackroff, J. M. Two types of auditory sequence perception. *Perception & Psychophysics*, 1976, *20*, 387–394.

Wiener, N., & Wiesner, J. Felix (sensory replacement project). *MIT Quarterly Progress Report*, Research Laboratory of Electronics, 1949–1951.

Willemain, T. R., & Lee, F. F. Tactile speech displays for the deaf. *IEEE Transactions of Audio Electroacoustics*, 1972, *AU-20*, 9–16.

Witcher, C. M. Vocotac (sensory replacement project). *MIT Quarterly Progress Report*, Research Laboratory of Electronics, Jan.–Oct. 1956.

Yeni-Komshian, G. H., & Goldstein, M. H. Identification of speech sounds displayed on a vibrotactile vocoder. *Journal of the Acoustical Society of America*, 1977, *62*, 194–198.

262

8. Social touching

STEPHEN THAYER

Stephen Thayer's chapter concerning social touching offers a unique perspective on tactual psychophysics. Most of the remainder of the book deals with more classical perceptual-cognitive functions of touch. That is, other chapters deal with obtaining information about the nature and characteristics of surfaces, objects, and such events as speech. Most of the sensory psychophysiology of the skin and the perceptual psychology of the haptic–tactual system concerns perception and the knowledge of the inanimate world around us.

However, we touch more than inanimate objects and inanimate graphic displays. We also touch surfaces and objects that touch us in return; we touch people and they touch us. Although relatively little is formally known about these commonplace activities (we have no social-haptic psychophysics), there are substantial scattered literatures bearing on them. Relevant information and data are seldom found in perceptual literatures. Rather, they are found in the literature of social psychology in general and nonverbal communication in particular. It is from these fields that Thayer brings his unique perspective.

Because social touching is so important to and so neglected by perceptual psychologists, this *Sourcebook* takes note of relevant questions and tentative answers in this area as a stimulus and guide to future researchers and model-builders.

Thayer reviews relevant literature from a great many sources, including biopsychological, psychological, and medical sources. He examines social functions of touch in infant bonding and attachment literatures, caretaking relationships, aggression, courtship and sexual relationships, first impressions, children's interactions, and psychotherapeutic and medical settings. These discussions provide a valuable survey of the data base forming the core of specific or general models of social touch emerging presently or in the future. This field is one greatly in need of both data gathering and model building, and future knowledge about the functional uses of the tactual system must take note of social touching. WILLIAM SCHIFF

Introduction

The chapter you are about to read is quite different from all of the other chapters in this book. It does not focus on sensory processes and discrimination tasks and skills but rather on what is known about the social and emotional correlates of touching between people. Beginning in the 1960s, a new research discipline emerged that sought to study a relatively neglected aspect of communication – nonverbal communication. This part of the communication process involves signs and messages that can accompany and substitute for words. It involves the way people look, stand, move, sound, and use space and touch to reflect and communicate how they feel about themselves, situations, and other people. A sourcebook on tactual perception would be incomplete if it did not consider the role of touch in social and emotional experience.

Touching things acquaints us with the world. And if what we touch is another person, then how, what, where, when, and why we touch lets this person know something about us. The impressions that we form about our world, including ourselves, may start out as simple sensory experiences, but as our knowledge grows, touch begins to assume a symbolic social meaning that transcends the information inherent in sensory experience. What do we know about touch as a form of social communication? What do we know about touching ourselves? What follows is a review of the development of social contact and the role of touch in human interaction.

Tactile communication, like other forms of nonverbal communication, can emphasize, qualify, or contradict spoken words. And perhaps because of its primitive and intense signaling value, the type, location, and quality of touching may even override other kinesic and paralinguistic signals. Even though the quality of touching may be monitored and intentionally modified to create a particular impression, it most likely will be trusted more by the person touched as a genuine reflection of feelings than all other forms of human communication.

Touch in language and imagery

Our language is filled with expressions that underline the importance of the sense of touch in communicating important subtleties of feeling and attitude. Consider the following expressions: keep in touch; a touching experience; he's touchy; a gripping experience; handle with kid gloves; deeply touched; be tactful or tactless; someone is a soft touch or has a soft touch; a clinging personality; how does that grab you?; a pat on the back; to press or push someone; a hands-off policy; get a grip or a hold on; holding my own; the personal touch; put on the finishing touches; the Midas touch; make contact with; rub someone the wrong way; to feel edgy; be on your toes; tickles my fancy; touched in the head; palpable lie; solid reputation; a rough character; rubbing shoulders with; cheek to jowl; nose to nose; makes my skin crawl; a slimy character; itching to go; touch and go; only scratched the surface; stretch the imagination; grasp an idea; get a handle on; able to handle something; only skin deep; like a slap in the face; a mere slap on the wrist; give elbow room; in a pinch; got by the short hairs; on pins and needles; walking on egg shells; like a kick in the teeth.

How is it that so many important social impressions and emotions are linked to touch and the different qualities of touch and physical contact? One reason may be that of all the sensory–perceptual systems, touch, the haptic system, is unique because touching not only gathers information but can also readily alter the world physically and emotionally.

As Frank (1957) noted:

Without tactile communication, interpersonal relations would be bare and largely meaningless, with a minimum of affective coloring or emotional provocation, since linguistic and much of kinetic communication are signs and symbols which become operative only by evoking some of the responses which were initially stimulated by the tactile stimuli for which these signs and symbols are surrogates. (Frank, 1957, p. 242)

Touch and perceptual subsystems

To think of our impressions of the world, based on touch, as being limited to the surface of the skin is naive to investigators of sensation and perception. Certainly, important information is transmitted by sensory receptors in the skin itself, whether by active or passive touch, but to have a fuller appreciation of the touch system, we must remember that the skin covers a body and that actions on the skin often stimulate other body parts. Gibson (1966), for example, divides the touch system into five perceptual subsystems. As you consider these subsystems, consider also how the experience and impressions of social touching, with all of its rich shadings, really depends on more than stimulation of the skin.

The skin and deeper tissue can be stimulated without movement of joints or muscles . . . *cutaneous touch*. The skin and deeper joints can be stimulated together with movement of the joints . . . *haptic touch*. The skin and joints together can be stimulated in combination with muscular exertion . . . *dynamic touching*. The combination of skin stimulation along with vasodilation or vasoconstriction . . . *touch temperature*. And the combination of inputs from the vestibular receptors and the joints and the skin together . . . *oriented touch,* that is, of objects in relation to gravity and the ground. (Gibson, 1966, p.109)

Consider also the perceptual capabilities of the haptic system, that is, the kinds of information available from touching or being touched. Keep in mind the role that these qualities might play as variables in the impression or impact of social touch: texture, temperature, shape, slope, curve, hardness–softness, weight, elasticity, pliability, resiliency, wetness. Now, consider the many qualities of touching, each of which may vary and contribute to the meaning of a touch: duration, frequency, intensity, breadth or extent of contact, continuity–discreteness, sequence of action or reciprocity. And finally, consider the different body parts involved, the different settings in which touch can occur, the relationship of touch to other social signals, and the relationship or roles of the individuals involved. All in all, this is rather complicated information to process. Yet touching is an activity that we all must do to function reasonably well in our social relationships. Where does this process begin, and what do we know about the role of touch in human relationships?

Touch, like all nonverbal behaviors, rarely has a unitary, unequivocal meaning. Whether it is a tap, a shove, or a caress, the meaning or message can vary profoundly depending upon a host of other factors. Because touching another's body generates an immediate demand for a response, as well as a special intimacy or threat unique among communicative behaviors, touch is probably the most carefully guarded and monitored of all social behaviors.

This chapter takes off from Frank's (1957) monograph on tactile communication published almost 25 years ago. Since then, research in nonverbal communication has burgeoned, generating a sizeable number of studies scattered throughout social-psychological, developmental, medical, and psychiatric journals. Cumulatively, these studies challenge the frequent complaint that touch is still a virtually neglected area of research in nonverbal communication.

The survey–review that follows is divided into several parts. It begins with infant origins and functions of the need for physical contact and then traces children's different experiences with and consequences of touch. Next, studies are reviewed that look at how the interpretation of touch is influenced by differences in types of touch, body parts touched, and the gender composition of the touching dyad. This is followed by studies on personality correlates of touching, cultural differences in touching, and outsiders' impressions of touching between others.

Origins of the need for contact

Reflexive aspects of touch

The need to hold or cling is biologically part of the human infant and an evolutionary remnant of our primate heritage still shown by infant monkeys and apes, who must cling to their mothers for safe transportation and protection. Although the human infant cannot use its toes and weak arms for sustained clinging, three reflexive behaviors, the grasp reflex, Moro reflex, and rooting reflex, show our biological disposition for physical contact. These reflexive behaviors would keep the human infant in clinging contact with its mother if human females still had extensive body hair. Ambrose (1966) suggests that the absence of maternal hair has been a major selection factor in the evolution of smiling and crying, which keep the mother in physical contact with her baby by holding, soothing, and carrying.

Fetal contact experiences

Even though it becomes elaborated and overlaid with special symbolic meaning, the sense of touch is very primitive. At approximately 8 weeks after conception, the fetus can respond to tactile stimulation because the underlying neurological system is among the first to myelinate. The importance of the touch–receptor system continues under the constant stimulation and pressure of the amniotic fluid, culminating in the birth process, during which the fetus is expelled via intense uterine contractions. Harlow's studies of infant rhesus monkeys emphasized the reinforcement value of physical contact for normal social bonding and later social and sexual development. He has even speculated that there is a "critical period" during which the absence of physical contact and stimulation may result in deep-rooted behavioral and social deficits.

Why physical contact should promote attachment and security in infancy and early childhood has been the subject of much speculation. Korner and Thoman (1972) offer a broadened perspective by arguing that most notions of contact are too simple. Almost all caretaking acts involve not only physical contact but movement of the infant as well. Six common caretaker soothing techniques were studied for their effect on crying time among 2- to 4-day-old infants. Procedures involved contact alone, vestibular-proprioceptive stimulation alone, and both kinds of stimulation in various experimental combinations. Although contact alone was

267

effective in soothing infant distress, vestibular-proprioceptive stimulation was more effective, both during and immediately after the soothing intervention. The most effective soothing for infants involves the kinds of rhythmic stimulation experienced in the uterus, a possible foundation for the later emotional impact of physical contact.

Contact and attachment bonding

To examine the role of contact for normal development, Harlow and his colleagues began a series of studies on maternal deprivation and its consequences (Harlow, 1958, 1960, 1963; Harlow & Harlow, 1962, 1965; Harlow, Harlow, & Hansen, 1963; Harlow & Zimmerman, 1959). Harlow (1960) reported that baby rhesus monkeys reared in isolation from their natural mothers preferred to spend more time in contact with a terry-cloth-covered "surrogate mother" than with an uncovered wire-mesh surrogate. Whether these infant monkeys had been nursed by the cloth-covered or plain-mesh surrogate, all babies spent 15 to 17 hr a day on the cloth surrogate and only 1 to 2 hr a day on the wire surrogate. Harlow (1960) also tested the strength and permanence of contact and attachment by separating baby monkeys from their mother surrogates at 6 months of age. After 18 months of separation, they still displayed the same powerful attachment to their cloth-covered surrogates.

Peer touching and child's play

Even though the cloth-covered surrogate mothers did give their monkey babies a refuge from fear, the security and comfort did not help them to deal with social situations when they grew up. In fact, Kohlberg (1969) places little emphasis on caregiver–infant contact security for later social behavior. Instead, he argues for the critical role of complementary sharing, via play, as a necessary precursor of effective adult social behavior. Although Harlow would agree that play is important for later social development, he emphasized the importance of early mother–child contact security as a necessary precursor of play itself.

> Intimate mother–infant contact comfort does transfer from maternal figure to age mates or peers. Play in all of its complex forms is impossible if bodily contact is looked upon as undesirable or loathsome . . . we simply accept reasonably basic security as an essential social antecedent to the formation of peer love. Without basic security, neither the human nor the monkey infant would be free to express physical contact and to explore the playthings and play-

mates that are essential for the formation of age-mate love. (Harlow, 1971, p. 35)

How does touch enter into children's play? Even for very young children, some of the subtle social–emotional distinctions in touching are conveyed by the behaviors in which play touch is embedded. Consider the healthy outlet provided by good, old-fashioned rough-and-tumble play. When children play, it is often difficult to distinguish between rough-and-tumble play and aggressive encounters. To understand the specific behaviors that comprise these two kinds of physical–social interactions, Blurton Jones (1972) recorded the specific behaviors and their morphological features that were associated with rough-and-tumble contact and aggressive contact in the play behavior of 2- to 4-year-old children.

Factor analysis indicated that rough-and-tumble play included laugh, run, jump, hit at, and wrestle, whereas aggression included visual fixate, frown, push, hit, and take–grab–tug. Although some of the behavioral elements comprising rough-and-tumble play involved seemingly aggressive physical contact (i.e., hit at, wrestle), their meaning for even these young children seemed to be understood as nonhostile and more playful mock fighting when they were accompanied by certain other behaviors that served as nonaggressive cues (e.g., laugh, run) and were not accompanied by certain other behaviors that served as aggressive threat cues (e.g., frown, visual fixate).

As for more general interaction involving touch between children, peer touching drops between 1 and 2 years of age (infants and toddlers) and is increasingly replaced by verbal interaction (Swift, 1964). At 1 year, infants touch their playmates more than toddlers do. At the later age, verbal contact begins to replace touch as a major channel of social interaction, and touch is less likely to be responded to than talking. Swift reported that the probability of looking at a child peer was five times greater when the interaction was initiated by talking rather than touching.

Willis and Hoffman (1975) and Willis and Reeves (1976) studied the frequency and nature of touching between children at different ages to examine in more detail the phenomenon of reduced social touching in public as children grow older. Between ages 5 and 15, there was a progressive reduction in touching throughout elementary and junior high school for the Kansas City children they studied. Touching occurred 50 percent as often for the junior high school students even though it was still more common for these teenagers than for adults. Most instances of contact in elementary school involved intentional touching with the hands, whereas in junior high school, most contact was accidental and involved shoulders and elbows. Lastly, similarity was a critical factor associated with touching; it was more frequent in same-sex and same-race pairs.

Touch, proximity, and survival

As children grow older, the kinds of affiliative and attachment behaviors they engage in with their caretakers begin to change. Touching and staying close, more proximal signals, come to be replaced by such behaviors as looking and vocalizing, more distal signals. With increasing age, physical proximity is greatly reduced in the absence of threat, although children may still "check in" visually or vocally under novel conditions (Rheingold & Eckerman, 1973). Part of this change comes from the child's increasing ability and interest in moving away from the caretaker to explore the environment and part from the caretaker's more permissive attitude toward the child's increasing competency to explore the environment safely. Additionally, with increasing age, responsibility for maintaining proximity and contact shifts progressively from the adult to the child (Hinde & Atkinson, 1970).

Whether there is, in fact, an attachment drive, one can consider the survival value of attachment behaviors. Individuals must live to reproduce their species, and proximity between infant and caretaker increases the likelihood that the infant will be protected from predators and injury. Any behavior that leads to caretaker–infant proximity will result in increased protection (e.g., clinging, smiling, crying, gazing; Bowlby, 1969). Such attachment behaviors appear to create an emotional bond between infant and caretaker that produces a sense of security in the growing child (Bischof, 1975). This feeling of security mediates exploration of the environment and develops increased physical and social problem-solving skills advantageous for species survival (Ainesworth, 1972). Infants who are insecurely or maladaptively attached to a caretaker need physical contact even when there is little environmental threat. When there has been a separation, such children may not explore their world even when they are reunited with their caretakers. Moreover, they may even avoid physical contact when they are reunited. Although such children may show intense attachment, the disruption of physical contact seems to break temporarily the emotional bond of primitive security (Sroufe & Waters, 1977), as shown by the distressed and tragic behavior of infants who have been separated from their caretakers for long periods of time (Bowlby, 1969).

Touch and responsiveness to the environment

Physical contact between infant and caretaker not only calms and soothes the infant but contributes to increased attention to the environment, a behavior likely to enhance learning and hence survival (White & Castle, 1964). Two groups of 6-day-old institutionalized infants were exposed to two different kinds of physical stimulation. One group received only the regular and minimal stimulation provided by the nursing staff during routine caretaking. The other group was given two 10-min periods of extra handling. This handling consisted of picking up the infant, holding it against the chest, and rocking.

Responsiveness to the environment was assessed beginning at 30 days of age, when the extra stimulation was stopped and continued at 2-week intervals until the infants were 120 days old. Each assessment period lasted 3 hr while the infant was awake and lying on its back. Responsiveness to the environment was recorded if the infant shifted its gaze within 30 sec. The results showed that the infants given extra handling were significantly more visually attentive throughout the assessment period.

Similar results were found by Korner and Grobstein (1966), who studied the relationship between physical stimulation and visual alertness in newborn female infants with an average age of 55 hr. Each infant's visual behavior was recorded for 30 sec immediately after each of six trials when the infant was placed in one of three positions while she was crying—picked up and placed against the shoulder, placed in a sitting-up position, and left alone in a supine position. In essence, this observation-experiment sought to assess the relationship between typical maternal soothing behavior and visual alertness.

When crying infants were placed against the shoulder, they opened their eyes and scanned the environment more than when they were put in the upright position. There was no difference in eye opening between infants in the nonhandled supine position and those in the handled upright position. The authors point out that because of the infants' relative motor helplessness, visual input was one of the few ways to make contact with and learn about the environment. They suggest that the soothing action of physical contact with the caretaker may lower the infant's state of physical arousal to one of alert inactivity, contributed to in part by the motor restraint of being held against the shoulder. As Casler's (1961) and Yarrow's (1961) reviews of maternal-deprivation studies indicate, early tactile stimulation is necessary for normal development. The studies of Korner and Grobstein (1966) and White and Castle (1964) suggest that activation of visual interest in the environment through tactile stimulation may be one of the means by which this early stimulation takes effect, because spontaneous visual scanning is quite low during the first weeks of life and increases only gradually over subsequent weeks (Wolff, 1965).

The role of contact in soothing and calming newborn babies is so powerful that some infants become distressed and cry when they are naked. Part of this may have to do with thermoregulation, which is a problem for most infant mammals, whose ability to maintain a constant temperature is poorly developed (Jonxis, Visser, & Troelstra, 1964). But temperature regulation is not the whole reason, as Wolff (1966) showed in a study of newborns. Half of the infants observed began to cry, from the third day on, when they were undressed, even when a comfortable temperature was maintained and the babies were awake and calm just before they were undressed. In order to calm down, these babies had to be swaddled or have a cloth put on their stomachs or chests. Covering them with a blanket was not enough to stop their crying.

Individual differences among infants

Comfort and soothing from physical contact are not things that all babies seek. Schaffer and Emerson (1964) studied individual differences in response to physical contact during the first year and a half of life. Some babies, it seems, can be described as *cuddlers* and some as *noncuddlers*. Both types showed strong, stable differences in how much physical contact they sought from the mother and how they reacted to close physical contact, a possible manifestation of more general differences in activity level.

Noncuddlers actively resisted being hugged and held tightly, even when they were upset, sick, or tired. They were more active and restless in response to restricting physical contact and embraces than cuddlers. These differences seemed to be inborn and dispositional, unrelated to how mothers actually handled their babies during the first weeks of life. All mothers, whether of contact-seeking or contact-avoiding infants, were sought out under fear or stress, but the cuddlers preferred holding contact whereas the noncuddlers preferred to maintain visual contact or minimal physical contact, such as holding on to their mother's skirt or hiding their face against her knee.

Patterns of touch between young children and their caretakers

Sex, age, and caretaker differences

Research on sex differences in child-initiated touching of the mother (frequency, latency, or duration) shows more studies in which there was no difference between boys and girls (10 to 18 months) (e.g., Ban & Lewis, 1971; Brooks & Lewis, 1974; Coates, Anderson, & Hartup, 1972; Maccoby & Jacklin, 1973; Rheingold & Samuels, 1969; Weinraub & Lewis, 1973) and fewer studies in which there was a sex difference favoring girls (e.g., Goldberg & Lewis, 1969; Messer & Lewis, 1972).

Goldberg and Lewis (1969) reported on instances of touch between mother and infant at two ages, 6 and 13 months, during 15 min of play in an open-field setting. At 6 months of age, girl babies were touched by their mothers more than boy babies. When these same infants were studied in a similar situation 7 months later for touch directed to the mother, girls touched their mothers more than boys did. Goldberg and Lewis suggest that differences in touching shown by children as they grow older may reflect differential modeling and reinforcement contingencies, often but not necessarily sex linked, that begin to influence the infant as early as the first 6 months of life.

Similarly, if we look at 3- to 5-year-olds at moments of physical separation from their caretakers (e.g., being dropped off at a day-care center), we find fewer instances of affectionate physical expression (e.g., kissing, cuddling, holding) between boys and their parents than between girls and their parents (Noller, 1978). Mothers are more affectionately expressive than fathers with children of either sex, a finding also reported by Kagan (1971). Fathers, in contrast, are less expressive with sons than with daughters. Noller suggests that boys are socialized to be less physically expressive:

> (a) A boy experiences less interaction with both parents than a girl does; (b) a boy sees his father, who is presumably an important model for him, express less affection than his mother; and (c) a boy experiences less affection in his relationship with his father than a girl does. It seems that a boy both experiences and observes that males are less expressive than females. (Noller, 1978, p. 318)

Similar results were reported by Lewis (1978) in a retrospective study of adult males.

Lamb (1977) studied the different ways mothers and fathers interact with their infants during the first year of life by observing instances of physical contact between parents and their infants at two different ages: 7 and 12 months. Although no differences were observed for the child's touching of the mother compared with the father, mothers and fathers held their babies for very different reasons. Mothers usually held them for caretaking purposes (changing, feeding, bathing), whereas fathers held them to play with them. These differences were observed at both age periods.

273

These differences in caretaker touching as a function of infant sex are further emphasized by the results of an observational study reported by Leiderman, Leifer, Seashore, Bartnett, and Grobstein (1973). There were no differences between male and female infants in the total amount of affectionate holding and touching by the mother during the first week after they came home from the hospital. The situation changed 3 weeks later, when mothers showed more affectionate touching of boys. Similar variations were documented by Lewis (1972).

Looking over the results of sex-linked differences in touching between parents and young children, we are forced to conclude that hard evidence favoring girls has not yet tipped the balance. Just where and why differences in touching appear in the behavior of males and females is an important research question that awaits further study.

Touch and premature infants

Premature infants are not only born before they are fully developed but are also deprived of the kinds of postnatal sensory stimulation available to normal full-term infants. Quickly isolated in special incubators, they are rarely handled by their mothers or hospital personnel because of medical concerns about infection. Rice (1975) taught a special stimulation procedure to the mothers of premature infants that consisted of stroking and massaging the infant's entire body. This stimulation lasted for 15 min, four times a day, for 30 days after release from the hospital. The mothers of a matched control group of premature infants received only routine infant-care instructions.

There was a significant enhancement of neurological development, enzymatic and endocrine functioning, and Bayley Scale test scores for the experimental group. Infants who received the special stimulation were also more socially adaptive and aggressive, and their mothers were more interested in and pleased by them. Similar results have been reported by other investigators (Bartnett, Leiderman, Grobstein, & Marshall, 1970; Williams & Oliver, 1969).

Another study of premature infants provided evidence about the importance of touch in the development of attachment from mother to infant. Leifer (1970) compared maternal responsiveness in two groups of premature infants. In the first group, mothers saw their infants only through the window of the hospital nursery. In the second group, mothers were allowed to touch and handle their infants. Even though there was actually only minimal contact for the second group of mothers, they showed stronger attachment behavior for several months after the infants were brought home compared to mothers who only saw their infants.

Children's impressions of touch

Do children interpret touch between others as a sign of caring? Raiche (1977) prepared videotapes of simulated counseling sessions to assess the impact of touch on impressions of caring, empathy, and readiness to self-disclose. Two variations were presented, with the counselor touching the 6-year-old client actor in one version but not in the other. After each pair of showings, the child subject was asked three experimental questions: Which of the grown-ups cared the most about the boy (girl?) (caring measure); Which of the grown-ups could best understand problems you might have and the way you feel? (empathy measure); With which of the grown-ups would you find it easiest to talk about yourself and the things that are important to you? (self-disclosure measure).

Both boy and girl subjects at ages 6, 7, 8, 9, and 10 preferred the touching counselor significantly more in response to all three questions. Even so, there was a slight drop that began at age 8 and increased until age 10, reflecting perhaps stereotyped notions about the "babyishness" of being touched. Although the sex of the counselor did not matter much, boys preferred the touching counselor significantly more than girls did.

Blindness and social aspects of touch

What role does touching play in the life of a child with a sensory handicap such as blindness or deafness? With regard to emotional security, we would expect that handicap or not, physical contact and nurturing are necessary and sufficient for effective caretaker–infant attachment bonding, with all of the attendant physiological and cognitive sequelae. Sensory handicap may mean deprivation of the redundant or contradictory messages relevant for the missing sense, but the primitive, soothing love bond engendered by physical contact seems so biologically embedded that touch and movement alone suffice to foster a strong sense of self and self-boundaries.

What seems to be missing from the life of a blind person are those qualifying visual cues about how other communicative signals, including touch, are to be interpreted, that is, metacommunications (Bateson, Jackson, Haley, & Weakland, 1956). There is enough research evidence to document the important role played by visually apprehended communications from various channels: postural (Mehrabian, 1972), spatial–prox-emic (Patterson, 1978), gazing (Argyle & Cook, 1976), gestural–kinesic (Dittman, 1978), and facial (Ekman, Friesen, & Ellsworth, 1972). What seems to be missing in the social experience of blind individuals is critical information about accompanying kinesic signals that communicate how one's partner really feels about the encounter (e.g., facial, postural, ges-tural, and gazing messages). From this point of view, we might expect that blind individuals would be more vulnerable to deceptive interactions be-cause, at the very least, they would be deprived of important nonverbal, primarily visual "leakage cues" (Ekman & Friesen, 1969a) about their partner's verbally and vocally unexpressed feelings and attitudes. Whether the blind develop compensatory skills to substitute for the ab-sence of affective visual messages is not known. One might hope that their vocal and tactile sensitivity would give them this information. But if we look at research on social–sensory compensation among the deaf for some precedents, we will be disappointed. Several studies have shown that visual social cues do not substitute for auditory cues (Schiff & Thayer, 1974; Sugarman, 1969). It seems that just as there is no eye for an ear, vocal and tactile messages usually do not substitute for the social–affective in-formation received by the visual channel. This does not, of course, suggest that blind individuals are robbed of important social cues from touch and sound, but it seems likely that touch as a social signal for the blind suffers unless visual cues are irrelevant in the situation.

We have only to look at the area of intimacy among the blind, espe-cially physical intimacy, to see how the absence of vision interferes with touching and physical contact. Although there have been no carefully designed, formal studies of social touching and blindness, there is some suggestive evidence from informal interviews of the blind reported at a symposium on haptic perception held in 1979 at the University of Louis-ville, and a preliminary study on the need for sex education for the blind (Foulke & Uhde, 1974). What seems clear is that although the blind obviously touch more to get through their daily activities, intimate social touching appears to be less frequent than among sighted people. On the one hand, this seems surprising, because one might expect that the blind would tend to overuse their sense of touch in social interactions, espe-cially when interacting with each other. After all, if touch is a major channel for acquiring information among the blind, they, of all people, should be most familiar, comfortable, accepting, and understanding of the need for contact both to transmit and to receive information. Touch-ing among the blind, however, occurs less often because they seem to fear that they will make mistakes and appear foolish and inappropriate, that they will "mess up" (N. Dotson, pers. comm., March 31, 1979). So, instead of touching more, they appear to be less comfortable about touching others and consequently touch less.

Foulke and Uhde's (1974) interview study sheds some light on why this is so. They started with the premise that the blind must actively seek out much of their information about the world because of the dysfunction of the relatively passive but highly informative visual sense. However, as children, the blind are often overprotected and prevented from exploring the world as freely as sighted people. Similarly, residential schools for the blind are careful to segregate the sexes, once again acting as a reasonable but overprotective parent surrogate to control tactile sexual misconduct. The blind child is deprived of important information about other people through touch, one of the most important channels of information. Blind children can smell and hear others but cannot explore them through touch. By the time blind children reach adolescence, they are extremely ignorant about the bodies of friends of the opposite sex and almost completely uninformed about the bodies of adults of either sex (even though it has been anecdotally suggested that blind people do "people watch" with their bodies rather than with their eyes). Foulke and Uhde note that although blind children are relatively well informed about their own bodies through self-exploration, "in terms of the evidence [they] can collect, many of the people with whom [they interact] tend to be disembodied spirits" (p. 194).

Blind children are not immune to the emphasis on sex, at least not in American society. They are as caught up in sexual curiosity as are sighted children and adolescents. But the blind child's combination of sexual curiosity and sexual and anatomic ignorance results in the creation of bizarre theories about human anatomy and sexual behavior. Left uncorrected, "the blind child's lack of opportunity to gain the experience that informs his sighted peers, and the misconceptions resulting from this lack of experience, predispose him to sexual maladjustment in adult life" (Foulke & Uhde, 1974, p. 194). On the threshold of sexual maturity, blind young adults are likely to be overly shy or aggressive. They generally lack the self-confidence and sensitivity to the shadings of social interaction that contribute to the development of a mature sexual relationship.

Foulke and Uhde reported the first systematic attempt to assess the blind child's accurate awareness of sexual anatomy and function. They presented 15 sex-related words to their blind subjects, such as *clitoris, orgasm, masturbation,* and *lactation,* and asked them to define each one. Responses were scaled according to the subject's accuracy about the anatomic location and function of each sexual term or concept. Subjects were

277

divided on the basis of having received some sex education or no sex education in school. The results showed that 92 percent of the subjects who had received some sex education gave responses that indicated a good or adequate conception of sexual anatomy and function. In contrast, only 60 percent of the subjects who had received no sex education showed a good knowledge of sexual anatomy and function. Conversely, anatomic and functional ignorance was shown by only 8 percent of the students who had received some sex education but by 40 percent of those who had not.

Interestingly, this sensory handicap of experience for the blind can generate an almost opposite reaction for sighted individuals who have worked intensively and extensively with the blind. After a period of time, they begin to feel more and more comfortable about touching as they work in the world of the blind. This feeling begins to generalize to the workers' social experiences in their own world of the sighted. It is as if they become more comfortable with physical contact after going through a kind of desensitization regarding inhibitions about touch.

Touch in a medical context

Are there situations in which adults are returned to a dependent state like that of the helpless infant? Being sick or disabled is such an experience in which doctors and nurses function like our mothers, vital caretakers of our survival.

Seriously ill patients who were touched by their nurses had more positive reactions than those who were not (McCorkle, 1974), and there is evidence that shows direct biochemical change as a consequence of touch. Krieger (1975), for example, reported that hemoglobin values changed significantly when patients were touched.

Touch and the medical status hierarchy

Even though touch in a medical setting may be positive, there is a status hierarchy that influences which staff members touch patients when there is no immediate medical reason for this contact. Watson (1975) observed the circumstances and frequency of touching by personnel in a geriatric nursing home. He also recorded how staff member status (nurse, nurse's aide, orderly) was related to touching. He divided his observations into two categories, instrumental (touching necessary for nursing tasks, such as treating a burn or helping a patient to stand) and expressive (spontaneous emotional touching not necessary for nursing tasks).

In general, instrumental touch occurred twice as often as expressive touch and depended primarily upon the nursing duties of the three nursing roles. In contrast to task-dictated touching, differences in expressive touching depended upon the occupational status of staff members; higher staff (i.e., registered nurses) touched their patients more. These results are reminiscent of Henley's (1977) studies, which found that touching was often a reflection of status and power differences between the toucher (usually a man or superior) and the person touched (usually a woman or subordinate); freedom to touch another person is one of the privileges associated with, and at times possibly abused by, individuals with higher rank or status.

Interpretation of touch in a medical setting

Although we have some evidence about the frequency and types of touching as well as the motives for it in a medical setting, there is little systematic information about what it means to patients. Stolte (1976) interviewed 150 maternity patients who had a normal pregnancy, labor, and delivery. All patients were interviewed one day after delivery to determine their experiences of being touched during labor.

Most women felt that the touch they received was positive or fairly positive; only a small number (26) felt it was negative, fairly negative, or neutral. The strongest positive meanings of touch fell in the interpersonal domain. Touch communicated caring, reassurance, companionship, comfort, help, and relief from pain. Negative experiences of touching related primarily to uncomfortable medical procedures (e.g., pelvic examinations, abdominal palpations). These results suggest that when an individual is stressed, a caring touch, even from a concerned and competent stranger, is very reassuring.

Behavioral and physiological responses to touch in a medical setting

Most studies follow the classic research tendency of looking only at the immediate effects of being touched. Are the consequences limited to transient and momentary effects, or does the impact of touch persist for some time? This question was addressed in an experiment on the impact of touch in a hospital setting (Whitcher & Fisher, 1979). What marked this study as special were (1) assessment of the effects of touch over many hours; (2) assessment of multiple responses to touch, behavioral and physiological responses as well as the more traditional affective and evaluative reaction; (3) assessment in a nonreactive setting; the impact of touch was measured as part of expected hospital procedures, and the patients were unaware that their reactions were being studied.

Before discussing the research results, a qualifying note about the emotional context of this experiment is necessary. All the subjects had been admitted to the hospital for elective major or minor surgery (e.g., orthopedic, eye, thoracic) and were anxious about their operation and recovery. Any generalizations from this experiment must consider the surgical-patient role of these subjects, with its inherent features of dependency and anxiety, as well as the uncontrolled variations in other communicative behaviors that may have accompanied touching. Finally, although the subjects were both male and female adults, the nurses who administered the various experimental touches were all females.

The investigators were interested in how natural and minimal touch affected pre- and postoperative attitudes and behavior. In fact, the touching was so restricted and subtle that *any* outcome differences are impressive. Similar powerful consequences of limited touch were obtained by Pattison (1973) with psychotherapy patients (discussed later). All subjects received the typical physical ministrations given to all patients. During a preoperative surgical-instruction period, the nurse touched the experimental subjects twice – once on the hand for a few seconds after introducing herself and then again for 1 min on the arm toward the end of the instruction period, while she and the patient reviewed a surgical-information booklet that was to be read at the patient's leisure. At the end of this meeting, the nurse extended her hand in a manner inviting contact and noted how the subject responded.

Patients who had been touched tended to judge their hospitalization experiences more positively, were less worried about surgical complications, and had lower systolic and diastolic blood pressure that was measured over seven 4-hr intervals before surgery. Responses to touch by males and females, however, were quite different. Relative to control subjects, males reported *more* anxiety about surgery, whereas females reported *less* anxiety. Females who were touched also reported reading more of the preoperative booklet, tended to like their nurse more, felt more interest from their nurse, and responded more with touch to the nurse's touch invitation. Males did not show these touch–no touch differences. Sex differences in response to touching were also obtained in the recovery room on physiological measures taken after surgery. Females tended to have lower systolic and diastolic blood pressure, whereas males tended to have higher readings on these measures taken at five different times.

These results show the range of persistent effects, generally more positive for females than males, as a consequence of being touched by a kind, skilled female caretaker while in a state of apprehension and dependency. Whitcher and Fisher attributed their results to socialization differences for males and females with regard to the experience and expression of affiliation and dependency needs. Females, they claim, are socialized to be more comfortable with dependency and males more uncomfortable. Additionally, as other research has shown, females are typically touched more often by people who are close to them (Henley, 1977; Jourard, 1966; Jourard & Rubin, 1968).

Patterson's (1976) intimacy model would explain these sex-linked results by noting that an increase in intimacy (touching) produces an increase in arousal. The individual interprets and evaluates this aroused state by drawing, in part, on sex-role beliefs about touch and dependency (see also Ellsworth & Langer, 1976, Kleinke, 1977).

Touch between healthy adults: accidental, friendly, and erotic

We have discussed the powerful role of touching in physically dependent infants and ailing adults. All of us spend most of our lives between the cradle and the hospital bed. What part does touch play in the mundane and erotic portions of our lives? How do we respond to instances of casual, accidental, and erotic touch?

The impact of casual touch

Even a fleeting, impersonal touch between strangers can have a powerful emotional impact. Clerks working at the checkout counter of a library were trained either to touch or not to touch a student's hand as library cards were being returned (Fisher, Rytting, & Heslin, 1976). The impact of this brief contact (0.5–1.0 sec) was assessed under the guise of a questionnaire about the quality of the library's staff and facilities.

Students who were touched reported feeling in a better mood and rated the library's staff and services more positively than students who were not touched. Apparently, as long as the social setting seems safe and physical contact is extremely limited and perhaps even accidental, a momentary touch enhances a person's feeling of well-being and promotes positive feelings toward other aspects of the situation.

Touch and prosocial behavior

Does a touch momentarily break down the barriers between strangers in a situation in which touching is clearly more intentional and not an accidental part of some other activity? Does the intimacy of touch make others behave more positively toward us? Kleinke (1977) created an experiment with two variations. In the first, female confederates approached people who were leaving a telephone booth and asked whether they had found a dime there (which had been intentionally left on the shelf by the experimenter). In the second variation, female confederates approached people in a shopping mall and asked to borrow a dime.

When the requests for a lost or free dime were accompanied by a touch, there was more compliance. There was almost 100 percent compliance in returning the dime when touched as opposed to 65 percent compliance when there was no touching, and almost twice as many dimes were offered when the confederate touched the subject while making the request. Similar positive effects of touch were reported by Silverthorne, Micklewright, O'Donnell, and Gibson (1975).

Touch and self-disclosure: sexual, cultural, and generational differences

Research on sharing important personal feelings with others indicates that physical contact may also be related to self-disclosure (e.g., Pedersen, 1973). Being open to another person physically or verbally is a way of being close or intimate because both modes of expression are signs of vulnerability and trust. Crosscutting this perspective, however, are cultural norms that differentially sanction or inhibit physical contact. Jourard and Rubin's (1968) correlational study, for example, found no relationship between being touched by another and disclosing personal information to that person. In contrast, Lomranz and Shapira (1974) found a strong relationship between these two intimate modes of expression for both same-sex and opposite-sex friends. These contradictory findings may be due to the fact that their subjects were Israelis, whereas Jourard and Rubin's were American, two cultures described as "contact" versus "noncontact," in which physical distance and touching are supposed core cultural differences (Hall, 1966). The Israeli researchers suggest that "a person who tends to be highly self-disclosing will also display a high degree of touching behavior, given a culture supportive of touching behaviors" (Lomranz & Shapira, 1974, p. 224). Thayer and Alban's (1972) research on similarity and proximity found equivalent cultural factors.

Is there reciprocity in body touching between people in different relationships? Although Henley (1977) reported that touching liberties were more one-sided, from higher-status to lower-status individuals, Pedersen (1973) found that body accessibility was generally mutual, with an almost perfect correlation between the extent to which a male college student was touched and his touching of the other person. This was true whether the other person was the student's mother or father or his male or female friend.

Cultural changes regarding sexuality and attitudes toward the body have also influenced touching. Building on Jourard's (1966) body-accessibility mapping procedure, Rosenfeld, Kartus, and Ray (1976) examined changes in body contact for unmarried American college students 11 years after Jourard's study. Subjects were asked whether different people (mother, father, close friend of the same sex and opposite sex) had touched different body areas in the past 12 months. Although there were some minor differences in the body parts touched, mothers still touched sons and daughters equally, and fathers still touched daughters more than sons. Results for same-sex friends were also similar, but as one might expect, body accessibility for opposite-sex friends changed dramatically, lending some support to the notion of a sensual-sexual revolution during the 1960s. In the 1970s, Rosenfeld et al. reported that males were now touched more by their close female friends on the chest, stomach, and hip areas, and females were now touched more by their close male friends over the entire torso from chest to knees.

The encounter group revolution: putting people back in touch

The encounter group movement has incorporated physical contact as one of the key features of these group-based experiences that are designed to enhance one's sense of self and one's connection to others (Schutz, 1967, 1971).

Do encounter groups work? One study asked whether encounter groups that used exercises incorporating body contact increased self-disclosure among strangers (Cooper & Bowles, 1973). English college students took part in a 2-hr tape-recorder-led encounter group, before which each member completed Jourard's (1971) self-disclosure scale. A matched group of students merely listened to the same tapes. Students who had actually participated in the exercises showed a significant increase in willingness to disclose private and intimate details of their lives to the group, whereas the matched control group showed no change. What is surprising is that after only 2 hr of vigorous physical contact, feelings of intimacy and trust among a group of strangers could have been so radically altered.

How much of touching others has to do with making contact with their bodies and how much with the movement involved or the increased attention one pays to the person who is to be touched? Burley (1972) divided male–female pairs into five experimental conditions and one control condition to find out how feelings were influenced by different features of the touching experience. The experimental conditions were: (1) talk only, (2) actual touch, (3) imagine touching but no movement, (4) imagine touching and go through the motions but do not actually touch, (5) look at your partner, close your eyes, and imagine what your partner looks like. Pairs in the control condition merely spent time in the same room without any shared interaction. Compared with the control condition, all of the experimental conditions produced more positive changes in feeling for partners, with actual touch yielding the most positive statements regarding change in feelings.

Touch and the regulation of intimacy

Touch is also a powerful intimacy behavior that contributes to what has been called an *intimacy equilibrium* (Argyle & Dean, 1965). Basically, this hypothesis proposes that there is an appropriate and tolerable level of intimacy for any relationship that is maintained by adjustments in specific behaviors that communicate intimate feelings.

Among the behaviors that signal closeness and attraction, and are interpreted as such, are eye contact, proximity, body orientation, personal verbal disclosures, facial expression, and, of course, touch. If the display or expression of one of these behaviors in a particular situation increases or decreases the intimacy beyond acceptable limits, there will be compensatory adjustments among the other behaviors that signal intimacy. For example, if the physical distance between two people is reduced and the situation becomes too close or too intimate, the frequency of eye contact or the duration of mutual glances will drop. Touch should operate the same way. Because touch is probably the most intimate and immediate social behavior, we should expect that changes in touching should be among the most powerful behaviors that demand reductions in the intensity or duration of the other intimacy behaviors.

Although this last hypothesis has not been tested experimentally, a number of social situations suggest that it is true. Consider any socially dense or physically crowded situation, such as a bus, train, or shopping crowd. The participants are often unintentionally forced to make physical contact with others. If during these accidental contacts they do not studiously avoid and monitor the expression of other intimacy behaviors, there is likely to be a sense of intrusion and unseemly liberties taken. If two strangers are pressed together in an elevator, they must be careful not to look for too long into each other's eyes, lest the physical contact be seen as an insensitive, intentional maneuver. In a word, each must signal via other behaviors that the physical intimacy was unintentional and merely tolerated, not enjoyed.

The need to monitor and control signals that accompany touch can be seen in the various distancing or intimacy-reducing behaviors between male doctor and female patient. Rather than place his ear to the chest area of a sexually mature female to listen to her heart or lungs, the physician was originally obliged to distance this intimate act by using a listening tube or stethoscope. This procedure not only enhanced auditory information but also neutralized the intimacy inherent in such examinations. Similarly, the male physician was historically forbidden to see the genital region of a woman during birth. Respecting her sexual privacy, he had to deliver the baby while the woman was covered with a sheet, using only his sense of touch, not his eyes, as an aid.

For most of us, our bodies are too private to allow others immediate liberties without a sequence of prior, mutually monitored, escalating intimacy behaviors. This motive is so strong that most of us do not even want to make contact with the traces of another's body. In submarines, for example, there are only so many sleeping bunks available to the entire crew. Men must take turns using these limited bunks. Many sailors dislike the sensation of "hot bunking," lying down in the thermal residue of another's body. Or consider the sensation of sitting down on a public toilet seat that is still warm. Body contact, whether direct or indirect, is carefully guarded.

The power of touch taboos is accentuated by a study of how groups of strangers behave in the dark (Gergen, Gergen, & Barton, 1973). Mixed-sex groups of eight American college students were left alone with no instructions in a dark or lighted room for 1 to 1.5 hr. Ninety percent of the subjects in the dark room touched someone else, whereas almost none of the light-room subjects touched. Although this was not spelled out in the research report, one is led to believe that most of the touching was erotic and took place between people of the opposite sex (e.g., stroking the face and body, hugging). The authors interpreted their results as showing that anonymity enhances whatever potentials are strongest in the situation – in this case, the potential for intimacy. People, it seems, and perhaps not just Swarthmore college students, seem to have a hunger for physical-sensual intimacy that is usually held in check by social norms that inhibit its expression. In the absence of factors that maintain or enhance these normative pressures, people seem to express their primitive needs for contact.

Touch in the sequence of intimacy

Morris (1971) proposed a 12-step sequence of escalating physical intimacy shown in most human courtship patterns, a sort of flow chart of body accessibility that elaborates on the work of Jourard and his colleagues. Although culture and personality may alter the sequence, Morris maintains that courtship typically moves from less to more physical intimacy and demonstrates the powerful role of touch in social bonding in infant–caretaker as well as adult–adult relationships. For whatever reason, it is typically the male in most societies who initiates the transition between steps.

The first three stages may be described as pretactile. They include (1) eye-to-body, to assess attractiveness and appeal, (2) eye-to-eye, to establish a mutuality of interest, often signaled by smiling and/or prolonged eye contact, and (3) voice-to-voice, to permit verbal signs of interest and further evidence of attraction. The next stages move through steps of increasing physically intimate contact and are signs of special interest, testing the growing attraction between the potential partners.

In stage 4, hand-to-hand or hand-to-arm contact, the male briefly guides or aids the female as they walk together. This, in a sense, gives the female a chance to signal her responsiveness to the male's first "safe" contact with her. Stage 5, arm-to-shoulder or side-to-side contact between their bodies, is the first instance of trunk contact with all of its inherent promise of later intimacies, and Stage 6, arm-to-waist contact, is the first direct physical statement of romantic intimacy. The next six stages cross the threshold from friendly attraction to erotic and sexual contact. They include (7) mouth-to-mouth, which, if prolonged, generates sexual arousal, (8) hand-to-head, erotic and tender caresses of the face, neck, and hair, which may signal that one's partner is more than a mere sexual object, (9) hand-to-body, the first private sexual contact that involves fondling, squeezing, and stroking that can serve as a signal about the desirability of the other's body, (10) mouth-to-breast, an analog, in many ways, of a special, feeding, mutually nurturing affection, (11) hand-to-genitals, evidence of total body accessibility, and finally (12) genitals-to-genitals, the opportunity to reproduce and potentially form a permanent family bond of transcending affection.

In Morris's scheme, each stage of intimacy seems to depend somewhat upon the couple's passing through earlier stages, although Morris acknowledges that sometimes one or more stages may be omitted or several stages may be collapsed. As a couple moves toward greater physical intimacy, we might expect that each comes to assume that certain touch liberties are not only acceptable and desirable but expected as a confirmation of the relationship. With this assumption, we can look at Morris's sequence from another point of view. What happens when a touch is not reciprocated or an expected touch or type of touch does not happen? Certainly the absence of a touch can communicate just as much as a touch itself. When people have come to expect certain types, qualities, durations, or frequencies of touch from another, their absence may be interpretcd as signaling something negative about the nontoucher's state of mind or attitude toward the relationship. This might be just as true for parents and children, and friends, as it would be for lovers.

The interpretation of touch in close relationships: differences in types of touch, body parts, and gender

The interpretation of different kinds of touch has received little research attention. One exception is the work of Nguyen, Heslin, and Nguyen (1975) whose research was based on the assumption that accurate decoding depends upon the *quality* of touch as well as the body area touched, an important research innovation. Unmarried college students were given a body map and asked to consider how they would interpret four different kinds of touch (pat, squeeze, brush, stroke) to 11 different areas of their bodies from a close friend of the opposite sex. They were asked to keep the same person in mind for each judgment and to consider only the meaning they would attach to each touch, not the possible intention of their friend. Five interpretations were available: pleasantness, playfulness, friendship/fellowship, warmth/love, and sexual desire.

Considering type of touch, the pat was rated most playful and friendly, whereas the stroke was rated most warm or sexual. As for the areas of the body touched, legs were rated most playful and hands and face most warm and friendly. For messages of sexual desire, the obvious was found: thighs, buttocks, and genitals. Types of touch, more so than areas touched, influenced judgments of playfulness, warmth/love, and pleasantness. In contrast, the area touched rather than the kind of touch was more influential for interpretation of friendship and sexual desire.

The way males and females interpreted touch was dramatically different. For males, the more a touch was associated with sexual desire, the more it was interpreted to mean playfulness, warmth, friendship, and pleasantness. For females, the exact opposite was true. Nguyen et al. (1975) wrote, "The same touch to an area which signifies sexual desire to the man is viewed by the woman as unpleasant and lacking in playfulness, warmth/love, and friendship/fellowship . . . ; a touch to an area which communicates warmth/love to him conveys nothing more than sexual desire to her" (p. 99).

The Nguyen et al. study was limited in the range of interpretations available to the subjects; there was no possibility of negative interpretations. This is an unfortunate research bias because all of the options were restricted to positive, affectionate interpretations (Henley,1977). For the subjects in this study, there was no opportunity to describe a touch as offensive, insulting, and so on.

A later study corrected this bias and included a negative interpretation, "invasion of privacy" (Nguyen, Heslin, & Nguyen, 1976). Unmarried subjects were more likely to interpret touches to sexual areas from their lovers as an invasion compared with the same touches from a spouse among married subjects – even though married men associated sexual touching with significantly less pleasantness and love than married women.

Touch as a stressor

Nicosia and Aiello (1976) studied sex differences in the reaction to accidental touching between strangers in a physically crowded situation. Skin conductance was used as an index of emotional arousal to assess the reactions of crowded groups of same-sex subjects who were separated by a transparent physical barrier or who actually made physical contact with each other. In general, subjects who were in touching contact reported more arousal and annoyance regardless of sex. But crowded men, especially those who touched each other, showed more arousal than men who were not in physical contact. Women, in contrast, showed more arousal when *not* touching. This suggests that men became more uncomfortable when they were touching in a crowded situation, whereas women were relatively more comfortable.

Negative reactions to being touched have also been observed among hyperactive children (Bauer, 1977a; Strauss & Lehtinen, 1947). The common expression that someone is "very touchy" implies that he or she is very sensitive and must be approached and dealt with in an especially cautious and gentle way. Hyperactive children certainly fall into this category. Bauer (1977b) investigated the reactions of 5-year-old hyperactive and normal boys to a test of tactile discrimination (Ayres, 1966). They found behaviors such as negative verbal responses to being touched, rubbing or scratching the skin area touched, and physical withdrawal. The social implications of this extreme negative sensitivity are profound. Bauer noted that "this reaction may affect their interaction with peers and parents, as well as their ability to integrate sensory information and to respond appropriately to motor and cognitive demands" (p. 358). Equally sad, she also proposed that such children might be "unable to inhibit the sensation of clothing on their skin, hair brushing the face, or being bumped in a crowd, thus contributing to their increased activity state" (p. 358). The mechanisms responsible for this hypersensitivity have been related to a deficit in the inhibitory processes of the central nervous system (Alabiso, 1972).

Classification of types of touching

The first attempt to classify the various types of touch according to their meaning was made by Heslin (1974). He developed a taxonomy of touching by considering the relationship between the people involved and how the type of touch both reflects and influences the relationship. He proposed five categories:

(1). *Functional-professional.* Performed by a person doing a task while in a special role and must not be accompanied by other verbal, vocal, or kinesic signals that communicate sexuality or disrespect.
(2). *Social-polite.* Performed by strangers, people meeting for the first time, or casual acquaintances; more formal and cordial than warm or intimate.
(3). *Friendship-warmth.* Occurs between people who have shared personal information about themselves and includes some personal concern and affection in their relationship.
(4). *Love-intimacy.* Occurs when the relationship includes strong affection and intimacy. Typically, there is deep concern for the other's welfare, and there would be great distress if the relationship were broken.
(5). *Sexual arousal.* Touching in its most physically intimate, sexual context.

Looking over these touching categories, we can see that they assume a likelihood of escalating intimacy with (1) more body parts becoming accessible, (2) longer and more frequent instances of touching, and (3) an increasing variety of the types of touch involved (e.g., stroke, pat, tickle).

Personality correlates of touch

The idea that being able to touch another person reflects a stronger sense of self received support in a study of the relationship between self-esteem and tactile communication (Silverman, Pressman, & Bartel, 1973). College students were asked to communicate nonverbally the emotion of love to an experimental confederate as if that person were a real friend. The higher a subject's self-esteem score, the more likely it was that intimate physical contact would be included in the expressive display, regardless of the sex of the subject or the confederate. Moreover, self-ratings indicated that those with higher self-esteem found the task significantly easier than those with lower self-esteem.

Dominance is another aspect of personality that has been linked to the likelihood of touching others. Henley (1977) reported that lower dominance scores were obtained by Harvard College students who said that they touch others less than most people do. Moreover, this dominance–touching relationship was sex linked. Low-dominance females, but not males, reported that they felt hesitant about touching others even though those others had touched them or the situation made touching appropriate.

Another sex-linked aspect of touching has to do with the number of body regions of a person touched in different relationships. Jourard (1966) reported that for the Protestant students he tested at the University of Florida in the early 1960s, females were touched more similarly in different relationships than were males (i.e., by mother, father, same-sex friend, and opposite-sex friend). According to Jourard, these results might be due to lower discrimination among females about accepting or rejecting touch from others, a point that is echoed by Henley's (1977) perspective on the subordinate role of females in a status-oriented society.

Physical attractiveness is another correlate of body accessibility. One might expect that more attractive people are more desirable and therefore are touched more. Jourard (1966) categorized college students into "attractive" and "plain" groups on the basis of self-ratings about their physical attractiveness. Attractive subjects reported being touched on more body areas than plain subjects, whether the toucher was mother, father, same-sex friend, or opposite-sex friend. Apparently, more attractive people are touched more in close relationships. Or, considering another perspective, perhaps those who rate themselves as more attractive do so because they have been touched more by people important to them. The relationship between touch experiences and attractiveness might be clarified by future research that includes independent ratings of attractiveness.

Sexuality and the wish to be held

It has been suggested that sensual needs (the wish to hold and touch and be held and touched) are more basic than sexual-genital needs (Hollander & Mercer, 1976). Because sexual relations are usually the occasion for physical intimacy, women who want to hold and be held may have to have their needs gratified only in a sexual context, with possible consequences of promiscuity and pregnancy. It is a sad comment on societies that legitimize physical intimacy *only* as part of sex. This problem has been addressed by the so-called encounter group movement, which has tried to recognize and encourage appreciation of these two different needs.

Hollander, Luborsky, and Scaramella (1969) examined how often women use sex in exchange for being held or cuddled – an experience that may reduce anxiety and loneliness and promote relaxation and a sense of security. Imagine, if you will, a person asking another to spend the night with them, just to hold them, without trading sex for this favor. For many people, sex and physical intimacy are inseparable. Hollander et al. write that "the wish to be cuddled and held in a maternal manner is felt to be too childish; to avoid embarrassment or shame, women convert into the longing to be held by a man as part of an adult activity, sexual intercourse" (p. 190). Their sample was composed of female patients, ages 18 to 59, married or formerly married, who were admitted to the psychiatric unit of a university hospital. All had come for treatment of acute emotional disorders, primarily depression.

All patients were given a five-point, self-rating, body-contact questionnaire that asked about their need to be held under different circumstances (e.g., trouble falling asleep, upset, depressed). They were also asked about their reactions to not being held under these different circumstances (e.g., feeling hurt, sad, depressed). Scores from both sets of questions were correlated with the response to two questions: "Do you use sex to get another person to hold you?" and "Do you make a direct request to be held?" (p. 189). The results showed a highly significant relationship between the need to be held and the use of sex to achieve this goal. Interviews with the women indicated that although they could generally separate the wish to be held from the desire for sexual intercourse, their husbands usually felt they went together. Consequently, some of these women would give up the wish to be held because they wanted to avoid sexual intercourse or would reluctantly engage in intercourse in order to be held. More to the point, Hollander et al. reported the results of an unpublished study of frigid women, more than half of whom engaged in intercourse in order to be held despite feelings of distaste, revulsion, disgust, or nausea. Similar findings have been reported by Blinder (1966) with patients suffering from depressive disorders.

The extent to which this phenomenon may be observed in other cultures was the subject of a study by Huang, Phares, and Hollander (1976). They examined the influence of cultural attitudes on the wish to be held among 20- to 40-year old married Chinese and Malay women living in Malaysia. Using a body-contact questionnaire on feelings about being held, they found that Chinese women educated in English schools were less likely to use sex to obtain holding, compared to Chinese women educated in Chinese schools. Their results indicated that a Chinese education fostered the inhibition of sensual needs and personal sexual gratification and caused these women to withhold from their husbands their desire to be held. This wish was gratified during sexual intercourse, which was necessary in exchange for holding. Is this holding–intercourse conflict limited to women? This question deserves further research.

Cultural differences in touching

Much has been made about the supposed ease with which people of certain cultures touch each other (e.g., Latin Americans: Baxter, 1970, Montagu, 1971; Morris, 1971). To assess the generalizability of this assertion, Shuter (1976) studied the tactile behavior of adults in three different Latin American countries: Costa Rica, Colombia, and Panama. In general, female pairs both touched and held each other more than male or male–female pairs. As for national differences, Costa Ricans both touched and held their partners more than pairs in the other two countries. This research emphasizes the error of overgeneralization and underscores the need for more systematic, empirical evidence about assumed cultural differences in touching. Cultural differences in touching also found no support in a study by Watson and Graves (1966) among native-born groups of Arab and American men studying at the University of Colorado. Although Arab students showed greater proximity, direct eye contact, and a more face-to-face orientation, the expected differences in touch behavior did not appear. However, because of the small size and questionable representation of the two samples, these results must be classified as suggestive findings that need further verification.

Touching and impressions about relationship qualities between others

What role do various intimacy cues play in creating impressions about the quality of a relationship? Kleinke, Meeker, and LaFong (1974) manipulated three intimacy behaviors between videotaped couples who were supposedly engaged – gaze, use of name, and touch. College students were asked to rate various qualities of the relationship. Touching couples were seen by both male and female judges as significantly more emotionally close, relaxed, and attentive toward each other than nontouching couples.

Not only do observers make inferences about closeness when couples touch, but actual measurement of videotapes of male-initiated touching between college-age engaged and dating couples showed that the duration of such touches was correlated with independent measures of romantic love and intimacy (White, 1975). Similar results have been found for married couples; it was observed that those couples who were happy with their marriage sat closer together and touched each other more than they touched themselves, whereas less happily married couples sat farther apart and touched themselves more than they touched their mates (Beier, 1974).

The results of the videotaped studies of couples by Kleinke et al. (1974) and White (1975) did not attempt to determine whether judgments of touching were influenced by the sex of the person touched and the person touching. If one observes a male–female couple and is asked to form personality impressions about each individual, do these impressions differ depending upon the sex of the person who initiates touching? In other words, how do sex-role expectations influence judgments of touching initiated by females as opposed to males?

Forden (no date) asked college students to evaluate a couple shown on videotape. Three tapes were prepared showing a male and female talking. Each tape was identical except for the beginning and end, where different touching variations had been attached. At these two points, either the man patted the woman lightly on the shoulder, the woman patted the man, or there was no touching. Subjects rated both persons on the one tape that they viewed.

Identical touches by a man or woman were judged differently. When the female touched the male, she was rated as more dominant or masculine than when the man touched her or there was no touching. In contrast, when the male was touched, he was seen as more passive or feminine than when he touched her or there was no touching. Despite research suggesting that males and females interpret touch differently (e.g., Nguyen et al. 1975), the sex of the viewer did not matter in Forden's study; males and females shared the same sex-role stereotypes about the very limited touching shown in the videotapes; touching was seen as a male behavior and being touched as a female behavior. Her results support Henley's (1973, 1977) arguments about men's greater power, status, or assertive privileges relative to women. That there was no significant difference between the male touch and no–touch conditions for viewers of either sex further supports the idea that it was seen as more natural for males to touch females and that judgments of personality changed only when the female did the touching.

In contrast, Major and Heslin (1978) reported that a touch recipient was seen as less dominant and assertive than a toucher regardless of gender.

The different results of Forden's videotape study and Major and Heslin's static study may be due to the more realistic, time-extended, or frequent touches in Forden's study.

Self-touching: origins and social functions

Not all of the touching that goes on in therapy is between therapist and patient. Often patients touch themselves, and these moments may provide valuable clues to the therapist about deception, discomfort, and other emotional states.

Ekman and Friesen (1972) describe a category of hand movements that they call *adapters*. They define these gestures as "movements first learned as part of an effort to satisfy self needs or body needs, or to perform certain bodily actions, or to manage and cope with emotions, or to develop or maintain prototypic interpersonal contacts, or to learn instrumental activities" (p. 361). Of interest to us is their subcategory of *self-adapters*, movements that are not used intentionally to communicate information to another. These movements have no intrinsic relation to ongoing speech tempo or emphasis, although they usually are influenced by the motives or feelings that are being spoken about or by discomfort with the conversational partner. The movements involved, according to Ekman and Friesen, "are relevant to facilitating or blocking sensory input . . . ingestive, excretive, or autoerotic activity . . . grooming, cleansing, or modifying the attractiveness of the face and body . . . facilitating or blocking sound making and speech . . . [or] aggression directed against the self" (p. 362).

For most people, these self-adapters (self-touchings) are performed more readily when alone because, from a conventional point of view, they may communicate bad manners or nervousness. When these actions are performed, the actor, like an ostrich with its head in the sand, will avoid visual contact with the other until the activity is completed. One exception to this perspective comes from the work of Scheflen (1965) who has described a category of social behaviors, *quasi-courtship movements*, that involve self-touching as well as other gestures that present the self in a more attractive and engaging way. These behaviors serve to capture the attention and participation of withdrawn or unresponsive individuals in a social situation and thereby maintain their involvement in the encounter. In many respects, these quasi-courtship behaviors resemble the kinds of activities that sexually interested individuals display to potential partners, although they are present in all interactions, even between members of the same sex, when the people know each other and are engaged in a common activity (e.g., party, business meeting, classroom, psychotherapy).

Foremost among these quasi-courtship gestures is preening – actions that seem to signal both a readiness and a bid for more personal involvement by accentuating the communicator's apparent interest in his or her appearance and attractiveness. Typical behaviors include adjusting or stroking the hair, slowly stroking the thigh, and adjusting the clothes. Such behaviors must be accompanied by other qualifying verbal and nonverbal behaviors, lest they be interpreted as inappropriate sexual advances. In fact, Scheflen suggested that unskilled management or understanding of these behaviors may be used by psychotherapists as evidence of emotional disorder, although he cautioned that different ages and social classes may have acceptable and entirely normal subcultural variations in quasi-courtship behaviors.

In contrast to Freedman and his colleagues (Freedman, Barroso, Bucci, & Grand, 1978), who believe that self-adapters or, as they call them, *body-focused movements* function to lower emotional arousal for cognitive processing, Ekman and Friesen (1972) believe that certain self-touchings reflect *particular* affective states. Thus, they write that "picking or squeezing part of the body is aggression against the self or aggression toward others temporarily displaced onto the self; covering the eye with a hand is relevant to preventing input, avoiding being seen, and shame" (p. 363). From one point of view, it is irrelevant what internal states or unconscious processes are being experienced, as judged by expert body-language researchers. For the naive person in everyday social encounters, there are social stereotypes and conventions about what certain body movements mean. Whether we like it or not, these gestures seem to signal particular attitudinal or affective states, and we guide our own immediate behavior by these naive assumptions. An example of this situation comes from a study by Ekman and Friesen (1974). They found that judges attributed more deception to people when they displayed many self-adapters (and appeared anxious, fidgety, and nervous) and more honesty when they displayed fewer self-adapters.

Similar results were discussed by Harper, Wiens, and Matarazzo (1978), who reported the results of an unpublished study of psychiatric patients by Kiritz, Ekman, and Friesen (p. 138). Psychiatrists were shown films of patients made at the time of admission and discharge and rated their emotional mood at both times. The results showed that patients who picked or scratched at themselves were judged to be more hostile or suspicious, and the total amount of self-touching was positively correlated with the judges' impressions of emotional upset.

The role of self-touching in emotion and cognition

The functions of self-touching have been systematically studied by Freedman and his colleagues. Beginning with his early research distinction between object-focused and body-focused movements (Freedman, 1971; Freedman & Hoffman, 1967), the functions of these different kinds of hand movements have been connected to speech production, attention focusing, and arousal regulation. Freedman describes object-focused movements as gestures away from the body that are connected to speech production. Body-focused movements, in contrast, are gestures on the body that are not related to speech but rather appear to reflect emotional arousal.

For Freedman, body movement is critical for cognitive activity in that it sustains what he describes as the processes of representing and focusing. "Representing fundamentally involves connecting image to symbol, and always entails some intervening activity which sustains the connection . . . Focusing, on the other hand, does not imply that an image has already been selected for representation, for before a thought can be shared, it must first be retrieved, ordered, and sorted. There must occur a reduction of multiple alternatives" (1977, p. 2). More generally, he maintains "that bodily action evokes a *kinesic experience* which serves to confirm existing schemata, and may even help to 'bind' image to word . . . It does not imply that action causes thought to occur, but rather that it is felt by the speaker to be an integral part of his communicative structure" (p. 2).

Recalling Freedman's description of representing and focusing, we can now connect them to his two major categories of hand movement. He suggested that body-focused gestures are physical manifestations of focusing, whereas object-focused gestures are physical manifestations of representing (p. 5). As to the origins of these processes, Freedman felt that the role of physical activity as a necessary building block for the formation of cognitive schemata begins in infancy and continues throughout life in the encoding and organization of thought. One recent study that demonstrates the operation of these processes was conducted by Barroso, Freedman, Grand, and Van Meel (1978). They designed an experiment with 10-year-old boys to assess the kinds of hand movements (object-focused vs. body-focused) evoked by two tasks calling for representing or focusing. One task was a series of oral water jar problems in which the child had to figure out how to obtain a particular amount of water by using two containers that could hold different amounts of water. A second task involved word definitions of objects and actions designed to evoke strong visual images (e.g., knowledge, nervous). The final task used the Stroop (1935) interference test, which required the subject rapidly and accurately to name a series of ink colors that were used to print different words. Confusion usually results from this last task, because the words shown are names of colors different from the ink used to print them (e.g., the word *red* is printed with *blue* ink).

Their results showed that body-focused movements were used significantly more during the interference test (when focusing would be expected), whereas object-focused movements were used significantly more in the water jar tasks and more for the word definitions that readily evoked visual images (when representing would be expected). This research demonstrated that touching oneself appeared during cognitive tasks in which an individual's attention was interfered with or distracted by irrelevant information. Freedman and his colleagues maintained that self-touching lowers or regulates arousal generated by distracting or stressful information and thus helps the individual to narrow and sustain attention – the process of focusing. In fact, in the Barroso et al. (1978) experiment, subjects who made fewer errors in the interference test touched themselves more.

Self-touching correlates of psychopathology

Mental patients who have been diagnosed into different categories show different kinds of kinesic activity, including several variants of self-touching, that have been connected to their particular underlying emotional pathology related to disturbances of cognitive processing. Using the construct of *filtering*, evidenced as movements of the feet and torso, but especially the hands, Freedman (1977) argued that particular types of self-touching reflect different emotional–cognitive tasks for individuals suffering from different psychiatric problems. Basically, filtering represents the individual's attempts to cope with thoughts, prior to encoding them, by cognitive processes that involve retrieval, selection, screening, and so on. These mental activities supposedly regulate attention and arousal and are reflected by gestural activity.

All of these filtering strategies are used by everyone but are especially important for understanding psychopathology, in which thought processes are severely disordered. Freedman and his colleagues maintained that these attempts to integrate thought become visible in kinetic behavior, especially the way that people touch themselves (Freedman et al., 1978; Grand, Freedman, Steingart, & Buchwald, 1975; Steingart &

Freedman, 1975). Scoring the body-focused activity of different diagnostic groups showed that schizophrenic patients had a significantly higher incidence of finger-to-hand movements involving both hands; depressed patients showed significantly more continuous movements of one hand on the other or on the body; and borderline patients showed significantly more discrete movements of one hand on the other or on the body.

The kind of self-touching shown by schizophrenics apparently regulates a hypothesized chronically high level of arousal by shielding the patient from stimulus overload, which then permits more focused attention. At the same time, this self-touching appears to affirm the schizophrenic's fragile sense of ego–body boundaries, a point echoed by Fisher (1973), who also reports that schizophrenics use self-touching to reassure themselves that their body boundaries are there and intact. The kind of continuous, soothing self-stroking shown by depressives apparently heightens awareness of body sensation and the retrieval of affect. For borderline patients, self-touching typically follows a tension-discharge movement (e.g., foot kick, posture shift) and supposedly represents a contrasting cognitive–affective oscillation that establishes a sense of ego boundary from threatening, intrusive primary processes.

Conclusion

This chapter has traced the appearance and impact of touch from early infancy through childhood into normal adult casual, friendly, and courtship encounters, as well as medical and psychiatric situations. Obviously there is still much to be learned about the role of touch in human relationships. It is hoped that further research will fill in the gaps now occupied by speculation. With the partial exception of studies of infancy and early childhood, most of the research on touch has appeared only in the past 10 years. It provides a significant beginning on a previously neglected channel of human communication.

In many ways, touch represents a confirmation of our boundaries and separateness while permitting a union or connection with others that transcends physical limits. For this reason, of all the communication channels, touch is the most carefully guarded and monitored, the most infrequently used, yet the most powerful and immediate.

Note

The author is grateful to Colette Thayer and Andrew Thayer for their valuable discussions on the meanings of touch, and to Silvana Pizutti for able library research.

References

Ainesworth, M. Attachment and dependency: a comparison. In J. Gewirtz (Ed.), *Attachment and dependency*. Washington, D.C.: Winston, 1972.

Alabiso, F. Inhibitory functions of attention in reducing hyperactive behavior. *American Journal of Mental Deficiency*, 1972, *77*, 259–282.

Ambrose, J. A. Ritualization in the human infant–mother bond. *Philosophical Transactions of the Royal Society of London, Series B*, 1966, *251*, 359–362.

Argyle, M., & Cook, M. *Gaze and mutual gaze*. New York: Cambridge University Press, 1976.

Argyle, M., & Dean, J. Eye-contact, distance and affiliation. *Sociometry*, 1965, *28*, 289–304.

Ayres, A. J. *Southern California kinesthesia and tactile perception tests manual*. Los Angeles: Western Psychological Services, 1966.

Ban, P. L., & Lewis, M. Mothers and fathers, girls and boys. attachment behavior in the one-year-old. Paper presented at the meeting of the Eastern Psychological Association, New York, April 1971.

Barker, R. G. *Ecological psychology*. Stanford, Calif.: Stanford University Press, 1968.

Barroso, F., Freedman, N., Grand, S., & Van Meel, J. Evocation of two types of hand movements in information processing. *Journal of Experimental Psychology: Human Perception and Performance*, 1978, *4*, 321–329.

Bartnett, C. R., Leiderman, P. H., Grobstein, R., & Marshall, K. Neonatal separation: the maternal side of interactional deprivation. *Pediatrics*, 1970, *45*, 197–205.

Bateson, G., Jackson, D. D., Haley, J., & Weakland, J. Toward a theory of schizophrenia. *Behavioral Science*, 1956, *1*, 251–264.

Bauer, B. A. Tactile sensitivity: development of a behavioral response checklist. *American Journal of Occupational Therapy*, 1977, *31*, 357–361. (a)
Tactile-sensitive behavior in hyperactive and nonhyperactive children. *American Journal of Occupational Therapy*, 1977, *31*, 447–453. (b)

Baxter, J. C. Interpersonal spacing in natural settings. *Sociometry*, 1970, *33*, 444–456.

Beier, E. G. Nonverbal communication: how we send emotional messages. *Psychology Today*, October 1974, pp. 52–59.

Bischof, N. A systems approach toward the functional connections of fear and attachment. *Child Development*, 1975, *46*, 801–817.

Blinder, M. G. Differential diagnosis and treatment of depressive disorders. *Journal of the American Medical Association*, 1966, *195*, 8–12.

Blurton Jones, N. Categories of child–child interaction. In N. Blurton Jones (Ed.), *Ethological studies of child behavior*. New York: Cambridge University Press, 1972.

Bowlby, J. *Attachment and loss*. Vol. 1.: *Attachment*. New York: Basic Books, 1969.

Brooks, J., & Lewis, M. Attachment behavior in thirteen-month-old, opposite-sex twins. *Child Development*, 1974, *45*, 243–247.

Burley, T. D. An investigation of the roles of imagery, kinesthetic cues, and attention in tactile nonverbal communication. Unpublished doctoral dissertation, University of Tennessee, 1972.

Casler, L. Maternal deprivation: a critical review of the literature. *Monographs of the Society for Research in Child Development*, 1961, *26*, whole no. 80.

Coates, B., Anderson, E. P., & Hartup, W. W. Interrelations in the attachment behavior of human infants. *Developmental Psychology*, 1972, *6*, 218–230.

Cooper, C. L., & Bowles, D. Physical encounter and self-disclosure. *Psychological Reports*, 1973, *33*, 451–454.

Dittman, A. T. The role of body movement in communication. In A. W. Siegman & S. Feldstein (Eds.), *Nonverbal behavior and communication.* Hillsdale, N.J.: Erlbaum, 1978.

Dotson, N. Pers. Comm., March 31, 1979.

Ekman, P., & Friesen, W. V. Nonverbal leakage and clues to deception. *Psychiatry,* 1969, *32,* 88–106. (a)

The repertoire of nonverbal behavior: categories, origins, usage and coding. *Semiotica,* 1969, *1,* 49–98. (b)

Hand movements. *Journal of Communication,* 1972, *22,* 353–374.

Nonverbal behavior and psychopathology. In R. J. Friedman & M. M. Katz (Eds.), *The psychology of depression: contemporary theory and research.* New York: Wiley, 1974.

Ekman, P., Friesen, W. V., & Ellsworth, P. C. *Emotion in the human face.* New York: Pergamon Press, 1972.

Ellsworth, P. C., & Langer, E. J. Staring and approach: an interpretation of the stare as a nonspecific activator. *Journal of Personality and Social Psychology,* 1976, *33,* 117–122.

Fisher, J. D., Rytting, M., & Heslin, R. Hands touching hands: affective and evaluative effects of an interpersonal touch. *Sociometry,* 1976, *39,* 416–421.

Fisher, S. *Body consciousness.* Englewood Cliffs, N.J.: Prentice-Hall, 1973.

Forden, C. *The influence of sex role expectations on the perception of touch.* Unpublished manuscript, University of California, Santa Cruz, undated.

Foulke, E., & Uhde, T. Do blind children need sex education? *The New Outlook,* May 1974, pp. 193–209.

Frank, L. K. Tactile communication. *Genetic Psychology Monographs,* 1957, *56,* 209–225.

Freedman, N. The analysis of movement behavior during the clinical interview. In A. Siegman & B. Pope (Eds.), *Studies in dyadic communication.* New York: Pergamon Press, 1971.

Hands, words, and mind: on the structuralization of body movements during discourse and the capacity for verbal representation. In N. Freedman & S. Grand (Eds.), *Communicative structures and psychic structures: a psychoanalytic interpretation of communication.* New York: Plenum Press, 1977.

Freedman, N., Barroso, F., Bucci, W., & Grand, S. Varieties of splitting: a comparative study of kinetic and linguistic behavior in the communication of schizophrenic, borderline, and depressed patients. Paper presented at the Second National Conference on Body Language, New York, October 1978.

Freedman, N., & Hoffman, S. P. Kinetic behavior in altered clinical states: approach to objective analysis of motor behavior during clinical interviews. *Perceptual & Motor Skills,* 1967, *24,* 527–539.

Gergen, K. J., Gergen, M. M., & Barton, W. H. Deviance in the dark. *Psychology Today,* October 1973, pp. 129–130.

Gibson, J. J. *The senses considered as perceptual systems.* Boston: Houghton Mifflin, 1966.

Goldberg, S., & Lewis, M. Play behavior in the year-old infant: early sex differences. *Child Development,* 1969, *40,* 21–31.

Grand, S., Freedman, N., Steingart, I., & Buchwald, C. Communicative behavior in schizophrenia: the relation of adaptive styles to kinetic and linguistic aspects of interview behavior. *Journal of Nervous and Mental Disease,* 1975, *161,* 293–306.

Hall, E. T. *The hidden dimension.* Garden City, N.Y.: Doubleday, 1966.

Harlow, H. F. The nature of love. *American Psychologist,* 1958, *13,* 673–685.

Primary affectional patterns in primates. *American Journal of Orthopsychiatry,* 1960, *30,* 676–684.

The maternal affectional system. In B. M. Foss (Ed.), *The determinants of infant behavior.* New York: Wiley, 1963.

Learning to love. San Francisco: Albion, 1971.

Harlow, H. F., & Harlow, M. K. Social deprivation in monkeys. *Scientific American,* 1962, *207,* 136–144.

The affectional systems. In A. M. Schrier, H. F. Harlow, & F. Stolnitz (Eds.), *Behavior of nonhuman primates,* vol. 2. New York: Academic Press, 1965.

Harlow, H. F., Harlow, M. K., & Hansen, E. W. The maternal affectional system of rhesus monkeys. In H. F. Rheingold (Ed.), *Maternal behavior in animals.* New York: Wiley, 1963.

Harlow, H. F., & Zimmerman, R. R. Affectional responses in the infant monkey. *Science,* 1959, *130,* 421–432.

Harper, R. G., Wiens, A. N., & Matarazzo, J. D. *Nonverbal communication: the state of the art.* New York: Wiley, 1978.

Henley, N. M. Status and sex: some touching observations. *Bulletin of the Psychonomic Society,* 1973, *2,* 91–93.

Body politics. Englewood Cliffs, N.J.: Prentice-Hall, 1977.

Heslin, R. Steps toward a taxonomy of touching. Paper presented at the meeting of the Midwestern Psychological Association, Chicago, May 1974.

Hinde, R. A., & Atkinson, S. Assessing the role of social partners in maintaining mutual proximity as exemplified by mother–infant relations in rhesus monkeys. *Animal Behaviour,* 1970, *18,* 169–176.

Hollander, M. H., Luborsky, L., & Scaramella, T. J. Body contact and sexual enticement. *Archives of General Psychiatry,* 1969, *20,* 188–191.

Hollander, M. H., & Mercer, A. J. Wish to be held and wish to hold in men and women. *Archives of General Psychiatry,* 1976, *33,* 48–51.

Huang, L. T., Phares, R., & Hollander, M. H. The wish to be held: a transcultural study. *Archives of General Psychiatry,* 1976, *33,* 41–43.

Jonxis, J. H. P., Visser, H. K. A., & Troelstra, J. A. (Eds.), *The adaptation of the newborn infant to extra-uterine life.* Nutricia Symposium 1964; Leiden: Stenfert Kroese, 1964.

Jourard, S. M. An exploratory study of body accessibility. *British Journal of Social and Clinical Psychology,* 1966, *5,* 221–231.

Self-disclosure. New York: Wiley, 1971.

Jourard, S. M., & Rubin, J. E. Self-disclosure and touching: a study of two modes of interpersonal encounter and their interrelation. *Journal of Humanistic Psychology,* 1968, *8,* 39–48.

Kagan, J. *Change and continuity in infancy.* New York: Wiley, 1971.

Kleinke, C. L. Compliance to requests made by gazing and touching experimenters in field settings. *Journal of Experimental Social Psychology,* 1977, *13,* 218–223.

Kleinke, C. L., Meeker, F. B., & LaFong, C. Effects of gaze, touch, and use of name on evaluation of "engaged" couples. *Journal of Research in Personality,* 1974, *7,* 368–373.

Kohlberg, L. Stage and sequence: the cognitive developmental approach to socialization. In D. A. Goslin (Ed.), *Handbook of socialization: theory and research.* Chicago: Rand McNally, 1969.

Korner, A. F., & Grobstein, R. Visual alertness as related to soothing in neonates: implications for maternal stimulation and early deprivation. *Child Development,* 1966, *37,* 867–876.

Korner, A. F., & Thoman, E. B. The relative efficiency of contact and vestibular-proprioceptive stimulation in soothing neonates. *Child Development*, 1972, *43*, 443–453.

Krieger, D. Therapeutic touch: the imprimatur of nursing. *American Journal of Nursing*, 1975, *75*, 784–787.

Lamb, M. E. Father–infant and mother–infant interaction in the first year of life. *Child Development*, 1977, *48*, 167–181.

Leiderman, P. H., Leifer, A. D., Seashore, M. J., Bartnett, C. R., & Grobstein, R. Mother–infant interaction: effects of early deprivation, prior experience and sex of infant. *Early Development*, 1973, *51*, 154–175.

Leifer, A. D. Effects of early, temporary mother–infant separation on later maternal behavior in humans. Unpublished doctoral thesis, Stanford University, 1970.

Lewis, N. State as an infant–environment interaction: an analysis of mother–infant behavior as a function sex. *Merrill-Palmer Quarterly*, 1972, *18*, 95–121.

Lewis, R. A. Emotional intimacy among men. *Journal of Social Issues*, 1978, *34*, 108–121.

Lomranz, J., & Shapira, A. Communicative patterns of self-disclosure and touching behavior. *Journal of Psychology*, 1974, *88*, 223–227.

Lowen, A. *The betrayal of the body.* New York: Macmillan, 1966.

Maccoby, E. E., & Jacklin, C. N. Stress, activity and proximity seeking: sex differences in the year-old child. *Child Development*, 1973, *44*, 34–42.

McCorkle, R. Effects of touch on seriously ill patients. *Nursing Research*, 1974, *23*, 125–132.

Major, B., & Heslin, R. Perceptions of same-sex and cross-sex touching: it's better to give than to receive. Paper presented at the meeting of the Midwestern Psychological Association, Chicago, May 1978.

Mehrabian, A. *Nonverbal communication.* Chicago: Aldine-Atherton, 1972.

Messer, S. B., & Lewis, M. Social class and sex differences in the attachment and play behavior of the year-old infant. *Merrill-Palmer Quarterly*, 1972, *18*, 295–306.

Montagu, A. *Touching: the human significance of the skin.* New York: Columbia University Press, 1971.

Morris, D. *Intimate behavior.* New York: Random House, 1971.

Nguyen, M. L., Heslin, R., & Nguyen, T. The meaning of touch: sex and marital status differences. *Representative Research in Social Psychology*, 1976, *7*, 13–18.

Nguyen, T., Heslin, R., & Nguyen, M. L. The meanings of touch: sex differences. *Journal of Communication*, 1975, *25*, 92–103.

Nicosia, G. J., & Aiello, J. R. Effects of bodily contact on reactions to crowding. Paper presented at the meeting of the American Psychological Association, Washington, D.C., September 1976.

Noller, P. Sex differences in the socialization of affectionate expression. *Developmental Psychology*, 1978, *14*, 317–319.

Patterson, M. An arousal model of interpersonal intimacy. *Psychological Review*, 1976, *83*, 235–245.

Patterson, M. L. The role of space in social interaction. In A. W. Siegman & S. Feldstein (Eds.), *Nonverbal behavior and communication.* Hillsdale, N.J.: Erlbaum, 1978.

Pattison, J. Effects of touch on self-exploration and the therapeutic relationship. *Journal of Consulting and Clinical Psychology*, 1973, *40*, 170–175.

Pedersen, D. M. Self-disclosure, body accessibility, and personal space. *Psychological Reports*, 1973, *33*, 975–980.

Raiche, B. M. The effects of touch in counselor portrayal of empathy and regard, and in the promotion of child self-disclosure, as measured by videotape simulation. Unpublished doctoral thesis, University of Maine, 1977.

Rheingold, H., & Eckerman, C. Fear of the stranger: a critical examination. In H. Reese (Ed.), *Advances in child development and behavior*, vol. 8. New York: Academic Press, 1973.

Rheingold, H. L., & Samuels, H. R. Maintaining the positive behavior of infants by increased stimulation. *Developmental Psychology*, 1969, *1*, 520–527.

Rice, R. D. Premature infants respond to sensory stimulation. *APA Monitor*, 1975, *6*, 8–9.

Rosenfeld, L. B., Kartus, S., & Ray, C. Body accessibility revisited. *Journal of Communication*, 1976, *26*, 27–30.

Schaffer, H. R., & Emerson, P. E. Patterns of response to physical contact in early human development. *Journal of Child Psychology and Psychiatry*, 1964, *5*, 1–13.

Scheflen, A. Quasi-courtship behavior in psychotherapy. *Psychiatry*, 1965, *28*, 245–257.

Schiff, W., & Thayer, S. An eye for an ear?: social perception, nonverbal communication, and deafness. *Rehabilitation Psychology*, 1974, *21*, 50–70.

Schutz, W. C. *Joy*. New York: Grove Press, 1967.

Here comes everybody. New York: Harper & Row, 1971.

Shuter, R. Proxemics and tactility in Latin America. *Journal of Communication*, 1976, *26*, 46–52.

Silverman, A. F., Pressman, M. E., & Bartel, H. W. Self-esteem and tactile communication. *Journal of Humanistic Psychology*, 1973, *13*, 73–77.

Silverthorne, C., Micklewright, J., O'Donnell, M., & Gibson, R. Attribution of personal characteristics as a function of touch on initial contact. Paper presented at the meeting of the Western Psychological Association, Sacramento, April 1975.

Sroufe, L. A., & Waters, E. Attachments as an organizational construct. *Child Development*, 1977, *48*, 1184–1199.

Steingart, I., & Freedman, N. The organization of body-focused kinesic behavior and language construction in schizophrenic and depressed states. *Psychoanalysis and Contemporary Science*, 1975, *4*, 423–450.

Stolte, K. M. An exploratory study of patients' perceptions of the touch they received during labor. Unpublished doctoral thesis, University of Kansas, 1976.

Strauss, A. A., & Lehtinen, L. E. *Psychopathology and education of the brain-injured child*. New York: Grune & Stratton, 1947.

Stroop, J. R. Studies of interference in serial verbal reactions. *Journal of Experimental Psychology*, 1935, *18*, 643–662.

Sugarman, I. R. The perception of facial expressions of affect by deaf and non-deaf high school students. Unpublished doctoral thesis, Columbia University, 1969.

Swift, J. W. Effects of early group experience: the nursery school and day nursery. In M. L. Hoffman & L. W. Hoffman (Eds.), *Review of child development research*, vol. 1. New York: Russell Sage Foundation, 1964.

Thayer, S., & Alban, L. A field experiment on the effect of political and cultural factors on the use of personal space. *Journal of Social Psychology*, 1972, *88*, 267–272.

Watson, O. M., & Graves, T. D. Quantitative research in proxemic behavior. *American Anthropologist*, 1966, *68*, 971–985.

Watson, W. H. The meaning of touch: geriatric nursing. *Journal of Communication*, 1975, *25*, 104–112.

Weinraub, M., & Lewis, M. Infant attachment and play behavior: sex of child and sex of parent differences. Princeton, N.J.: Educational Testing Service Research Bulletin, 1973.

Whitcher, S. J., & Fisher, J. D. Multidimensional reactions to therapeutic touch in a hospital setting. *Journal of Personality and Social Psychology*, 1979, *37*, 87–96.

White, B. L., & Castle, P. W. Visual exploratory behavior following postnatal handling of human infants. *Perceptual & Motor Skills*, 1964, *18*, 497–502.

White, G. T. The mating game: nonverbal interpersonal communication between dating and engaged couples. Paper presented at the meeting of the Western Psychological Association, Sacramento, April, 1975.

Williams, C. P. S., & Oliver, T. K., Jr. Nursery routines and staphylococcal colonization of the newborn. *Pediatrics*, 1969, *44*, 640–646.

Willis, F. N., & Hoffman, G. Development of tactile patterns in relation to age, sex, and race. *Developmental Psychology*, 1976, *12*, 91–92.

Willis, F. N., & Reeves, D. L. Touch interaction in junior high school students in relation to sex and race. *Developmental Psychology*, 1976, *12*, 91–92.

Wolff, P. H. The development of attention in young infants. *Annals of the New York Academy of Sciences*, 1965, *118*, 815–830.

The causes, controls, and organization of behavior in neonates. New York: International Universities Press, 1966.

Yarrow, L. J. Maternal deprivation: toward an empirical and conceptual re-evaluation. *Psychological Bulletin*, 1961, *58*, 459–590.

9. Haptic pictures

JOHN M. KENNEDY

John Kennedy's chapter is concerned with apprehension of the environment via haptic pictures. Kennedy notes the skepticism among perceptual scientists, educators, and even blind people themselves regarding the possibly informative role of pictures to be touched rather than seen. He develops a general theory of representation that transcends purely visual information as a prerequisite for grappling with traditional definitions of pictures. These definitions seemingly preclude the possibility of rendering objects located in three-dimensional space on two-dimensional surfaces for perception by blind observers. Kennedy then reviews literature bearing on this possibility and summarizes his own program of cross-cultural research on drawings made by and for blind children and adults. This research suggests substantial spatial comprehension – even by those who have never seen their environments – of spatial meanings of pictorial representation.

Kennedy's unorthodox treatment of a controversial topic provides considerable evidence that blind people can comprehend three-dimensional spatial representations given appropriate questions and materials. If this is so, the possibility of useful haptic pictures for blind people emerges as a reality most psychologists and educators have dismissed – perhaps prematurely.

WILLIAM SCHIFF

On haptics and pictures

What is a haptic picture? It is a tangible picture whose function is to depict objects for a blind person. For a long time, it was thought that pictures for blind people were a contradiction in terms, that tangible versions of visible pictures were doomed to failure because they would be based on visual principles and optic geometry, neither of which could be appreciated by the blind without advanced education. However, recent research and thinking on the blind, geometry, and pictures are at a turning point. As a result, this chapter reviews the possibility that haptic pictures may be quite useful to the blind, including the congenitally blind, with little or no previous experience or training with depictions.

Haptics is a discipline in parallel with optics and acoustics that studies the tangible world just as optics studies visible energies and acoustics audible vibrations (Kennedy, 1978b). If there were a Haptics Society, as there is an Optics Society, its members would meet to discuss the properties of the world that make it tangible and the properties of the body that make it able to explore the tangible world, obtaining information about its surfaces, media, objects, and events.

Haptic pictures are part of the tangible world just as photographs are part of the visible world. Haptic pictures are generally flat plastic or paper sheets with markings on them in the form of raised lines, patterns of raised dots, or grooves. The purpose of haptic pictures is generally to inform the blind perceiver about a layout of tangible surfaces other than the pictorial display itself. If haptic pictures were effective, the blind perceiver would accept the markings as representing edges, corners, wires, and foreground and background relationships even though, of course, the display is basically flat and has no slanting surfaces, curved surfaces, or abrupt steps in depth to the background between its lines and grooves. Also, if the blind perceiver were to make a haptic picture, he or she would have to intend it to stand for a layout of surfaces other than just the particular set of markings created.

Thus, if the blind person makes or is given a drawing of a long, thin rectangle and says that it represents a cylindrical water pipe, the flat display is interpreted as depicting a rounded object.

Research on haptic pictures was rare until very recently, probably in part as a direct consequence of the discouraging theories of major writers on haptics.

If Berkeley's (1948) view that touch teaches vision had prevailed, more attention might have been paid to touch. But in fact, this century's thoughts on touch are closer to those of von Senden (1960). His theory is that the blind achieve something approximating perception of form only by secondary means. The primary percepts of a blind person were said to include duration of movement and the feel of the textures or the solidity of the object being touched. From the primary percepts, von Senden wrote, the blind person may slowly and deliberately, with effort, extract information about the relative location of the parts of an object, its size, and its shape. The blind person cannot grasp an object with one hand at either end and, spanning the object in this way, obtain an immediate impression of its length, he contended. Instead, the blind person has to engage in a circumlocution such as running a finger along the length of the object at a steady rate to become aware of the time required to get from one end to the other. Whereas the sighted person is immediately aware of length, in von Senden's theory the blind person is supposed to be aware of time taken (cf. Kennedy & Fox, 1977).

306

Révész (1950) too argued that understanding how features fit together in a whole object often depended on a skill that lay outside of haptics, namely, the skill of *visualization*. If one is passive and inactive, Révész thought, space seems diffuse, whereas if one intends or undertakes actions, the direction and sequence of the movements bring a firm order to perceived space. For Révész, an orderly, stable space arises only in connection with action. An abstract Cartesian space containing three-dimensional bodies with an origin or central focus but no reference to action is not a haptic space, in Révész's theory, but instead is a kind of geometry for perceived space that can arise because of vision and the capacity for visualization, or internal visual imagery.

Haptic pictures are designed to present shapes and to refer to forms other than the ones on the depicting surface. Neither von Senden nor Révész would expect much success for such pictures for the blind. The mastery of shape requires visualization, for Révész, which can hardly be expected in the congenitally blind. There is nothing in von Senden's theory about the world of the blind that would readily allow the blind person to detect a simple shape and understand how it would refer to a somewhat different layout of surfaces. Indeed, if the blind person were to rely on the perception of textures and materials, pictures would be deeply confusing, because the pictorial surface is irrelevant whether it be paper or plastic or metal. The adventitiously blind might cope quite well, but the congenitally blind would lack visualization and efficient form perception. As Marks (1978) put it, in space perception "both tactile and visual information are referred to a single spatial representation and that representation is fundamentally visual in nature" (p. 333).

In this connection, it is worth noting that the kind of information referral discussed by Marks would have been deemed impossible without language by some psychologists as late as the 1960s (Ettlinger, 1961), and a popular view in the 1970s was that kinesthetic information is difficult to store in memory even for a matter of seconds (Wilberg & Girouard, 1976), a serious matter when haptic pictures can take more than 10 sec to explore. Thus a reasonably eclectic view, in line with much in recent psychology, would be that the blind use secondary means to obtain form information, and the information has to be coded in language before it can be transferred to a stable modality (visual imagery) in which it can be integrated into a unit or percept of an object.

By extension, the reverse process would presumably be required were one to want to create a drawing, and presumably language would be necessary once again.

This eclectic view is too pessimistic. Language does not seem to be necessary for picture comprehension and cross-modal transfer of pictorial information, for it occurs in the higher apes at least in rudimentary form (Davenport & Rogers, 1970). And some perceptions of shape and distance are accurately made and remembered by the blind (Shagan, 1970).

Further, the Révész and von Senden theories are hardly tight, cohesive, and unequivocal. To say that some percepts are primary and others are derived leaves open the possibility that the derived percept can be quite accurate and stable once it is achieved. Also, the distinction between primary and derived is never clearly stated. The criteria may boil down to the idea that some percepts are more difficult to achieve than others, which may be a matter of taking a little more time and paying a little more attention. If so, the distinction is not serviceable. One could never apply it wholesale, saying that any information about spatial layout was more difficult to use in perception than any information about texture. Obviously, it would take a short time to tell two curved objects apart by touch if one had many gentle curves and the other many pronounced curves, whereas two textures would be hard to tell apart if they were similar in many features.

Révész's notion of visualization, too, is easy to criticize. Perhaps its greatest single weakness is its closeness to pure circularity, for it may boil down to classifying the capacity to appreciate configurations as visual, and then calling perceiving or imaging form visualization without having any independent way of checking whether shape perception was visual or haptic.

However carefully collected the evidence, no theory need be taken seriously if it has the formal logical problems evident in those of von Senden and Révész. Unfortunately, as Fletcher (1981) documents, the thesis that the blind do not have a stable, integrated perception of space and shape, and rely on sequences of movements to get from A to B, dominated thinking for several decades and is still held to be true of the blind child by some advisors. In 1980, for example, I was told of a blind person who could not appreciate that a figure 8 route he had walked many times had a crossover in the middle. If this is true, I suspect that problems other than blindness were responsible. For as Warren (1978) argues at length, the blind are not a uniform group. They are diverse and individualistic, and the mere fact of having blindness in common, from birth or not, may not be a powerful leveling influence that renders them all uniform.

In my experience, some blind people are very mobile and read maps skillfully; they navigate familiar buildings and cities confidently and set about learning their way in strange buildings without hesitation. They have a good grasp of the layout of objects and furniture in familiar rooms, and they apprehend the shapes of objects quickly. Others are much more sedentary, abhor maps, and dislike novel surroundings. They may have a limited awareness of their own surroundings and are inept at manual exploration of objects.

Logically, a low ability in space and form perception could follow from low motivation or, vice versa, low motivation could follow from a lack of ability. Which comes first is a chicken-and-egg question. What is sure is that blind people are heterogeneous, and one should not generalize to all blind people on the basis of a limited sample. Instead, one can establish the range of abilities of a sample and determine whether one condition (such as early blindness) seems to be an important or necessary factor in limiting the range of abilities. In tasks such as making drawings, one might be wise to prepare for wide variations in skill. Even sighted people seem to range from the high shown by those who have the knack from childhood to the low shown by those who feel they have never been able to draw, and a middle range occupied by people who can draw a recognizable house or person but who stop short when they try to sketch a horse or dog.

In contrast to von Senden and Révész, some writers on haptics such as Katz (1925) and Gibson (1962) have contended that haptics is quick and accurate in space perception, with Gibson strongly defending a realist's position that haptics extracts the required information efficiently across a wide range of conditions. However, even Gibson recoiled when considering haptic pictures, and he predicted that they would fail to be meaningful to the blind.

Gibson's theory, unlike Katz's, contained distinctions and definitions that led him to rule out haptic pictures as impossible. For Gibson, a picture is a display treated so as to project to a point of observed light that contains the same kind of optic information that would arise from a natural environmental origin. Pictures are optic by this definition on two grounds. First, they have to project light; second, they have to capitalize on the laws of optic information. Blind people are not capable of sensing the projected light, and even if they were granted some device that translated optic energy into palpable energy, why should they be capable of using the principles of optic information if they have never seen?

Gibson's definition, however, is not the last word. Though some pictures fit his definition, others escape it (Kennedy & Ostry, 1976), and if a broader definition or a different basis for one can be found, there may be judicious hope yet for haptic pictures for the blind.

To begin a reappraisal, consider the fact that some pictures involve forms that are congruent with their referent, a simple transformation, for instance, of a solid form into an outline one. A coin, being a circular disc with a solid interior and space around it, can be depicted by a circle. A book could be depicted by a rectangle. A fish can be drawn in outline. These outline pictures need not depend on projection to a point of observation. To be sure, the outline could have been created by means of projection, but it could also have been done by imprinting the object on a flat, yielding surface or tracing around it. Imprinting and tracing transformations should not seem as difficult as projection to the blind. A remaining problem for the blind might be the outline transformation, in other words, the use of a line to stand for different kinds of edges, solidity represented on one side of the line and space on the other, the step from foreground to background across the line.

Can outlines serve the same kinds of depiction functions for the blind as for the sighted? Research is required to answer this question. The research should begin by listing the pictorial functions of a line. Then examples can be prepared and blind people can be given tasks that require understanding of the pictorial functions, to determine whether they understand these functions without explicit training.

As a second step in reappraising Gibson's definition of a picture, consider whether optic information is necessary for a display to function as a picture. Strict criteria must be satisfied in order to claim that a display is presenting optic information on a particular object.

Optic information is present if and only if the optic patterns *specify* the object, that is, the pattern must be specific to that object and no other. However, the human eye can take an outline sketch that does not specify any particular foreground/background layout of surfaces and, though depth is not given, see a coherent, stable, particular foreground/ background relationship. We can look at a *U* and see a tongue (or a valley or a handle for a bag) or at a *Z* and see the prow of a ship cutting through calm water (or a slash of lightning, or a winding road). Hence Gibson's definition applies only to a restricted class of displays, and pictorial perception is not restricted to that class.

If, even for the eye, pictorial perception is more flexible than Gibson allows, then it may be worth testing the limits to assay what can be available to the hand.

A third point in this reassessment of Gibson's analysis of pictures is the possible utility of optic information.

Even if optic information is being used by a pictorial display, it may not be entirely foreign to haptics. There is some common ground between haptic and optic information. Notably, the geometry of direction is identical, whether it is being dealt with by touch or vision. Pointing is useful for both blind and sighted people. Both point to objects and locations, showing that they understand directions. Many of the important principles of optic information can be considered in terms of direction. A receding object projects a narrower cone of light because of the change in direction of its periphery from the point of observation. The shape transformation of a rotating disc, projecting first a circular cone, then an ellipse, and finally a line, can be described as a set of changes in direction of its periphery from the point of observation.

The optic principles of form and space from a fixed point of observation, including perspective transformations with change of distance and rotation, are present in haptics as principles of direction. The principles apply to pointing outward as readily as they do to rays traveling inward. Hence, there may be a basis for a blind person to understand some haptic pictures that conform to optic information. (Later, some further problems in the use of optic information in haptic pictures will be discussed.)

As a fourth point in this reassessment, consider aspects of pictures rooted in intentional communication rather than in physical optics. In some everyday pictures, a running dog might be shown with extra legs, a busy mechanic might be given extra arms, or a hard-pressed executive may have 10 telephones nearby. These are *metaphors*, for the literal referent is not supposed to have sprouted extra limbs (Friedman & Stevenson, 1980; Kennedy, 1978a, 1980a, b, c). Similarly, in pictures showing emotions, the husband's hair flies off in surprise when the wife shows him the price tag on her new coat, or spirals may appear in Linus's woebegone, anxious eyes. These graphic devices transcend optics. They are not literal; they are metaphoric.

The fact that the artist and the audience can invoke metaphor comprehension so that not all the picture has to be taken literally is useful in avoiding a purely physical approach to pictures. Pictures have cognitive principles as part of their functional role. They are devices for communicating in which artist and receiver understand each other's roles and intentions (Kennedy, 1980b; Korzenik, 1977). Intention is, of course, a psychological concept distinct from the optics of pictures, and there is nothing in blindness per se that would prevent one from understanding intention, the role of a communicator, and metaphor.

In sum, Gibson's optical definition may be useful for some pictures, but it is not complete and should not preclude haptic pictures. The object–picture transformation may result in either a congruent form or a perspective version without leaving the realm of haptics entirely; whether the edge-to-outline change is understood by the blind is an empirical question; optic specification is not always necessary in depiction; and metaphoric aspects of depiction introduce cognitive matters, beyond optics, that the blind and the sighted share. (For other arguments on haptics and representation, see Kennedy & Fox, 1977.)

What definition of a picture would be broad enough to admit haptic pictures without straining? An appropriate approach is included in the following: A flat display on which there are elements making up a configuration is said to be a picture if the elements can be taken to represent the features of the layout of surfaces that structure the perceptible world, and the elements are so taken in the absence of training or specific instruction in a code to that effect.

Notice how this definition contrasts to ones based on other possible approaches.

Gibson's definition emphasized optic information, stressing the patterns that are specific to certain origins. The present definition emphasizes the elements, that is, the lines and sets of dots, because it acknowledges the possibility that the elements act in a pictorial manner even though the pattern is not specific to the referent. When the pattern is specific to a referent, it is still appropriate to say that the elements are acting pictorially. For example, in both a simple sketch and a detailed drawing of a face, the line for the silhouette of the nose acts to show the foreground/background step. The present definition also contrasts to Gibson's by mentioning the perceiver and, sidestepping the purely optical criteria of Gibson, setting conditions on the naive perceivers required to test haptic pictures.

Another popular approach to pictures, one that might readily be confused with the present definition, with unfortunate consequences, is a phenomenological approach (Kennedy & Ostry, 1976).

If the definition were to rest on phenomenological criteria, the test of a picture would lie in the kinds of experiences it evokes. Does the display give rise to a kind of double perception, of a flat surface physically present and a set of depicted surfaces not really present, seeming to slant this way and that, some foreground, some background, all in a virtually pictorial space? This is what happens in vision. Is there anything comparable in touch – perhaps a set of virtual directions?

At present, the only sure claim one can make is that no one is sure how to inquire about possible pictorial experiences in the blind. No one has formulated the issues, the proper questions, the key unambiguous terms, the exact comparisons with vision.

The day may come, but at present the time is not ripe for a phenomenological inquiry into haptic pictures. On the other hand, it is perfectly possible to investigate haptic pictures by asking questions such as, What can be recognized by blind people in haptic pictures? and What do blind people intend by the lines they make when they are asked to draw objects? The question of what is experienced can be finessed.

At this point, it is worth noting that Guarniero (1974, 1978) found many perceptions of depth and location that he, a blind person, achieved by means of a sensory prosthesis to be ambiguous or at least difficult to put into words. His account makes one all the more hesitant to ask questions about experience when one is not sure what words to use.

A definition that rests on recognition and intention need not become enmeshed in how a display is experienced. All that matters is whether the blind person can tell what a picture is representing and can indicate what the lines of his or her own sketches mean. Of course, if that were the sole criterion, the blind child who makes a mark haphazardly and calls it "a horse – no, a goose – no, an igloo" would have to be deemed as depicting in turn the horse, the goose, and the igloo. (And the child who feels a haptic picture casually and incompletely, and then pronounces it to be the Toronto City Hall, would have to be said to be taking it as a picture of the City Hall, instead of just guessing wildly.)

Something more is needed. The person must identify the elements, not just the overall mass vaguely, and the identification of the elements must follow a system that has not been taught. The underlying hypothesis is that pictures conform to a universal human capacity not restricted to those who have been taught the code but available, at least in a rudimentary way, even to those who have never had the opportunity to exercise it (Kennedy, 1974a; Kennedy & Ross, 1975). The hypothesis, then, is that the corners and edges depicted in sketches for the eye to examine are seen because of an untaught visual aptitude. Haptic pictures for the hand to examine may lead blind persons to identify the same kinds of layout features without the intervention of a teacher to teach them the possible referents for the elements in the sketch.

In fine, a definition of pictures broad enough to include haptic pictures can be based on the understanding of the naive subject.

Practical work on haptic pictures

Despite the discouraging theories of haptics prevalent in this century, haptic pictures have occasionally been made for the blind.

Libraries in institutions for the blind are sometimes offered books prepared by volunteer groups. One I have seen has the story of Little Red Riding Hood. The road to Grandma's house is indicated by a double row of tiny sea shells. Little Red Riding Hood's hair is a fibrous material, her dress is a vinyl material, and her legs are cloth, all the materials being shaped like silhouettes and glued to the page. The end result is a mix of vaguely suitable materials, collage, bas-relief, and depiction.

The librarians and teachers I have spoken to say that these books are accepted graciously, although they are of little or no use. They confuse the blind, take a long time to explain, are misleading at times, are frustrating rather than motivating, and are no substitute for real objects, which are what the blind really need. Accordingly, the books are stored and not used.

Some publishers have included a few illustrations in occasional books. The *Expectations* series, for example, includes some drawings made of lines of raised dots. Some Peanuts books have appeared with plastic pictures in relief. I know of no formal program to test these drawings and help design them. Reports from educators and occasional blind persons who have tried them indicate that they are impossible to understand. I have tried them with 9-year-old children in Toronto who also found them extremely difficult; no picture was identified without hints and clues. I myself have tried them and found them baffling. Once I succeeded while blindfolded in identifying a picture of a lion, and my experience may be worth recounting. I knew the picture was of an animal and isolated a tail with a lump on the end. That made me guess "lion" correctly, although I could not make any sense of the rest of the picture. Finally, I looked at the picture. The mane was large and curly, and the curls were comparable in size and length to the ears, teeth, and claws. The mouth was gaping, and the limbs were partly tucked around the body. The whole was a mass with many curls around the silhouette; there were so many curly prominences that one did not know how to isolate one set (teeth), another set (mane), and the third set (claws). I believe it would have been easier if the artist had not chosen a gaudy cartoon-caricature style, but instead had drawn a simple profile, with the limbs distinct from the body and mane and the mane distinct from the teeth.

This point – that the drawing could be kept simple, without ornate decoration of the silhouette, and the separate units drawn so as to be easy to distinguish – was made repeatedly by several blind people who tried a few pictorial aids at the Louisville Workshop on tactual graphics in 1979. However, it should be noted that some of the highly educated and articulate blind people there argued that the pictorial material was bound to fail whatever style was used because, they said, concepts such as point of view and overlap would not be understood by most blind readers.

Fukarai (1974), a teacher in Japan, has had considerable success encouraging his children to make pictures. The students began by making pottery, including statuettes. Then they were introduced to dance and mime. As part of miming, the children would outline, say, the shape of a tree in the air with their hands. Once this kind of tracing in air was understood, Fukarai had the children hold a paintbrush so that they could leave a record of their hand movements on a large sheet of paper held vertically before them. Fukarai himself would then glue sand to the brush marks on the paper to make the trail tangible.

The children's drawings reproduced in Fukarai's books are truly remarkable – as substantial and powerful as a haiku. Fukarai's gradual, step-by-step approach to drawing is useful for teachers. He does not claim, it should be noted, that his approach is the sole route to depiction by the blind, nor does he offer a theory of the underlying abilities of the blind. He simply offers his end results as testimony to the value of his methods.

Vincent (1977), working in the United Kingdom, has also been able to teach blind students complex drawing skills including three-point perspective. He taught them the concepts of vanishing points, points of observation, and the horizon, and employed a drawing board with T squares of his own devising, one that makes raised lines. He believes blind subjects are capable of visualizing objects before being taught, but they have no knowledge, he states, prior to his instruction of drawing objects in three dimensions.

Vincent begins by explaining the coordinate system of his drawing aid to students and then relates the coordinates to distance in space. Next, he explains three-dimensional perspective terminology. After the terms are understood, he takes his students through a booklet of three-dimensional drawings of common objects on perspective grids, beginning with simple pictures and moving to more complex ones (an exercise that he repeats at intervals of about 1 month). Next, the students measure familiar objects and employ the measurements to create drawings. Then they make drawings following step-by-step instructions. Eventually, Vincent says, the students do not need step-by-step instruction.

Vincent contends that his procedure teaches his students the rudiments of freehand drawing. "The ultimate goal would be reached when equipped with portable . . . drawing boards they could by free hand drawing communicate their ideas and designs in a visual form" (1977).

In one study, teaching five students, with an average age of 17 years, Vincent reports that after 10 weeks all of them were able to make raised-line drawings of their own design unaided. Vincent's drawing boards have been used in several West German schools for the blind. In an anecdote, Vincent notes that a 10-year-old blind girl (age and degree of blindness unstated) was able to identify 11 of 12 raised-line pictures presented in 5 min.

Vincent has reproduced neat, efficient, and quite complex recognizable drawings made by his students, including exercises, drawings made under dictation, and drawings of objects from memory. His work is encouraging in that it indicates that proficiency can be achieved with a short training course in drawing.

It should be noted that Vincent's theory of the blind person's ability has not yet been tested directly by his work. He holds that the blind can visualize objects in some three-dimensional way as a mental image, but they have to be taught to take a point of view and to draw. He offers no independent test of their ability to have a three-dimensional mental image other than the fact that they profit from his instruction. A critic might conclude that the instruction was inculcating the ability to have a three-dimensional image. In addition, Vincent is unclear about his students' capabilities before receiving instruction. He notes some attempts, before learning, to draw views that he thinks would arise prior to the realization that objects have more than one plane. But yet he claims that visualization of an object in three dimensions is an untaught ability in the blind! His views seem to be contradictory at times.

Vincent and Fukarai are convincing on one point: The blind can be taught to draw. However, surely this should be no surprise. No one claims the blind are uneducable. Perhaps the most useful lesson, therefore, ought to be the methods Vincent and Fukarai used. Their end result was an ability to turn the training to any object, so that the system is not some paint-by-numbers procedure that is tied to a restricted set of prototypical schemas for pictures. There are other teachers (e.g., Wally of Puerto Rico) who have sometimes taught students to make "formula" pictures, such as a landscape with a horizon, road, setting sun, and clouds. Vincent and Fukarai leave students able to turn their hand to any subject.

Jensen and Haller (1978), of the International Children's Book Service, Denmark, have produced a prize-winning little book, *What's that?*, for blind children (it is popular with sighted children too). The heroes are Little Rough, Little Shaggy, and their friends. They are depicted by patches of embossed textures in rounded, angular, but not realistic forms. Jensen is convinced that blind children can understand more realistic drawings, but many European educators of the blind told her she was wrong. However, she has now met a few people in Scandinavia who work with the blind and are optimistic about pictorial materials, and the Book Service hopes to design some books with realistic representations.

In Lausanne, Switzerland, Monique Gapany of the Centre Pedagogique pour Handicapes de la Vue is undertaking research on pictures from a Piagetian point of view. Pictures, she suggests, are a useful indicator of some aspects of mental images, and in the Piagetian theory the mental image is an important intermediary between mime and pretense, on the one hand, and true interior schemes of thought, on the other. Gapany considers pictures to be semiotic instruments of a class between words and objects. Her present research is designed to determine if there is a development of pictorial skills in the blind child to parallel developments in the sighted child. Four drawings she sent me by blind children (10 to 12 years of age, onset and degree of blindness unstated) show the human figure drawn quite plainly in stick-figure style.

In the United States, a notable research effort on haptic pictures in the 1930s by Merry and Merry (1933) began optimistically but ended in pessimism. Their blind subjects were able to recognize some drawings at the start of their testing, but after practice they identified fewer of them. This may have been due to a drop in motivation, but Merry and Merry did not check this possibility and drew unfavorable conclusions about the ability of the blind to understand haptic pictures.

Merry and Merry's pessimism is echoed in the Nuffield Foundation Report (1973) on education for the blind, which concluded that pictures would not be helpful or motivating. These conclusions are curious because the appendix to the report mentions blind students who say that pictures are recognizable and interesting.

Millar (1975) of Oxford University supports the idea that blind children should be taught to draw. Her own work is concerned with the cognitive process, but as part of her research she had blind children draw people, which they did quite recognizably on many occasions.

In sum, there are some striking reports on successful teaching of drawing and some leads suggesting that the untrained abilities of the blind in depiction may not be as meager as some pessimistic reports have concluded. The issues are certainly not closed, and the appropriate action now is to define cogent issues and examine them in detail, evidence in hand. The issues are best addressed with studies on the congenitally blind, but comparisons with the later blind should be drawn. Bearing in mind the definition of a picture reached above, the issues to be addressed here are: the line element in outline pictures, the role of perspective in haptics and depth in depiction, and the more cognitive factors in

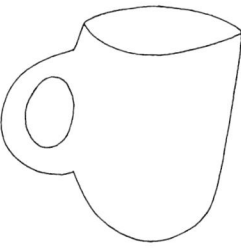

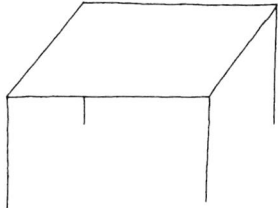

Figure 9.1. Two raised-line illustrations identified by blind adults. (From Kennedy, 1980c)

metaphoric devices in depiction. Later, aids for removing ambiguity in pictures will be mentioned briefly.

A program of research on haptic pictures

Since 1970 (Kennedy, Fox, & O'Grady, 1972), a line of investigation has been undertaken on the hypothesis that blind people can understand depiction without training. The major points of the first two steps in the research program can be summarized as follows:

Kennedy and Fox (1977) reported 15 blind adults examining eight raised line drawings of familiar objects (Figure 9.1). They noted, first, that six of the eight drawings were identified by at least one blind person. Second, some of the drawings were identified much more often than others. Third, on the average, the blind were not as adept as blindfolded subjects. Fourth, some of the blind were much better than most of the blindfolded subjects. Fifth, the criterion of success – the blind must respond with the same term used by a sighted person who saw the display – could be broadened to include the question, does the blind person's response make pictorial sense to the sighted? If the criterion for

318

success were broadened in this way, the blind would score much higher. Sixth, the blind made sense of the drawings in detail once a general label was given to the drawing (e.g., cup, table). Seventh, overall, congenitally blind people can understand the medium of outline depiction, although particular pictures may be easy or difficult.

Kennedy (1978, 1980a) describes an evaluation of stories with raised-line illustrations and raised-line drawing tasks undertaken by 17 blind adults, including eight congenitally blind subjects – totally blind or with slight light sensitivity – with little or no pictorial experience prior to the study. The drawing aid was a Sewell kit, using a plastic sheet that makes a raised line when one writes on it with a ballpoint pen. (The same kit was used in later studies with children in Phoenix, Tucson, & Haiti.)

All of the subjects, whether congenitally or later blind, totally blind or light perceivers, were able to understand almost all of the illustrations, and were able to make drawings that conform to the style used in standard outline drawings for the sighted. Occasionally stick-figure drawings were made, but usually the drawing depicted objects by enclosed spaces. Many of the subjects had never drawn before and were surprised at their latent talent (one was so interested that he continued the first interview, at his behest, continuously for 9 hr).

The subjects often realized that there was more than one way to portray an object, depending on the point of view, and indicated the point of view for their drawings. For some drawings, the parts of the object were connected accurately but without a point of view. The subjects often recognized ambiguities or problems in their portrayals and many times suggested effective ways to counter them. Appropriate rules for showing depth and overlap were invented.

Overall, the blind adults in Kennedy's studies succeeded in drawing in the outline style and recognized outline drawings without training.

More recent research has resulted in a videotape on blind adults drawing bowls, boxes, and other objects (Kennedy & Heywood, 1979) and studies (Kennedy, 1980c) on 13 blind adults depicting objects in depth, with specific orientations, or in movement, as well as studies with blind children aged 5 to 17 from Phoenix (11 subjects), Tucson (8 subjects), and Port-au-Prince, Haiti (15 subjects).

The drawing tasks are a graded series, useful for diagnostic and teaching purposes as well as research. They were given in their entirety to some of the Phoenix children and in part to the other children. They involved drawing, identifying pictures, and examining illustrations for a story in each of four rounds.

Round 1
Drawing: Coat hanger, ring, cubic box, hexagonal box
Pictures: Hand, mitten, place setting, cup, teapot, face, page of fruit (apple, pear, banana)
Story: Duckling story (see Kennedy, 1980a)
Round 2
Drawing: Man, man walking, man running
Pictures: Man, front view or profile view, with the pictorial surface oriented in different positions
Story: Tricycle story (see Kennedy, 1980c)
Round 3
Drawing: Cubic objects
Pictures: Car, boot, telephone, hammer
Story: Elephant story (see Kennedy, 1980a)
Round 4
Drawing: People in a circle, glass, table
Pictures: House drawn from different vantage points
Story: Guitar story

The results of the latter steps in the Kennedy research program can be summarized under three headings – outline, depth, and movement metaphors (see Kennedy, 1980c, for the full presentation).

Outlines

In outline drawings the length and shape of the line is significant, unlike, say, a drawing with cross-hatch lines, in which density is paramount. Vision readily takes lines in outline drawings as depicting features of surface layout involving changes in depth or slant, and because these features are tangible, it is a simple matter to ask if they are used by the blind person deciphering a haptic picture. (There are other features of visible environment, such as change of color or texture or brightness, that may be depicted by outline, but such depictions are uncommon, work much less well for vision than changes of depth or slant, and in the case of color and brightness are intangible; therefore they will be neglected here.) The list of features includes corners, occluding edges of flat-faced objects, occluding bounds of rounded objects and "parallel features," where corners, edges, and bounds are close together, elongated, and parallel, forming indentations (grooves), ridges (tracks), and cylinders (wires).

The tasks mentioned above were designed to bring out different uses of line. The coat hanger was depicted with lines showing *parallel features*, in this case a wire. The ring was drawn with lines depicting the inner and outer perimeters or *occluding bounds*. The box tasks were successful in obtaining uses of lines standing for *corners* and *occluding edges* (see Figures 9.2, 9.3, and 9.4).

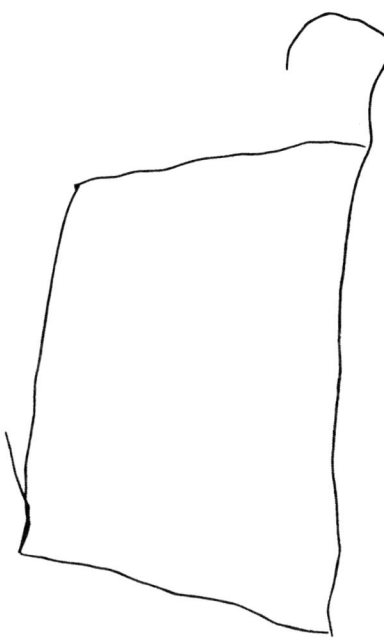

Figure 9.2. A raised-line drawing of a coat hanger, by Cel (Haiti, age 6, totally blind at age 1 to 2 years). (From Kennedy, 1980c)

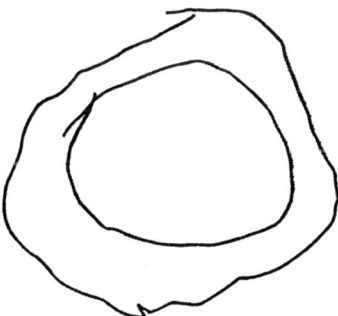

Figure 9.3. A raised-line drawing of a thick ring, by Ol (Tucson, age 14, congenitally blind, with some light perception). (From Kennedy, 1980c)

In some cases, it is difficult to judge whether pure outline drawing is being used or not; the answer depends on the vantage point and the accuracy of the drawing. With these doubts in mind, it is important to ask whether there was anyone in any of the four testing sites who never

321

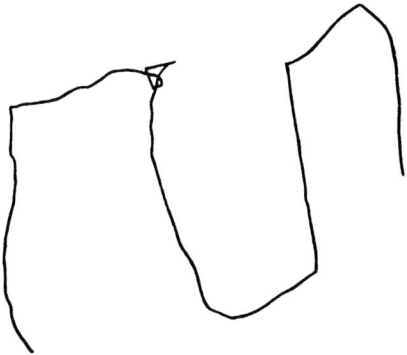

Figure 9.4. A raised-line drawing of the front of a hexagonal box, including lines depicting corners and occluding edges, by Ram (Phoenix, age 8, congenitally totally blind). (From Kennedy, 1980c)

used or understood the outline style in any drawing. The key facts are as follows. First, the youngest subjects all used the outline style on occasion, if not always. Second, the only subject who failed to make an outline drawing or to identify a picture unaided has extremely severe attentional problems that are probably the cause of his performance. Third, in one site (Haiti), few pictures were identified, but all subjects made outline drawings. The Haitian subjects rarely explored pictures thoroughly, which may be the cause of their low recognition performance. Fourth, no adults failed to use the outline style.

In sum, there is strong evidence for an untrained predisposition in the blind to employ haptic lines to stand for the features of the environment that outline drawings depict to the eye.

Depth

When asked to draw objects (such as those made of stacked cubes), the blind mentioned many techniques. Kennedy (1980c) lists a number of them. Here, three of the techniques will be considered because they were offered by children as well as adults and were obtained in every testing locale, suggesting that their comprehension may be universal. The techniques will be called the *bulky line*, the *enclosing line*, and the *fold-out*. After they have been described, a brief mention of perspective is in order.

The bulky line is obtained by thickening the outline, raising it more than usual, or repeating it several times to suggest the height of the edge being shown above the background. The initial outline "is just the sur-

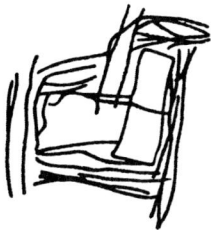

Figure 9.5. A raised-line drawing of an L made of cubes, using a bulky line technique to show depth, by Na (Toronto, adult, congenitally totally blind). (From Kennedy, 1980c)

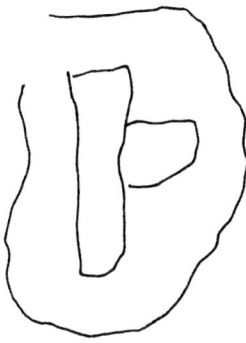

Figure 9.6. A raised-line drawing of a T made of cubes, using an enclosing line to show depth, by De (Toronto, adult, congenitally totally blind). (From Kennedy, 1980c)

face," said Na (early, totally blind adult), "and because I couldn't go through the page, I showed the depth with four or five lines. If it were only slightly thick, I would have used just one or two lines" (Figure 9.5).

The enclosing line is obtained by drawing one face of the object and adding a single bordering line that runs around the drawing of the face to enclose it (Figure 9.6).

The fold-out is obtained by drawing each face of the object as though it were frontal, preserving some of the order, for example, the way the faces are arrayed around a central face. The result often resembles a cardboard box that has been folded out and laid flat (Figure 9.7).

In one study, adults were asked to indicate orientation, that is, what was near and what was far (Kennedy, 1980c). Six people offered pointers on this problem. Besides conventional solutions such as an arrow pointing to the nearest spot, four people offered general solutions that are all similar. For example, Cl (early, totally blind) said that one could vary the

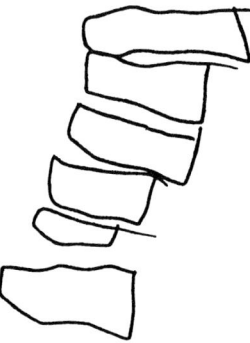

Figure 9.7. A raised-line drawing of a hexagonal box, using a fold-out technique, by Ha (Phoenix, age 10, totally blind since age 2). (From Kennedy, 1980c)

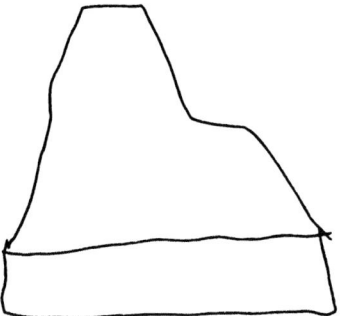

Figure 9.8. A raised-line drawing of an L made of cubes showing near and far edges, in perspective, by Ra (Toronto, adult, congenitally blind, with some light sensitivity as a child). (From Kennedy, 1980c)

"intensity" of the lines and ended by describing the denser (thicker) line as the most suitable for nearness. Na (early, totally blind) suggested that the line should get thinner as it moves farther back, toward the far end. "You can tell if you substitute near for thick and far for thin." Ra (late, totally blind) suggested narrowing the lines or having "a narrower point" at the far end instead of making a rectangle. He added, "There's another way – by showing the depth you see at the bottom [a visible side] but not at the top [an occluded back side] . . . because you can't see *through* the top to the vertical part . . . you'd see the top and then [past the top you'd see] the surface it was on . . . The sides are something like the top, you can't really see them." Then he drew Figure 9.8, which fulfills his description perfectly.

Four of the six adults who used narrowing to indicate recession said that the idea came from hearsay and did not originate with them. Two did not. None of the children used narrower enclosures or thinner lines to convey slant. However, this is not to say that the technique is alien to haptics. It may be that children appreciate that a distant object subtends a smaller angle than a same-sized nearer object.

To test the blind children's perception of the change in angle subtended with distance, a pointing task was attempted with the Tucson and Haitian children.

The children were guided to the center of a wall of the testing room. The interviewer then guided each child along the wall, in contact with it, to one corner of the room and commented, "here is a corner." The child was then guided back to the center of the wall and on to the other corner of the wall with the comment, "here is another corner." The child was then guided back to the center of the wall, again maintaining contact with it. The child was then asked to step back a pace and point with both arms outstretched to the corners of the room. The distance between the fingers was measured. He or she was then guided straight back approximately 5 m (15 ft) and asked to point again to the corners. The distance between the fingers was again measured.

In every case, the children pointed with a narrower angle when asked to point from the farther distance. This is true for the Haitian as well as the Tucson children (Table 9.1). Hence, in the pointing behavior of blind children, there is evidence for an intuitive sense of convergence, the basis of perspective. This, it is hoped, may prove an important basis for learning to draw complex configurations.

Movement and metaphor

The Toronto, Phoenix, and Tucson studies (Kennedy, 1980c) involved depicting a man walking or running and a wheel revolving. The Toronto adults' work will be shown briefly here to indicate the range of devices, their nature, and the breadth of subjects from whom they were obtained. Kennedy (1980c) notes that blind children offer the same range of devices, and the adults offer the devices in other drawing tasks.

Three kinds of devices were used by the Toronto adults to indicate movement: postural or shape ones, context-of-the-object clues, and "additional graphics" in the form of trailing lines and others (see Kennedy, 1974b). The postural devices were most common with depictions of a person in movement, and for a rolling wheel settings such as a hillside were used most often. However, the additional graphics deserve espe-

Table 9.1. *Distance between fingertips while pointing to the corners of a wall, measured in centimeters and inches, for Tucson and Haitian children*[a]

Vantage point		Tucson children									Haitian children							
Close to the wall	(in)	55	57	57	54	36	40	56	40	38	47	44	44	58	51	65	46	57
	(cm)	140	145	145	137	91	102	142	102	97	119	112	112	147	130	165	117	145
Twelve feet from the wall	(in)	44	34	55	37	8	19	22	22	18	33	40	40	38	33	42	36	33
	(cm)	112	86	140	94	20	48	56	56	46	84	102	102	97	84	107	91	84

[a]Pilot testing with one adult in Toronto and four children in Phoenix obtained the same results: All pointed with a smaller angle when the wall was farther away.

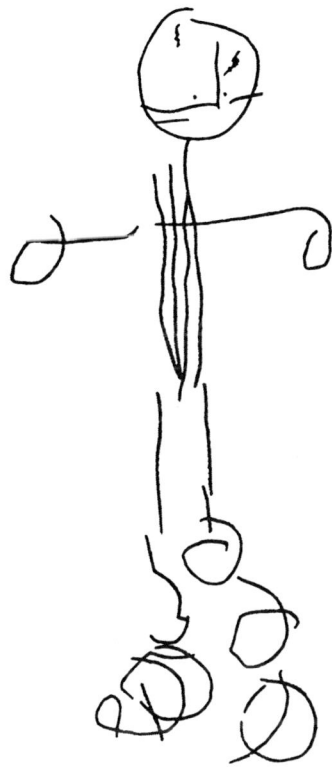

Figure 9.9. A raised-line drawing of a man walking, with graphic additions to show the steps, by Ly (Toronto, adult, congenitally totally blind). (From Kennedy, 1980c)

cially close attention, being both striking manipulations of the pictorial medium and as nonliteral as some of the postural devices.

The two added graphics used in portraying a man walking were from Ly (early, totally blind), who used small circles, each standing for a foot, to indicate "steps he's taking . . . as if walking towards me" (Figure 9.9), and from Pau (late, totally blind), who used lines at neck level as a sign of the direction of movement.

In drawing the man running, Ly continued to add swirls below the feet, now more densely packed, "very quick as if the feet were moving." Pau also added circles for footsteps. Na (early, totally blind) put a curved line behind one foot that "shows how fast he's running."

To distinguish a spinning wheel from a static one, one cannot just freeze the movement and portray it. More needs to be done.

The various devices depicting the spinning wheel can be classified as devices of context, modified shape, and additional graphics. Context was

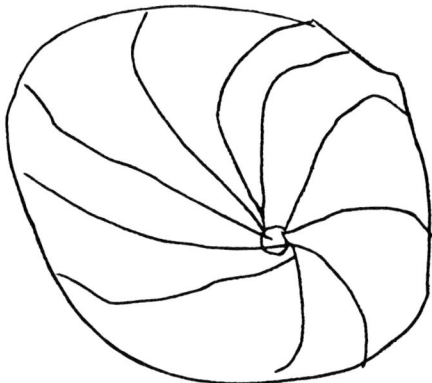

Figure 9.10. A raised-line drawing of a spinning wheel, by Pa (Toronto, adult, congenitally totally blind). (From Kennedy, 1980c)

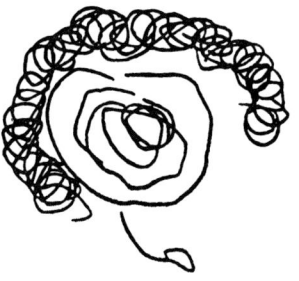

Figure 9.11. A raised-line drawing depicting a spinning wheel, showing movement by means of a dense spiral exterior to the wheel and interior circles, by Pau (Toronto, adult, totally blind after age 5). (From Kennedy, 1980c)

employed once, modifications of shape six times, and graphic indicators three times.

The context device is Ro's (late, totally blind), who drew the wheel held by a bicycle fork and a boy's hand pushing the wheel. Shape modifications included curving the spokes, as in Figure 9.10 (Pa, early, totally blind; Mau and Ra, both late, totally blind), putting the hub off center (Na, early, totally blind), and making the spokes more crossed and mixed up (Ji, early, totally blind).

The added graphics were circles added to the one for the circumference of the wheel from De, Ly (both early, totally blind), and Pau (late, totally blind), who drew the dense spiral shown in Figure 9.11 and some interior circles.

Similarly, to show the wheel rolling, shape modifications were used on five occasions, context was used seven times, and added graphics appeared four times. Related devices were used to show a moving car.

If one were to take all the lines in all of these drawings literally and try to find an outline feature for each, the intent would be lost. The artists do not believe that spokes curve or lengthen, that hubs leave the center of the wheel, that back wheels are small, or that there are spirals of substance left in the wake of turning wheels or moving feet. On the assumption that the use of the outline system to depict the depth and slant features of the environment realistically is *literal*, the modifications of shape and added graphics to show a revolving wheel are *metaphors;* in this sense, the blind adults here are inventing pictorial metaphors.

Discussion

This research program is unique in proposing a universal, untutored picturing ability in the blind. Thus the main hypothesis of this chapter is that the blind person raised with experience of the ecological, tangible environment of solid surfaces has an untutored ability to understand and make raised-line depictions. In particular, the blind person, it is hypothesized, may understand pictures made in outline style and deploy raised lines in literal and metaphoric ways.

Each group tested has some advantages and some disadvantages, so far as the basic hypothesis is concerned.

It is easier to communicate with adults than with children. Adults do not tire so readily in interviews, and they are likely to be more familiar with representational displays such as graphs, charts, and diagrams, with a possible spillover when trying pictures. However, as their own reports of their experience suggest, they have usually not been taught the outline style and methods for depicting depth and movement.

The American children are not as familiar as the Toronto adults with sophisticated, conventional displays. Some of them may have notable difficulties in handling tasks in a structured interview and in communicating with the interviewer. And they become noticeably less motivated toward the end of an interview.

The Haitian children are even less accustomed to representational displays, except for braille text. Their general intellectual achievement is low, and communication with them takes place across a cultural barrier. Their previous experience with the kinds of plastic sheets and styles involved in the drawing tests is minimal or nonexistent.

However, these cautions have to be weighed against the convergence

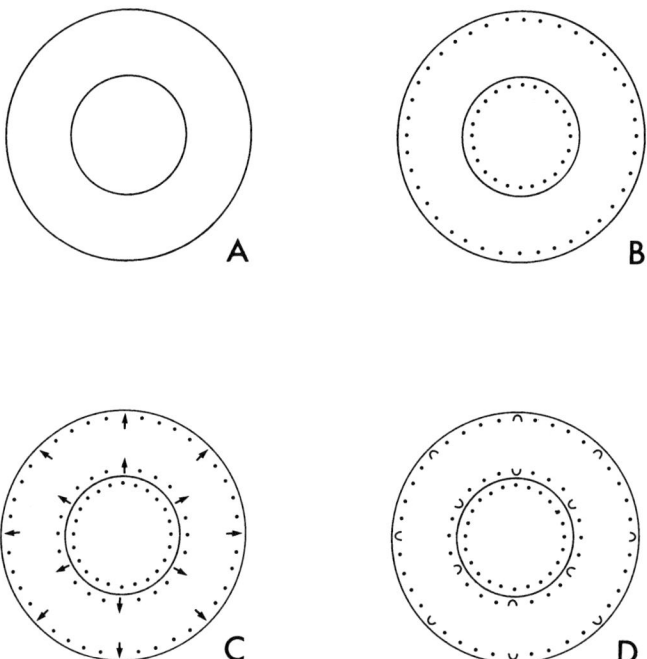

Figure 9.12. *A* is ambiguous, for it could depict, for example, a penny on a plate or the sun seen through a porthole. *B* uses dots to indicate the foreground side of the line and shows a flat disc on another flat disc. *C* uses arrows to indicate a slant and shows a cylinder with a flat bottom – a bucket. *D* uses arcs to indicate concavity and shows a bowl. (from Kennedy, 1980c)

of the results, the way in which comparable patterns are produced by the various types of subjects, whether congenitally or later blind. The fact remains that each group contains a number of individuals who devise the same kinds of responses in drawing or react in similar ways to the pictures they attempt to recognize. Each of the quite disparate groups produced displays that used the outline style (depth puzzles), handled problems in comparable ways (buildup, lines surrounding outlines, and fold-out), and depicted movement with the same devices (context, metaphoric changes in shape, and graphic additions).

Outlines can stand for any of several features of a surface layout. But one must discover the configuration of which a line is a part to know which referent to call upon, and the discovery process can be time-consuming. Some help in clarifying particular lines would be beneficial. Accordingly, a system devised by J. Campbell and myself may be useful (Figure 9.12).

A series of dots to one side of the line could be used to indicate which side of the line depicts the near surface or foreground – the figure, to use Rubin's (1915) terms. The side with the dots is to be taken as foreground. If there are no dots on either side, the line is a wire. If there are dots on both sides, the foreground is on both sides (e.g., a corner). In addition, a small arrowhead to one side of the line could indicate which way the surface slanted – toward the observer in the direction of the arrow, we suggest. Thus two arrowheads on either side of the line pointing toward the line indicate that the line represents a convex corner. If both arrows point away from the line, it stands for a concave corner.

Finally, let the arrowhead be replaced by an arc where the surface is rounded rather than flat. If the arc is concave toward the line, the line shows a rounded surface like a ball. If the arc is convex toward the line, the line shows a rounded surface like the interior of a bowl.

In sum, dots, coupled with occasional arrows and arcs, could clarify corners, occluding edges, occluding bounds, and parallel features such as wires without requiring the subject to explore an entire configuration to untangle a particular line. Also, the display can be so simple that it is incapable of clarifying its lines and yet still be serviceable.

Acknowledgments

Assistance from the National Sciences and Engineering Research Council, Canada, is acknowledged.

References

Berkeley, G. Essay toward a new theory of vision, 1709. In A. A. Luce & T. E. Jessop (Eds.), *The works of George Berkeley, Bishop of Cloyne*, vol. 1. Toronto: Nelson, 1948, pp. 143–239.

Davenport, R. K., & Rogers, C. M. Perception of photographs by apes. *Behaviour*, 1971, *39*, 318–320.

Ettlinger, G. Learning in two sense modalities. *Nature*, 1961, *191*, 398.

Fletcher, J. Space processing in the blind. Unpublished doctoral thesis, University of Toronto, 1981.

Friedman, S., & Stevenson, M. Perception of movement in pictures. In M. A. Hagen (Ed.), *What then is a picture? The psychology of representational art*. New York: Academic Press, 1980.

Fukarai. *How can I make what I cannot see?* New York: Van Nostrand, 1974.

Gibson, J. J. Observations on active touch. *Psychological Review*, 1962, *69*, 477–491.

The senses considered as perceptual systems. Boston: Houghton Mifflin, 1966.

The ecological approach to the visual perception of pictures. *Leonardo*, 1978, *11*, 227–235.

Guarniero, G. Experience of tactile vision. *Perception*, 1974, *3*, 101–104.

The senses and the perception of space. Unpublished doctoral thesis, New York University, 1978.

Jensen, V. A., & Haller, D. W. *What's that?* London: Collins, 1978.

Katz, D. Der aufbau der tastwelt. *Zeitschrift für Psychologie*, 1925, *11*, 1–270.

Kennedy, J. M. A psychology of picture perception. San Francisco: Jossey-Bass, 1974. (a)

Pictures, perception and the etcetera principle. In R. B. MacLeod & H. Pick (Eds.), Perception: essays in honor of J. J. Gibson. Ithaca, N. Y.: Cornell University Press, 1974. (b)

Pictures and the blind. Paper presented at the meeting of the American Psychological Association, Toronto, August 1978. (a)

Haptics. In E. C. Carterette and M. P. Friedman (Eds.), Handbook of perception, vol. 8. New York: Academic Press, 1978. (b)

The blind can recognize and make pictures. In M. Hagen (Ed.), What then is a picture? the psychology of representational art. New York: Academic Press, 1980. (a)

Depiction considered as a representational system. In J. Furber (Ed.), Perceiving artworks. Philadelphia: Temple University Press, Philosophical Monographs, 1980. (b)

Haptic pictures. Papers in Language Use and Language Function. Toronto: Scarborough College, no. 13, 1980. (c)

Kennedy, J. M., & Fox, N. Pictures to see and pictures to touch. In D. Perkins & B. Leondar (Eds.), The arts and cognition. Baltimore: Johns Hopkins University Press, 1977.

Kennedy, J. M, Fox, N., & O'Grady, K. Can haptic pictures help the blind to see? A study of drawings to be touched. Harvard Graduate School of Education Bulletin, 1972, 16, 22–23.

Kennedy, J. M., & Heywood, M. Picturing the tangible world. Videotape documentary. Scarborough College Audio-Visual Centre, 1979.

Kennedy, J. M., & Ostry, D. J. Approaches to picture perception: Perceptual experience and ecological optics, Canadian Journal of Psychology, 1976, 30, 90–98.

Kennedy, J. M., & Ross, A. S. Outline picture perception by the Songe of Papua. Perception, 1975, 4, 391–406.

Korzenik, D. Saying it with pictures. In D. Perkins & B. Leondar (Eds.), The arts and cognition. Baltimore: Johns Hopkins University Press, 1977.

Marks, L. E. Multimodal perception. In E. C. Carterette and M. P. Friedman, (Eds.), Handbook of perception, vol. 8. New York: Academic Press, 1978.

Merry, R. V., & Merry, F. K. The tactual recognition of embossed pictures by blind children. Journal of Applied Psychology, 1933, 17, 148–163.

Millar, S. Visual experience or translation rules? Drawing the human figure by blind and sighted children. Perception, 1975, 4, 363–371.

Nuffield Foundation report on the education of the blind. London: Nuffield Foundation, 1973.

Olson, D. R. Cognitive development: the child's acquisition of diagonality. New York: Academic Press, 1970.

Révész, G. Psychology and art of the blind. Toronto: Longmans, Green, 1950.

Rubin, E. Synsoplevede figurer. Copenhagen: Gyldendals, 1915.

Senden, M. von. Raum- und Gestalt-auffassung bei operierten Blind geborenen vor und nach der Operation. Leipzig: Barth, 1932. (Translated by P. Heath as Space and sight. London: Methuen, 1960.)

Shagan, J. Kinaesthetic memory in blind and sighted individuals. Unpublished doctoral thesis, George Washington University, 1970.

Vincent, C. N. Pictorial recognition and teaching the blind to draw. The Communication of Scientific and Technical Information, 1977, 31, 8–15.

Warren, D. H. Perception by the blind. In E. C. Carterette & M. P. Friedman (Eds.), Handbook of perception, vol. 10. New York: Academic Press, 1978.

Wilberg, R. B., & Girouard, Y. Information sur les distances, effect de l'étendue les stimuli et mémoire motrice à court terme. *Canadian Journal of Psychology,* 1976, *30,* 63–71.

Willats, J. Development of perspective drawing in the child. Paper presented at the Concordia University Symposium on Perception, Cognition, and Representation, 1979.

10. Mobility maps

GRAHAME A. JAMES

Grahame James's chapter is concerned with the design, use, and improvement of mobility maps for visually impaired people. James's work at the National Mobility Center in Birmingham, England, and his earlier research at the Blind Mobility Research Unit, Nottingham, provide him with a wealth of firsthand information on the use of mobility maps.

He begins by introducing various types of tangible maps and discusses their relationship to maps in general. Maps are useful providers of several sorts of spatial information relevant not only to mobility but to knowledge of the spatial layout of the world. Traveling through this world is a major problem for many blind persons, and the importance of map scales, symbology, and training in the uses of maps is stressed in James's review of the relevant research literature. James introduces readers to some of the kits and other materials found to be successful by map producers and useful by blind travelers. Not all maps useful for blind people are tangible; verbal maps and verbal adjuncts to maps also play a role in mobility.

James's excursion through the world of mobility maps includes not only shopping centers and campuses, which seem to be heavily represented in maps for blind travelers, but also the more esoteric terrains of pedestrian subway travel, yachting, and orienteering. He concludes with recommendations regarding map making and future map research, all of which should prove useful for applied researchers concerned with representing terrestrial space and with education and rehabilitation of the visually handicapped.

WILLIAM SCHIFF

Introduction

A blind person traveling on foot or using public transport in a new area requires geographical information. This person may need to know the layout of streets in a city or town and the position of important landmarks. Details on the location of shops, public buildings, or public transport routes may be required. These types of spatial information can be provided by mobility maps.

Maps of the world, continents, climates, and so forth are necessarily small scale because of the large area represented. Conversely, mobility maps are large scale in order to include the details likely to be useful to the blind pedestrian. Often, two maps of different scales are used by a blind person – one to gain a general impression of an area and to orient the self, and a second to gain sufficiently detailed information to permit independent travel. For example, a general orientation map would display the position of a railway station within the context of major streets and buildings in the vicinity, whereas a more detailed map would show the actual station building.

Maps are commonly defined as representations on a flat surface of all or part of the earth's surface. This now embraces areas on other planets and includes other solar systems. Essentially, a map is a two-dimensional portrayal of spatial information, whereas a diagram or a model may be three-dimensional.

Differences between blind and sighted map readers

Consider a sighted person reading a map. He or she is able to obtain a simultaneous visual impression of the spatial relationships represented on the map's surface. For example, a regular street pattern in a town would be identifiable with no more than a brief inspection. The shape would have immediate visual impact, although identifying an actual street might require considerable searching. If a raised-line facsimile of that street plan were produced, it would need to be much larger in scale to be read by touch alone, and it would probably require considerable simplification before it was legible. No doubt many raised mobility maps are useless because the map maker attempted to transliterate from the printed map without considering the different information-processing ability of touch compared with vision. Moreover, the strategy for reading the raised-line street map would be quite different from that of reading the printed one. The reader would not gain a simultaneous impression of the map content from a brief inspection; instead, he or she would need to build up impressions by exploring the details section by section. The overall impression of the map content would, therefore, appear to consist of an accumulation of separate haptic experiences. Nevertheless, like the sighted map reader, the blind person should be able to gain an overall cognitive image from the information displayed on the map. The adequacy of this cognitive image, inasmuch as it corresponds to reality, may be tested by questions or tasks that might be answered or accomplished by sighted and blind map readers.

Maps as abstractions

It is important to emphasize that maps are abstractions of the real world. A simple aerial photograph, for example, may be identifiable visually because of the many recognizable features displayed. A map of the same area may be meaningless if the map reader is not familiar with the conventional symbols used to depict the salient features. Similarly, to use a mobility map successfully, a blind person needs to relate the abstract representation on the map's surface to reality. This requires not only the mastery of symbol interpretation but also the understanding of basic concepts such as geographical compass points, distance and scale, relative position, and so forth. Many sighted people never master these basic concepts, which are essential to reading even a simple street plan.

Once basic map-reading skills have been established, maps prove very rich in spatial information. Consider the fact that one location on a map's surface may be related to an almost infinite number of other locations. Consider the various frames of reference that can be used by the map reader: Relative positions may be defined as being north or south of each other, up or down, to the left or right, or at a certain distance. It is possible to make a variety of decisions or observations about the structure of an area not experienced directly, but with the aid of a single map. Ideally, raised-line mobility maps should present the blind person with spatial information that is not easily communicated through other means.

Verbal descriptions of a geographical area or a route through an area are often referred to as maps. A verbal description is the chief method by which blind persons gather information about a geographical area. Typically, they may ask a sighted friend or gain information from a professional mobility instructor. The information may be presented as a description familiarizing the blind person with a new locality or as a list of instructions. Further, it may be presented aurally on a tape recorder or in printed form (large print or braille). Verbal route maps, which convey the minimum information to allow a blind person to travel from A to B, may be presented in an abbreviated or code form.

Verbal maps appear to be most successful when the information is relatively simple or confined to single routes. For the skillful blind traveler, a route is adequately described by a series of instructions indicating the main choice points, landmarks, and additional information to confirm that the path is correct. Of course, for this type of route map, it is often difficult to reverse the instructions provided for a route from A to B in order to return from B to A. A separate map may be required. Because a list of instructions conveys information sequentially about a particular route as a blind person actually experiences it, verbal route maps may provide much useful information.

Verbal route maps cannot do much more than describe the main features of a narrow perceptual tunnel through which a blind person travels. However, they may attempt to provide a more extended representation of the environment than a single route through it. In such a map, a narrator would attempt to describe the boundaries of an area, its shape, its size, and the relative positions of the main features. This is a difficult task. The narrator is attempting to convey details of a spatial display through a sequence of words. Provided the area being described is relatively simple, the verbal map may be successful. However, if the area is complex, the listener may get lost in the wealth of detail; may forget previous information and fail to connect the components being described to an overall structure; may abandon the verbal map because it does not proceed at a suitable pace; and may fail to gain any Gestalt whatever from the display.

Despite their drawbacks, verbal maps have many advantages for the wide variety of potential users. When compared with tactual mobility maps, less new conceptual skill is required to understand an auditory display. Auditory maps may be easier to prepare and more cost-effective. In addition, many blind people have difficulty in reading tactually, although raised map displays have been dealt with quite successfully by nonbraille readers. Nonbraille readers should not, therefore, be precluded from using tactual mobility maps.

Rather than being conceptualized as separate entities, the various types of mobility maps should be viewed as complementary. A tactual map should be more meaningful if a verbal introduction is provided; a verbal map of an area might be more meaningful if a raised-line outline of that area is provided, no matter how rudimentary.

Research review

The majority of blind people have never used a mobility map for independent travel because only a small proportion attempts any kind of independent travel. For example, Gray and Todd (1968) found that only about 15 percent of the blind population added anything new to their repertoire of routes that would require a mobility map. Even for those few who might require mobility maps, only recently has progress been made in providing a variety of maps that are legible or understandable.

Little basic research is available indicating how spatial information is

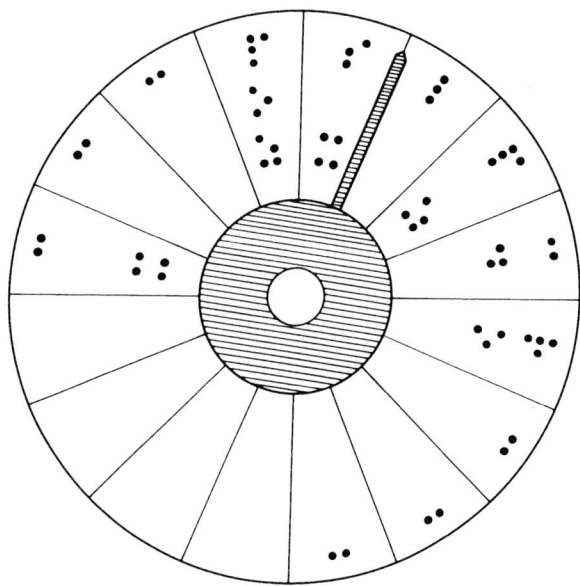

Figure 10.1. The plastic memory disc for the route used in the Leonard and Newman (1970) study. A cursor can be moved in 16 steps to indicate the person's place on the memory disc. Braille letters provide coded information: An outer ring on the disc indicates action to be taken at the end of the block (e.g., left or right turn); a middle ring provides information about the special features; an inner ring indicates the appropriate side of the street.

best presented nonvisually or for people whose vision is impaired. Maglione (1969) demonstrated that blind and blindfolded subjects who used a tactual map in addition to verbal instructions were able to travel a maze pattern more quickly and with fewer errors than subjects who used only verbal instructions.

At a more practical level, Leonard and Newman (1967) demonstrated that congenitally blind schoolchildren could travel a relatively simple but unfamiliar street route with only the aid of a tactual route map for navigation.

Leonard and Newman (1970) further established the viability of portable route maps when they compared the use of three types of maps for blind people: the tape-recorded route map, a memory disc (Figure 10.1), and a "spatial diagrammatic map." This study found that half of the subjects using the tactual maps were able to complete an unfamiliar test route (2 km [1.25 mi] long) with no errors.

Leonard and Newman's work centered on plastic maps produced by the Thermoform process from deposited masters devised by W. J.

Pickles, Worcester College for the Blind, England. Their experimental results of map use were confined to single street routes.

However, Bentzen (1971, 1972) was the first to demonstrate that blind subjects could successfully use a tactual map to plan their own routes to different objectives. She designed a map of Perkins School for the Blind, hand-produced it by inscribing a master of metal foil, and used depositions of wood and sandpaper to produce symbols. Plastic copies were then produced by the Thermoform process (a simple vacuum-forming process). Her choice of symbols was decided on the basis of previous research (Angwin, 1968; Leonard & Newman, 1970; Schiff, 1966; Wiedel & Groves, 1969). A novel feature of this map was the use of overlays to display braille and different classes of tactual information. After training in map reading, all subjects in this study were able to locate successfully three objectives on an unfamiliar Perkins campus.

Wiedel and Groves (1969) conducted a series of studies on problems of design, reproduction, reading, and interpretation of tactual maps for mobility. Their main conclusions, some influenced by Schiff (1966) were:

> Tactual maps must hold enough information to meet the needs of the user but not so much as to confuse him.

> Clutter can be partly eliminated by the use of elevation difference of symbols according to selected criteria: braille .02 in., line and area symbols .04, and point symbols .06 in.

> Symbolization must be standardized in order to facilitate design and use.

> The north edge of the sheet must be marked – a north indicator is not adequate.

> Braille need not be placed all horizontally.

> Multi-layered maps can be used. In fact they are desirable when large amounts or different types of information are needed.

> Selection of information to be mapped on Mobility and Orientation maps must be made by personal inspection. The landmarks and information required by the blind do not appear on existing map sources. (1969, passim, p. xviii)

Wiedel and Groves's work was notable for its inclusion of a list of suggested symbols to represent specific landmarks, although no criteria of acceptability were provided.

They reported that on one of their maps, a "red overprint was added to facilitate the sighted in helping the blind" (p. 11). The use of visual markings can also help low-vision or partially sighted travelers (Sherman, 1965).

Kidwell and Greer (1972, 1973), at that time architectural students,

339

designed and evaluated a tactual map of the Massachusetts Institute of Technology. The map was produced by Harry Friedman of Howe Press, in polyvinyl chloride by a process normally used for making table mats. The material was flexible, weather resistant, and durable.

One of the main features of the MIT map was the wealth of detail. Its high information density would probably make it a difficult proposition for all but highly skilled tactual readers.

Braille labels were placed on the underside of the MIT map, and print legends and symbols were provided for the sighted reader.

Prior to some of the research just described, a good deal of the groundwork on mobility maps had been covered by teachers and mobility specialists, although their efforts were not always documented. W. R. K. James (1972) emphasized the fact that the blind child is seldom trained to think in terms of spatial concepts, let alone representations of these concepts. His work on three-dimensional illustrations suggests that children have to be taught basic concepts by concrete experiences. James emphasized that blind children should gain experiences of known places, and then these may be represented in simple diagrammatic form. It is well known that the sighted child receives constant exposure to diagrammatic representation via news media, advertisements, and picture books. The blind child, in contrast, is relatively deprived of these kinds of experiences.

W. R. K. James produced some quite detailed maps, such as the one of Coventry Cathedral, England, and another to illustrate *Treasure Island*. However, he maintained that maps and diagrams are a means of organizing information and concepts; therefore, very simple representations of the known environment are essential stepping stones to the development of basic concepts that enable a blind child to understand mobility maps or any other haptic displays.

Congenital or early-onset blind children frequently develop conceptual distortions as a result of too many verbal instructions or descriptions of the environment that have never been reinforced or corrected through physical contact or direct experience. Gilson, Wurzburger, and Johnson (1965) reported that tactual maps could eliminate confusion and distortion of environmental concepts that may be responsible for the blind child's lack of confidence in traveling and reluctance to explore independently. Tooze (1978) verified these observations and developed a systematic program of map instruction aimed at improving navigational skills in blind schoolchildren. Pickles (1970) developed a similar program.

This chapter does not concentrate on production techniques for tactual mobility maps, but a few points require consideration because they directly affect the progress of previous research. For example, the Royal

National Institute for the Blind's (RNIB) map of the London Underground Railway is produced on manila paper. Many blind people prefer paper as a reading medium, but generally it is insufficiently durable and weatherproof for outdoor use. Wood, rubber, and linoleum have also been used to produce special-purpose maps, such as the one at the Leamington Guide Dog Centre in England.

Mass-production systems, both in the United Kingdom and the United States, have been confined largely to the production of world, continent, and regional maps. (An exception is the RNIB'S map of Central London and Birmingham City Centre.) Historically, mobility maps have been produced locally, often for specific blind people or special purposes. They have been produced by schoolteachers (Pickles, 1970; Tooze, 1978), mobility instructors (Mumford, 1972), or interested volunteers (Angwin, 1968). Local involvement and the fact that only a small number of blind people are potentially able to use maps for travel purposes prompted Leonard (1970) to comment that one should seek solutions in which standardized procedures can be applied locally at relatively low cost and without complex equipment.

Standardization of symbols

A conference held at Birmingham University, England, in 1968 was attended by 10 people concerned with research on mobility maps that they defined as "orientation," "mobility (neighborhood)," and "special-purpose types." Other conferences at the American Printing House (Louisville, Ky.) and Worcester College for the Blind in 1971 attempted to deal with dissemination of information and some standardization for mobility maps. The growing interest in mobility maps was reflected by the International Conference on Mobility Maps held at Nottingham, England, in 1972 and attended by 72 people.

At the Nottingham conference, agreement was reached on a list of environmental features that should be represented on tactual mobility maps. Appropriate symbols to match these features were subsequently produced using a computer-aided design system at Warwick University (Gill, 1974). The appropriateness of this matching was evaluated based on the long-term retention by blind children of the meanings of each symbol (James & Gill, 1974).

Another result of this conference was that current information on mobility maps was recorded in a handbook (Armstrong, 1973). When this information was disseminated in the United Kingdom, more mobility maps became available for blind people than at any time in the past.

341

Although the handbook acted as a fillip to mobility map makers, any kind of standardization of symbols for plastic Thermoform maps was severely limited by the variety of production techniques commonly used. Maps were produced by ingenious attempts at improvisation: Nuts, washers, string, and fabrics were used. Agreement on symbology for mobility maps was frustrated by lack of standard materials rather than other considerations.

The Nottingham Kit for making raised maps

The Blind Mobility Research Unit, Nottingham, then developed and marketed a complete kit of materials for map making by the Thermoform process. The Nottingham Kit for Making Raised Maps represented a considerable advance in providing standard materials to be used locally (James, 1975).

Figure 10.2 shows the contents of the map-making kit. Six different line symbols are produced from soft solder that is rolled into a suitably engraved die with the aid of a lathe. Point symbols are produced by injecting a mold with plastic to produce "trees" of symbols. Area symbols consist of quantities of linoleum tile, sandpaper, aluminum gauze, and tapestry canvas with suggestions that these should represent buildings, parks and open spaces, pedestrian ways, and areas of water, respectively.

In order to produce a map master with the kit, symbols are attached to a sheet of transparent cellulose covered with Twinstick to provide a sticky surface. Once completed, the sticky surface is neutralized by sprinkling the area with glass powder (ballotini). Copies are then vacuum-formed in plastic from the map master.

Figures 10.3 and 10.4 illustrate the key sheets provided with the kit to assist in standardization. Figure 10.5 illustrates a simple Thermoform street map of a quiet residential area produced by materials from the kit.

Now, with a generally accepted standard for symbols on mobility maps, it became possible for individuals trained to read maps made by a map maker in one part of the United Kingdom to read maps made elsewhere without the need to learn a new set of symbols.

Map-making courses were organized in England (James & Campbell, 1975) and in Sweden.

As the result of a number of new developments in types of maps, a new version of the maps handbook was published (James & Armstrong, 1976). This handbook was also translated into Swedish (Jansson, 1977) and Japanese.

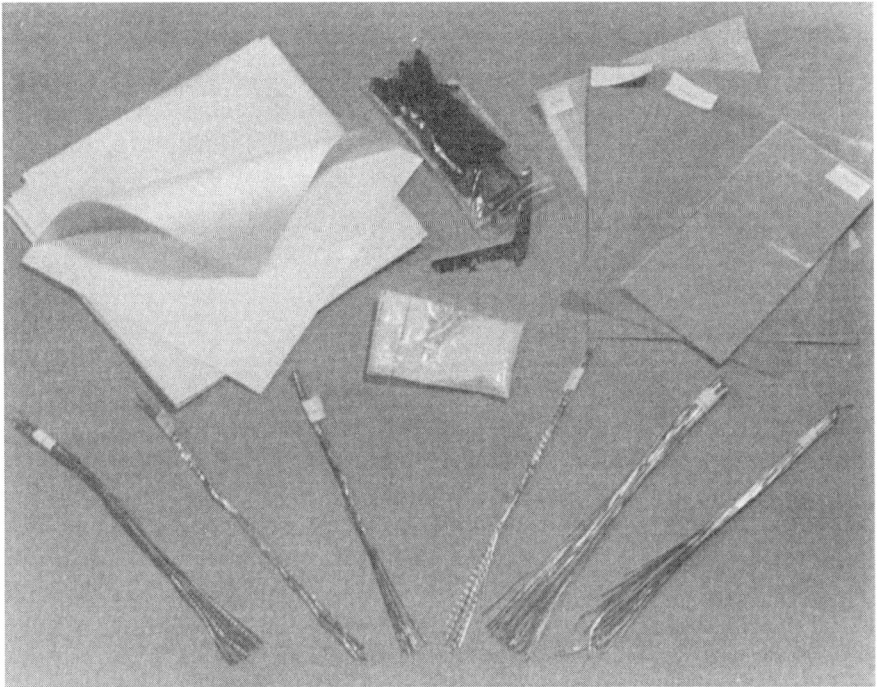

Figure 10.2. The contents of the Nottingham Kit for Making Raised Maps. (Courtesy of Sam Grainger)

After the publication of the new handbook, many new developments in the production of mobility maps were made by professional mobility instructors for use as teaching aids. New maps included ones of simple indoor areas, more complex shopping centers, railway stations, and university campuses, in addition to street plans.

A shopping center map

Blind people usually request area maps when there is a strong likelihood of becoming disoriented. The Victoria Shopping Centre in Nottingham, for example, is complex. However, James and Armstrong (1975) demonstrated that once blind people were taught to use a map of the shopping center, it proved very valuable for travel purposes. Pillars located in the shopping mall were labeled in braille with three types of information: (1) D or U indicating lower or upper floor, (2) E or W indicating east or west side of the mall, and (3) a numeral that was referenced on the map and allowed the map reader to locate and identify the names of shops. Figure

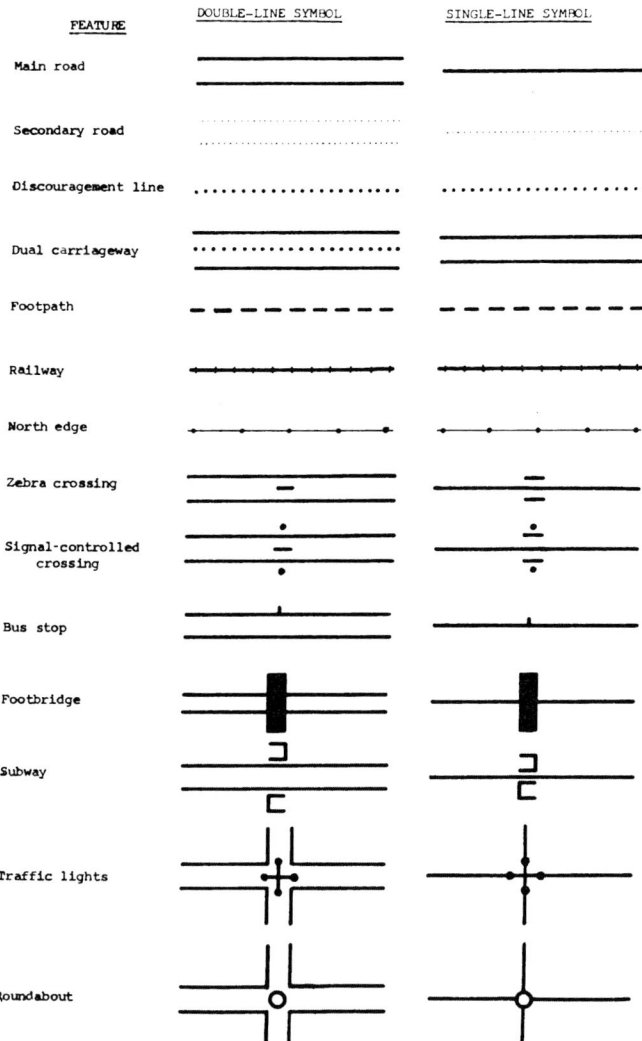

Figure 10.3. Printed key sheets provided with the map-making kit assist the maker in using standard symbols.

10.6 shows a blind person using the map. A detailed task analysis consisted of tasks ranging from easy to difficult. It was found that two congenitally blind people could use the map and shop independently without prior direct experience with the shopping center. Figure 10.7 illustrates one of the routes taken by blind people. The route may be conceptualized as a three-dimensional diagram. How might a congenitally blind person conceptualize it?

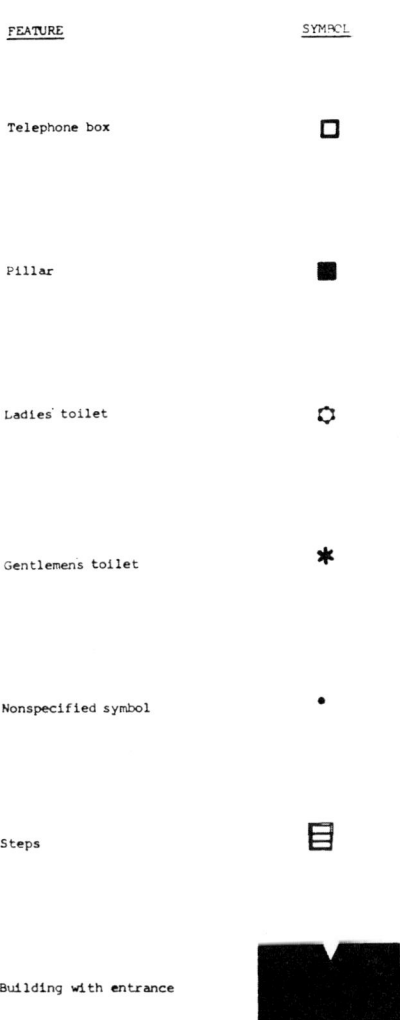

FEATURE   SYMBOL

Telephone box

Pillar

Ladies' toilet

Gentlemens toilet

Nonspecified symbol

Steps

Building with entrance

Figure 10.4. Printed key sheets provided with the map-making kit.

Pedestrian subways

Pedestrian subways are another example of difficult areas for blind people. Frequently, there is a shortage of nonvisual navigational clues. James, Campbell, and Armstrong (1974) demonstrated how blind people could be disoriented deliberately in a complex pedestrian subway system and then could find a destination independently using a braille compass and a tactual map. Another similar study (James, 1977) involved posi-

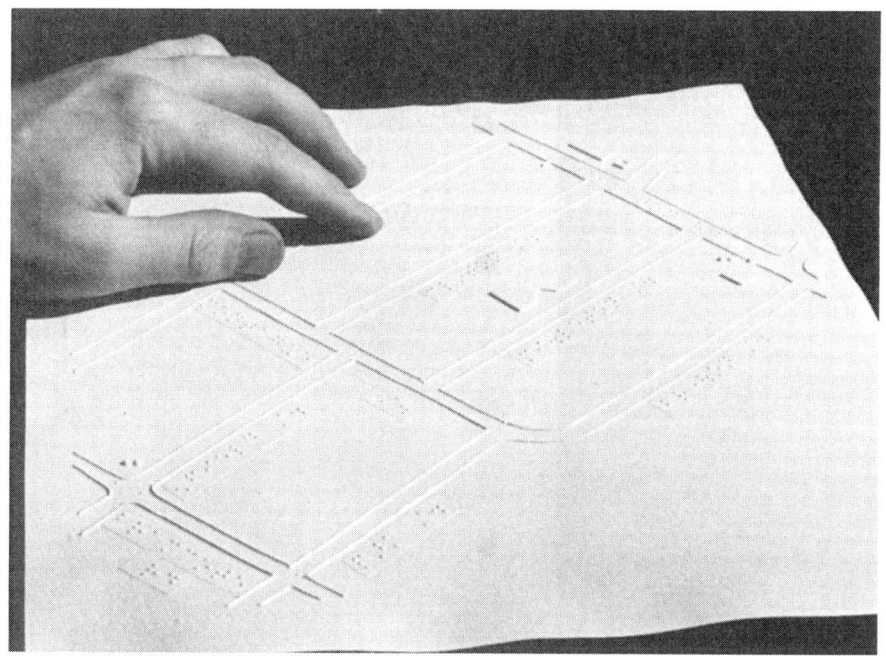

Figure 10.5. A Thermoform mobility map of a quiet residential area in England. The map was produced by a mobility instructor at the Blind Mobility Research Unit, Nottingham. (Courtesy of Sam Grainger)

tioning experimental tactual and large print labels on exit tunnels from a central subway concourse and observing that they were useful to blind people using a map or becoming disoriented.

Public transport maps

Information concerning public transport has also been provided through tactual maps. James and Swain (1975) produced a tactual map of the Nottingham City Centre. Four blind adults were taught to use the map, and all completed a map-reading evaluation consisting of questions to test their understanding of the map content. Finally, with the aid of the map, the blind people traveled as passengers on the buses. Observations confirmed that they could maintain a minute-by-minute record of their geographical position during travel.

Bentzen (1977) further illustrated how tactual maps could illustrate public transport routes. Two maps produced by different techniques were evaluated: first, a simple map of the Boston Rapid Transport Sys-

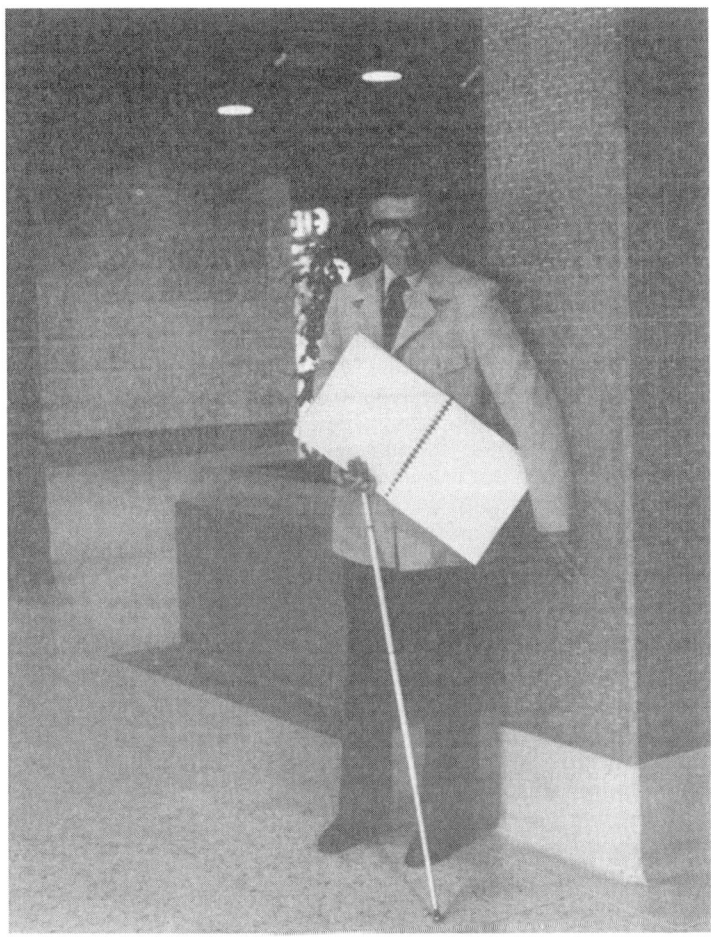

Figure 10.6. A blind person using the Victoria Shopping Centre map. The braille label fixed to the pillar in the shopping mall displays information about a person's geographical position, which can then be established by reading the tangible map. (Courtesy of Grahame James)

tem, and second, a detailed map of the Boston–Cambridge area. Eighteen visually impaired people planned and traveled an unfamiliar route using the maps and reported that they found the maps helpful in aiding understanding of the spatial relationships of the city and those of major transportation links.

Bentzen noted that not all visually impaired travelers in this study required instruction in map usage if an effective set of verbal instruc-

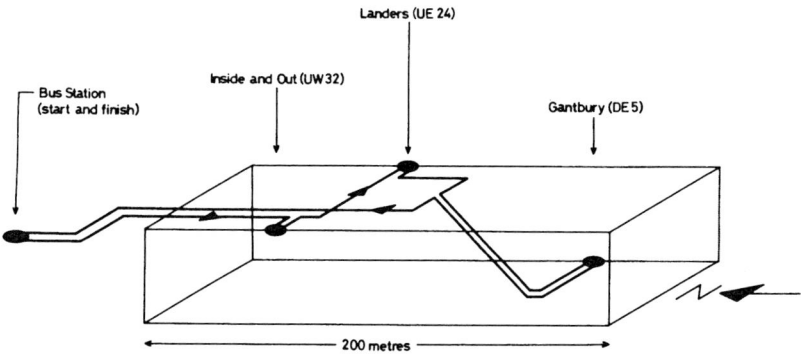

Figure 10.7. Route taken by blind people as part of the evaluation of the Victoria Shopping Centre map. Geographical information required to visit objectives on this route is obtained solely from separate maps illustrating the upper and lower floors of the shopping center. In this diagram, the route is conceptualized as a three-dimensional model. How might a congenitally blind person conceptualize the same route?

tions accompanied the map. She also noted that both tactual and visual coding systems were used by people with some usable near-point vision.

Verbal maps

Verbal mobility maps have received less attention in the literature than tactual ones. James, Armstrong, and Campbell (1973) surveyed the types of verbal instructions used by mobility instructors to give directions to blind people. Forty-five instructors, including chief instructors of the Guide Dogs for the Blind Association's Centres in the United Kingdom were sent a printed map showing a detailed street route. The instructors were requested to write down the instructions they would give to enable an imaginary blind person to negotiate the route on the map. The instructions were to be concise enough for the blind person to remember because no memory aids were allowed. The results of the survey showed considerable diversity in the terminology normally used. The instructions were analyzed on the basis of use of introduction or recapitulation, suggestions on where to seek public help at appropriate places, landmarks, use of traffic sounds, compass directions, methods of explaining distances, and whether or not street names were included. The survey concluded that although there is no such thing as an imaginary blind person, instructions *can* be presented in an organized form that is likely to be translated into action by the user.

Another study (Blasch, Welsh, & Davidson, 1973) reviewed the relative merits of auditory and other types of maps. They emphasized that auditory maps should be used by visually handicapped people already trained in mobility skills. Further, they distinguished between auditory *route* maps and auditory *district* maps and pointed out the advantages of both compared with tactual maps.

Recreational aids

Few studies have reported the use of any type of mobility maps as recreational aids for the visually handicapped. In 1977 and 1978 the Royal Yachting Association provided tactual charts for visually handicapped people participating in their sailing courses at Plymouth, England. The charts showed the position of dry land, major reference points such as lighthouses and buoys, and the boundaries of deep water. No formal observation of the efficacy of these charts was attempted, but some subjective reports confirm that they were useful.

James and Burnett (in press) organized an orienteering course for visually impaired schoolboys who competed in three separate teams rather than individually. *Orienteering* may be defined as a competitive sport that involves navigating from point to point with the aid of a special map and compass as quickly and efficiently as possible by whatever route one considers best. In this competition, navigational aids for each team consisted of braille compasses; tactual maps showing the major features of the course and the position of checkpoints; and braille descriptions listing checkpoints, compass directions and other topographical information, and a tape-recorded route map. The variety of navigational information ensured that each member could contribute to the team's progress. The results of the orienteering course confirmed that the boys worked hard physically and mentally and enjoyed an immense feeling of achievement as the result of participating in a challenging competitive sport. The study recommended that initially orienteering courses should consist of easily identifiable landmarks to ensure success, and emphasis should be placed on the development of navigational skill rather than speed.

During the past 10 years, research has contributed greatly to our understanding of how mobility maps may enable a visually handicapped person to gather geographical information about the immediate locality. Advances in standardized production techniques have enabled more people than ever to use legible, good-quality maps. The introduction of improved map-making materials and the dissemination of information about different types of mobility maps do not solve all the problems associated with producing maps or using them successfully. But at least we now have maps that can be supplied to people on demand, and we are able to evaluate their usefulness for the individual.

Map reading and training for map reading

It is difficult to be definitive about teaching map-reading methods because so much depends upon the interaction between teacher and student. Teachers use varying approaches, and their students respond in different ways depending upon age, experience, and ability. However, now that the use of maps is becoming a more common feature in the mobility program for blind people, a body of knowledge is quickly accumulating that permits the suggestion of teaching guidelines. This section presents guidelines to help teachers structure and develop their approach in using maps as teaching tools for mobility training.

Mobility skills

There is obviously a complex interaction between competence to travel safely and efficiently and the ability to utilize additional information for navigation. The two skills of competent travel and map reading cannot, therefore, be viewed in isolation.

The following basic mobility skills can be developed simultaneously with map-reading skills.

1. Straight-line walking without too much veering.
2. The use of auditory cues when moving: for instance, locating doorways, driveways, obstacles, ends of blocks, and landmarks, whether indoors or outdoors, and traffic directions.
3. Identification of textures underfoot.
4. Fairly rapid movement in travel; this leads to fewer errors in the location of landmarks.
5. Awareness or a mental picture of the environment through the use of different reference systems. This entails the development of considerable perceptual ability.
6. Knowledge of the structure of different environmental features: street crossings, types of road junctions and street patterns.

Map-reading skills

As stated previously, steps leading to competent map reading can be described only generally because age, degree and onset of blindness, and ability are influencing factors. An adventitiously blind adult may have a visual frame of reference from previous experience with printed maps that may facilitate learning. On the other hand, a congenitally blind child will need basic training in surface representation and geographical concepts, just as the sighted child needs this training for print maps and diagrams before he or she is able to understand them. The following broadly defined steps, leading to the competent use of mobility maps, will be expanded upon in this section:

1. Involve students in an active learning situation by encouraging them to make maps for themselves that represent the environment they know or can discover.
2. Teach the use of different geographical reference systems. Involve students in using these reference systems to describe areas and the locations of places.
3. Begin by using simple maps of known areas and ask students to solve problems that will improve their understanding of the relationship between map and environment.
4. Introduce more complex maps with greater detail and symbolism.
5. Introduce maps of unknown environments with detour problems or route-planning exercises. Use maps for planning journeys on public transportation and visiting unknown areas.

Early training

A basic starting point in teaching the use of mobility maps is the development of the student's body image (see Cratty, 1971, and Kratz, 1973). The ability to understand different personal and geographical reference systems is a necessary part of early training. Versatility should be developed in the use of different reference systems such as left and right, turning 45, 90, and 180 degrees, and using the points of the clock and compass points. The use of auditory cues for direction finding is an important aspect of developing the orientation skill of blind children. These kinds of skills can be approached through physical education and dance activities.

Combining reference systems

Geographical reference systems have to be taught separately before they are combined. But once the references have been firmly established, they may be used in combination. For example, teaching points can help establish that if one walks north and then changes direction to walk west this is the same as making a left turn. Or if one walks east after walking south, this again is the same as a left turn. Combining these reference systems greatly facilitates the ability to understand maps. A common problem with orienting maps is that the map reader cannot conceptualize the map from any other point of view except that of facing north (i.e.

351

when facing north, west is on the left, east on the right, and south behind). The problem arises when the map is oriented south, and west is now on the right, east on the left, and north behind the map reader. Many map readers suffer reversal problems with the position of east and west in this situation and become confused. A good early training exercise to reduce the likelihood of this happening is to ask the student to face each compass point and then to point to the others and describe their position. For blind children, this can form the basis of a game. General principles of physical geography fit in with combining geographical reference systems. For example, in the morning the position of the sun indicates the direction of east, at midday (in northern latitudes) it indicates south, and in the evening the sun sets in the west. Knowledge of prevailing winds may also aid orientation. The position of the sun or the direction and strength of prevailing winds may sometimes be unreliable cues. However, knowledge of and experience with these cues may permit a blind person to use them almost automatically when they are available.

Initial representation using raised symbols

As previously stated, it is unwise to develop map-reading and interpreting skills from abstract representations. Rather, early training should include demonstrations that the known environment can be represented in simple, abstract form. In schools this training can proceed in conjunction with surface representation used in mathematics, geography, and the sciences. Actual models, block representations, and outline plans can be used to develop understanding of surface representation. Students can begin by making simple maps or models of areas that are already familiar to them (e.g., the classroom) and then systematically progress to more complex maps of new areas. In the early stages, the students should be given only simple materials to ensure that they concentrate on the ideas involved rather than on the materials themselves.

Blind people drawing maps for themselves

Classrooms, corridors, or the rehabilitation center or grounds can be mapped by blind students themselves. For instance, as part of the mathematics program, blind children can measure the dimensions of their classroom and represent it to scale on a plan that they themselves draw. Blind adults may wish to draw outlines of the rooms in their homes so that they may experiment with the positioning of furniture. In this way, the concept of scale can be introduced in a practical manner.

Using a magnetic board to teach basic concepts

A magnetic board can be very useful for teaching basic concepts. Roads are represented by thin strips of magnetic rubber on a metal sheet. The strips can be moved around to build up different simple street layouts.

To begin with, blind students may explore a simple street in the environment. Then they can attempt to represent the street using the magnetic rubber strips. The rubber strip is a simplified representation of a road and includes no differentiation of pavements, curbs, or gutters from the street itself. Therefore, it has to be pointed out that the two sides of the strip represent the alternative pavements that could be walked on in real life. Students can run a finger down either side of the strip to establish this representation.

Next, students can explore and build up representations of more complex street layouts on the magnetic board. *T* junctions, *Y* junctions, crossroads, and cul-de-sacs on their own and, later, in combinations can be investigated.

Reinforcing knowledge of compass directions

Once a student is familiar with the idea that edges of the magnetic strip can represent two pavements, compass directions can be introduced. If the road runs from north to south, then the pavements will be east and west of the road line. At this stage, the convention of calling the top of the map "north" should be adhered to because this will provide a framework as more complex routes are constructed.

After a series of streets with different junctions have been investigated and represented on the board (e.g., *T* and *X* junctions or cul-de-sacs), a more complex street with side streets entering it should be chosen. For example, the street could run from north to south. Students can first walk north down the west pavement and investigate and name the corners of each side street they encounter. Then they can discover that each side street has two corners. The first corner will be the southwest corner, and the one on the other side will be the northwest corner. By exploring these corners in some detail, they can find some features whereby they can recognize them again. After this inspection they can return to the school and take notes on what they have discovered. They then walk to the next side street, where they repeat the exercise. Having investigated the four side streets, they return to school. By using their notes, they can make a map on the magnetic board using rubber strips that have street names in braille.

In the next lesson, students can walk down the east pavement. At each junction, they can cross the main street to determine its relationship to the streets on the other side. For example, there might be three side streets on the east side, one a crossroads with an opposite side street, one an "offset" crossroads, and the third forming a T junction. On returning to school, students complete their maps.

Tactual maps for blind people who do not read braille

In the early stages of teaching map reading, the map should be left clear of braille so that there is a low density of information to interpret. However, although over 60 percent of the blind population cannot read braille, this does not necessarily exclude them from using tactual maps.

Figure 10.8 shows a tactual map of the lounge of the RNIB Rehabilitation Centre at Clifton Spinney, Nottingham. It has proven useful in teaching blind people who read no braille about the layout of the lounge area and the position of furniture. Textures represent the seating areas around the edges of the room, and table and chairs are shown in the center. Other features such as the piano, sideboard, and telephone are also represented. The positions of doors from the lounge are shown by gaps in the line symbols representing the walls. As part of their indoor training, blind people are asked by the mobility instructor to locate objectives in the room after they have familiarized themselves with the map. If a mistake is made and the incorrect route is taken, the blind person can check the error on the map. This provides much faster and more immediate feedback than having to travel the route again and rely on the instructor's directions. By referring to the map, blind persons may explain any errors to themselves and their instructor and then take the correct route. Tasks can be made more difficult by asking map readers to sit in different places in the lounge so that they must reorient their map and therefore alter their perspective of the room. Extension of these kinds of exercises should ensure that blind persons become versatile in conceptualizing the immediate surroundings from different points of view depending upon where they are in the building.

A whole building can be mapped in this simple way so that blind persons undergoing rehabilitation will have a complete record of the building where they are staying. With adequate reinforcement and direct experience, this should assist them to be well oriented with respect to their surroundings.

Teaching the discrimination of raised print and raised numbers. It is valuable for congenitally or early blind children to be able to read raised upper-

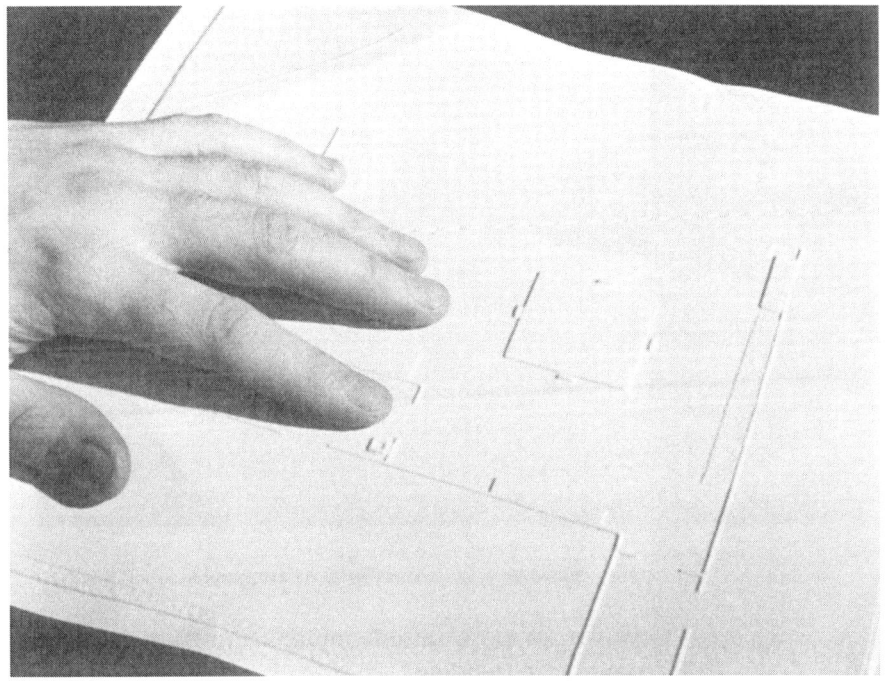

Figure 10.8. Map of the lounge at the Royal National Institute for the Blind (RNIB) Rehabilitation Centre, Nottingham. (Cartographer: Pauline James)

case letters of the English alphabet in order to identify embossed street names or car numbers. Additionally, reading and writing print letters is a worthwhile activity if it includes the ability to sign one's name. For the adventitiously blind person who reads no braille, raised letters and numbers can be used to label features on a map.

Figure 10.9 shows a complex map for nonbraillists of the Victoria Shopping Centre in Nottingham. The shops are numbered with large raised numbers. The verbal key to the map is provided on a tape recorder, and the number system is explained to the map reader. This idea could be used to map most areas for nonbraillists, although the scale of the map would have to be larger than normal to accommodate the large raised letters or numbers.

Using more complex maps

If braille labels need to be added to simple maps for the purpose of showing special streets or buildings, the name can be stuck on by using

355

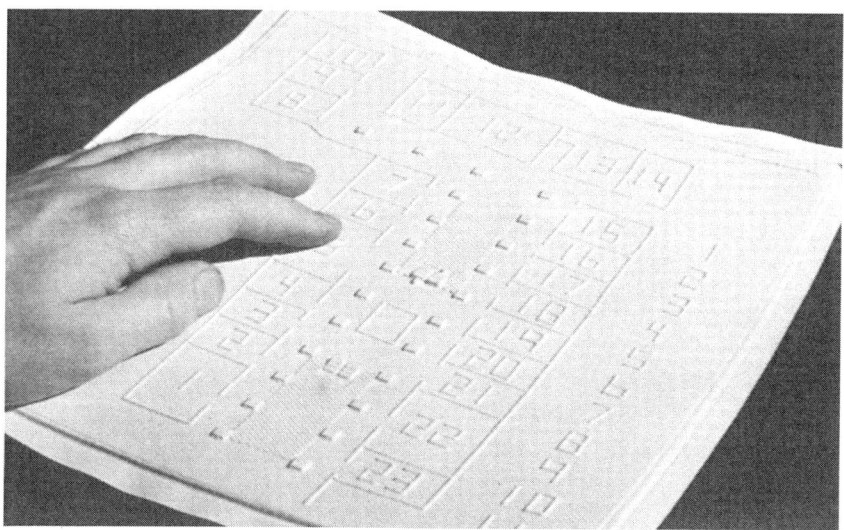

Figure 10.9. Shopping center map for nonbraillists. (Cartographer: Rick Swain)

embossing foil. However, as maps become more complex, various types of labeling will become more frequent.

Index numbers (or letters) or overlay and underlay systems can be used to present additional information later on.

A whole series of maps progressing from simple maps of familiar areas to more complex ones of unfamiliar areas can be presented in book form. Books can be produced in Brailon held in a ring binder and kept firm with a cardboard base.

Figure 10.10 shows a complex map of the City Centre of Nottingham incorporating two bus route maps as separate overlays. Braille initials of streets are shown on an underlay. The map book includes an introduction and a key at the front and a street index at the back.

The following systematic teaching approach was developed for adult blind people using this map:

Familiarization. Map readers were given adequate time to read the introduction, key, and maps. They were shown how to interleave the bus-route maps and to read the bus-route map with one hand and the city center map with the other. Practice was given with the location of braille initials on the underside of the street map.

The importance of a general scan. Before dealing with specific map content, it is wise to ensure that the map reader develops a systematic and

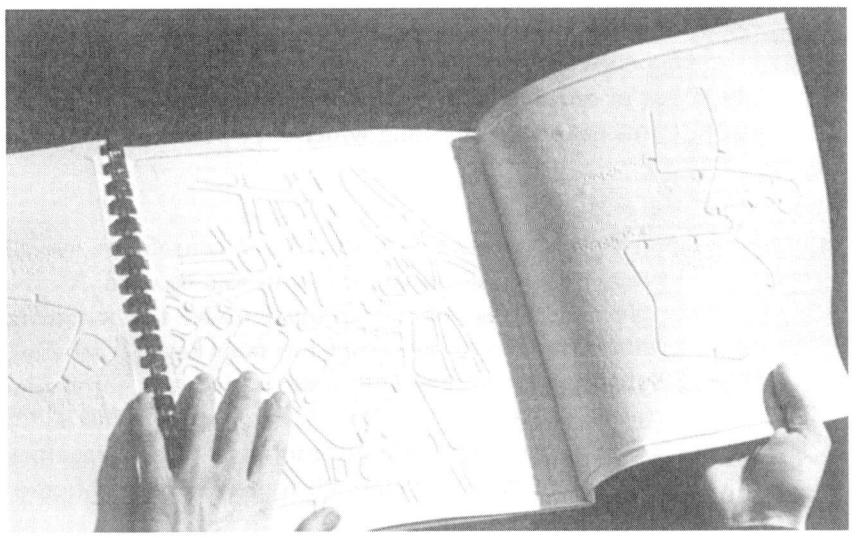

Figure 10.10. A multilayered map of the Nottingham City Centre. (Cartographers: Grahame James and Rick Swain)

efficient method of reading the map surface. A random reading pattern may mean that the reader misses important parts of the map. Instead, it should be impressed upon the reader that by moving the hands in rows or columns, or concentric circles, there is less likelihood of wasting time and missing significant parts of the map.

Orientation of the map. A check has to be made on the map reader's understanding of geographical reference systems, chiefly the relationship of the compass points. A question can decide whether training is required, for example, "If you are facing east, which directions are north, south, and west?" The significance of the north edge map symbol can then be explained.

Discussion of the map content. The map reader should be taught to identify the symbols on the map by referring to the key and should be given practice in the use of the braille underlay and indexing system.

Spatial distribution and relative location of features are then taught so that map readers can imagine journeys beginning at various easily found location points such as buildings or roundabouts (circular crossroads). Readers should be encouraged to develop their own preferred reference points as they gain experience in using the map.

357

The bus routes can then be discussed. It is important to locate and label bus stops and to assess the direction in which the buses travel.

Practice should be given in using the street map in conjunction with the bus-route maps in order to become conversant with the routes taken by the buses in terms of the streets along which they pass and the places where they stop.

Consolidating overall knowledge of the map. In order to consolidate overall knowledge of the map, a map-reading questionnaire can be used. For the map in this example, questions can be grouped under the following headings: (1) identification of symbols from the map key, (2) labeling features by use of the braille underlay and indexing system, (3) spatial distribution and relative location of features, (4) bus route questions, (5) use of bus stop labels and check on route directions, (6) putting together the bus-route map and the city center map, (7) route planning at home.

Using the map during travel. Once the blind person is fully conversant with the map, accompanied and then independent journeys can be attempted either on foot or by using the public transport systems illustrated on the maps.

Methods of using maps

Many sighted people enjoy reading maps for their intrinsic value. Blind people should be encouraged to do this too, even if the map has no immediate functional value. In the early stages, the map is best taken out. Routes can be indicated by pins stuck through the map into a stiff board. Later, the map can be taken out and kept close at hand in case it is needed for reference. On the other hand, the more experienced map reader may wish to keep the map at home and transfer relevant information from the tactual map to the tape recorder or memory disc as a series of sequential instructions. Ultimately, map readers will leave the map at home to memorize the main features of the route they wish to follow.

Conclusions and recommendations for future research

Hardware

There are various methods for producing tactual mobility maps; each should be considered for its value in a particular application. However, research should continue to explore production methods offering improved materials for use on mobility maps that are cost effective. Standardization should not necessitate stagnation of ideas for improving hardware.

Together with improving materials, efforts should be made to understand more clearly how the map reader processes information from these materials. What are the map–relevant capabilities of the haptic system?

User populations

What about user populations? It appears that most blind people travel only familiar routes. Indeed, professional mobility instructors spend most of their time teaching blind persons to travel safely and efficiently before considering the possibility of dealing with unfamiliar areas. It is essential that basic travel skills be established before advanced work is undertaken. In an unfamiliar area, it may be easier for instructors just to show blind persons around the area and supervise while they explore. Maps are rarely used. Could map work, no matter how basic, form a more useful and integral part of a mobility training program?

Survey techniques may help to define more clearly the user population. A representative sample of blind people might be asked: "Have you ever used a map?" or "Could you use a map like this one?" (example shown) or "What would you do if you wanted to visit an unfamiliar area?" Are some blind people limited in their independent mobility because of a lack of geographical information?

When blind people have access to different types of mobility maps over a protracted period, how do they use them? It is well known that if the fingers are cold it is difficult to read tactually. Can "map memory" be sufficiently developed with practice to enable some people to refer to maps at home and then attempt a journey? Why should mobility maps be portable? Can blind persons extract the information they require from a fixed map by making their own portable versions? Could blind people read maps successfully that are much larger than the span of two hands?

Mental mapping

Geographers, planners, and psychologists are becoming increasingly interested in how ideas and experience can influence the cognitive maps of individuals (Canter, 1977). Basic laboratory studies could be designed to compare the role of different types of maps in contributing to an individual's ability to relate *cognitive space* to *real space*. Cognitive space is essentially a learned mental representation of the environment, whereas real space is the actual environment. Tasks requiring a person's direct negotiation with the environment, or a simulated environment, could test the cognitive map learned indirectly through maps of various kinds. Thus, such experiments might indicate more clearly the potential or limitations of tactual or verbal maps or maps that have been systematically distorted in some way.

We know that people have conceptual deficiencies as the result of lack of spatial experiences or impoverished experiences. Recent work, such as that of Casey (1978), shows that congenitally blind children have a considerably impoverished and distorted map of their school campus compared with children who can see something of it. Research is required to highlight these deficiencies and to remedy them. Gilson, Wurzburger, and Johnson (1965) claim that tactual maps can help to eliminate confusion and distortion of environmental concepts. More research is required to substantiate this claim and to specify how maps can help to clarify environmental concepts for congenitally blind people.

Blind people have little chance to draw maps and diagrams for themselves. More studies could involve blind people in using specially designed apparatus to illustrate shapes and routes as part of concept development. Drawing should also be considered as a means of eliciting from an individual some representation of a cognitive image – although the ability to draw is always an unknown factor in this type of observation.

Tactual and visual displays

The vast majority of visually handicapped persons have some useful vision. Research has indicated the necessity of providing visual displays in addition to tactual ones. Some map readers may use both simultaneously. However, individual requirements for a visual map display vary enormously. The most cost-effective method of providing a visual display on a small number of Thermoform mobility maps may be simply to outline the main features with a waterproof pen in colors preferred by the individual. Can we be more systematic than this?

Improved training and dissemination of information

Training courses in map production and use should be developed for rehabilitation specialists or teachers involved in using maps with visually handicapped people. Blind people should have access to a variety of maps as teaching aids appropriate to their requirements.

Variety of maps

Only by experimenting with a variety of maps for different purposes will the full potential of mobility maps be realized. Many sighted people read maps for pleasure as well as information. Visually handicapped people should do this too. Registers should be established to stock maps that may be of general use to people visiting new areas. In this way, unnecessary duplication of mobility maps will be avoided, and it will be easier to monitor their quality and diversity.

References

Angwin, J. B. P. Maps for mobility. 1, 2. *The New Beacon*, 1968, *52*, 115–119, 143–145.

Armstrong, J. D. The design and production of maps for the visually handicapped. *Mobility Monograph No. 1*. Nottingham: University of Nottingham, Dept. of Psychology, 1973.

Bentzen, B. L. An orientation and travel map for the visually handicapped: hand production, testing and commercial reproduction. Unpublished master's thesis, Boston College, 1971.

Production and testing of an orientation and travel map for visually handicapped persons. *The New Outlook for the Blind*, 1972, *66*, 249–255.

Orientation maps for visually impaired persons. *Journal of Visual Impairment and Blindness*, 1977, *71*, 193–196.

Blasch, B. B., Welsh, R. L., & Davidson, T. Auditory maps: an orientation aid for visually handicapped persons. *The New Outlook for the Blind*, 1973, *67*, 145–158.

Canter, D. *The psychology of place*. London: Architectural Press, 1977.

Casey, S. M. Cognitive mapping by the blind. *Journal of Visual Impairment and Blindness*, 1978, *72*, 297–301.

Chang, C., & Johnson, D. E. Tactile maps with interchangeable parts. *The New Outlook for the Blind*, 1968, *62*, 122–124.

Cratty, B. J. *Movement and spatial awareness in blind children and youth*. Springfield, Ill.: Charles C Thomas, 1971.

Craven, R. W. The use of aluminum sheets in producing tactual maps for blind persons. *The New Outlook for the Blind*, 1972, *66*, 323–330.

Franks, F. L., & Baird, R. M. Geographical concepts and the visually handicapped. *Exceptional Children*, 1971, *38*, 321–324.

Gill, J. M. Tactual mapping. *Research Bulletin of The American Foundation for the Blind*, 1974, *28*, 57–80.

Gilson, C., Wurzburger, B., & Johnson, D. E. The use of the raised map in teaching mobility to blind children. *The New Outlook for the Blind*, 1965, *59*, 59–62.

Gray, P. C., & Todd, J. E. *Mobility and reading habits of the blind*. London: H.M.S.O., 1968.

Greenberg, G. L., & Sherman, J. C. Design of maps for partially seeing children. *International Yearbook of Cartography*, 1970, *10*, 111–115.

James, G. A. Problems in the standardization of design and symbolization in tactile route maps for the blind. *The New Beacon*, 1972, *56*, 87–91.

Problems of orientation and navigation in blind mobility with special reference

361

to maps. Unpublished doctoral thesis, University of Nottingham, England, 1973.

A kit for making raised maps. *The New Beacon*, 1975, *59*, 85–90.

Blind people and pedestrian subways. *The New Beacon*, 1977, *61*, 309–312.

James, G. A., & Armstrong, J. D. An evaluation of the "Silva" braille compass. 1. Static tests. *The New Beacon*, 1974, *58*, 225–229.

An evaluation of a shopping centre map for the visually handicapped. *Journal of Occupational Psychology*, 1975, *48*, 125–128.

Handbook on mobility maps. *Mobility Monograph No. 2.* Nottingham: University of Nottingham, Dept., of Psychology, 1976.

James, G. A., Armstrong, J. D., & Campbell, D. W. Verbal instructions used by mobility teachers to give navigational directions to their clients. *The New Beacon*, 1973, *57*, 86–91.

James, G. A., & Burnett, J. Orienteering for blind and visually impaired people. *The New Beacon*, 1979, *63*, 1–3.

James, G. A., & Campbell, D. W. A practical course in map making. *The Teacher of the Blind*, 1975, *64*, 4–6.

James, G. A., Campbell, D. W., & Armstrong, J. D. An evaluation of the "Silva"Braille compass. 2. Field trials. *The New Beacon*, 1974, *58*, 253–255.

James, G. A., & Gill, J. M. Mobility maps for the visually handicapped: a study of learning and retention of raised symbols. *Research Bulletin of the American Foundation for the Blind*, 1974, *27*, 187–198.

James, G. A., & Swain, R. Learning bus routes using a tactual map. *The New Outlook for the Blind*, 1975, *69*, 212–217.

James, W. R. K. Systems of illustration for the visually handicapped: psychological principles of design and usage. Cambridge, England: The Leonard Conference, 1972, pp. 78–84.

Jansson, G. Reliefkartor for Synskadade–en handbook av, Grahame James och John Armstrong. Uppsala: Uppsala University: Pedagogisk Forskning, Pedagogiska Instititionen, 1977.

Kidwell, A. M., & Greer, P. S. The environmental perceptions of blind persons and their haptic representation. *The New Outlook for the Blind*, 1972, *66*, 256–276.

Sites, perception and the nonvisual experience. New York: American Foundation for the Blind, 1973.

Kratz, L. E. *Movement without sight.* Palo Alto, Calif.: Peek Publications, 1973.

Leonard, J. A. Experimental maps for blind travel. *The New Beacon*, 1966, *50*, 32–35.

Leonard, J. A., & Newman, R. C. Spatial orientation for the blind. *Nature*, 1967, *215*, 1413–1414.

Three types of maps for blind travel. *Ergonomics*, 1970, *13*, 165–179.

Maglione, F. D. An experimental study of the use of tactual maps as orientation and mobility aids for adult blind subjects. Unpublished doctoral thesis, University of Illinois, 1969.

Mumford, D. O. The Leicester map project. *The New Beacon*, 1972, *66*, 231–233.

Nolan, C. Y., & Morris, J. E. *Tactual symbols for the blind* (Final Report No. RD-585). Washington, D.C.: Vocational Rehabilitation Administration, 1963.

Pickles, W. J. Raised diagrams, in R. C. Fletcher (Ed.), *The teaching of science and mathematics to the blind.* London: Royal National Institute for the Blind, 1970, pp. 118–154.

Schiff, W. *Manual for the construction of raised line diagrams.* New York: Recording for the Blind, 1966.

Using raised line drawings as tactual supplements to recorded books for the books for the blind (Final Report No. RD-1571-S). Washington, D.C.: Vocational Rehabilitation Administration, 1967.

Schiff, W., Kaufer, L., & Mosak, S. Informative tactile stimuli in the perception of direction. *Perceptual & Motor Skills*, 1966, *23*, 1315–1335.

Sherman, J. C. Needs and resources in maps for the blind. *The New Outlook for the Blind*, 1965, *59*, 130–134.

Tooze, D. W., In P. F. Portwood & R. T. Williams (Eds.), *Readings on the visually handicapped child*, vol. 2. Leicester: British Psychological Society, 1978, pp. 53–54

Wiedel, J. W., & Groves, P. A. *Tactual mapping: design, reading and interpretation* (Final Report No. RD-2557-S). Washington, D.C.: U.S. Dept. of Health, Education and Welfare, 1969.

11. Haptic perception of tangible graphic displays

EDWARD P. BERLÁ

In Chapter 11, Edward Berlá looks at problems concerning display legibility, related haptic skills necessary to obtain information from haptic displays, and the perceiver's knowledge of the subject of the display. All three seem to interact in the process of extracting information from tangible displays.

Berlá first points out that tangible displays for blind *children* are typically too difficult, and so are seldom used by their teachers. This omission in turn, leads to poor skill development and a vicious circle of underutilization of a potentially useful adjunct to learning – the tangible display. Berlá then examines the specifics of tangible graphics production (e.g., symbol size, figure–ground relations, spatial orientation, redundancy), reviews the research literature on these topics, and then recommends solutions to some general problems with legibility.

Professor Berlá also discusses haptic exploration and search processes, emphasizing the integration of fragmentary information. However, an invariant structure is typically identified despite highly variable sequential inputs. Whether this is so for unpracticed blind children is an interesting if moot point.

Berlá nicely summarizes a great deal of research concerned with the development of such haptic skills. This chapter is a must for teachers of blind children, those concerned with the utilization and design of tangible displays for blind children and adults, and researchers interested in haptic skill acquisition.

WILLIAM SCHIFF

The haptic reading of tangible graphic displays

The reading of tangible graphic displays is dependent upon three factors: the legibility of the symbols in the display, the tactual–motor skills necessary for exploring and reading the display, and the knowledge the reader brings to the task (Nolan & Morris, 1971). Although research on each of these factors has generated a small body of knowledge, in general the quality of tangible graphic displays has improved only slightly, and very little has been done to improve the skills and concept development of blind children who are supposed to use graphic displays in a variety of subject areas. The crux of the problem is the fact that the producers of tangible graphic displays know little of tactual perception

364

or the problems facing blind children. Consequently, the graphic displays that appear in braille books are generally reported to be difficult for blind children to read (Berlá, 1974; Nolan & Morris, 1971). Because the graphics are poorly designed, many teachers avoid using them to any extent in the classroom. Blind children, as a result, are not given the opportunity to use them and not only fail to develop rudimentary skills for reading them but also cannot acquire the information conveyed through these displays. For example, a common complaint of social studies teachers in the higher grades of residential schools for the blind is that the children lack even the simplest map-reading skills. Consequently, when they attempt to introduce a tangible map as part of a lesson, they are faced with the dilemma of either avoiding the use of maps altogether or teaching the basic skills, which would then take much time away from other subjects. Although attempts have been made in recent years to improve the quality of tangible maps (Nolan & Morris, 1971) and to delineate the concepts and skills necessary for reading maps (Berlá, 1974; Franks, 1974), very little of this information has been incorporated in commercially produced tangible maps or in the curricula for blind children. As a result, tangible maps and other graphics are of poor quality, and blind children lack the skills and knowledge to read them. Researchers who then attempt to test different map designs are faced with unskilled subjects. Research on graphic design and legibility thus becomes very difficult.

Legibility of graphic displays

Some early research on the legibility of haptic displays investigated blind children's ability to recognize raised-line representations of two-dimensional (e.g., square, cross, triangle, star, and circle) and three-dimensional (e.g., shovel, house, rabbit, chair, and table) figures (Merry, 1930, 1932; Merry & Merry, 1933). Blind children's ability to recognize raised representations of two-dimensional figures was much better than their ability to recognize those of three-dimensional figures. Although training and verbal clues improved their ability in both areas, three-dimensional identification remained very poor due to their inability to understand and perceive perspective via the tactual modality (but see Chapter 9).

Since Merry's early studies, research has focused on identifying (1) the factors that contribute to the legibility of tactile shapes and (2) a set of highly discriminable symbols that can be used on a variety of graphic displays.

Size

The size of tactual displays and the size of the symbols on them are of major importance in designing readable graphics. Because the resolving power of the fingertip is much less than that of the eye, it is often necessary to enlarge the symbols and the size of the display for the haptic reader. For example, a typical map in an ink-print text would need to be enlarged several times in order to provide the haptic reader with the same information that is available to the sighted reader. However, as the size of the haptic display is increased, it creates a much more difficult reading task for the haptic reader by enlarging the area to be inspected and requiring the integration of information from different parts of the display. For example, some commercially produced wall maps and globes for the blind are several meters in diameter. Typically, when graphic displays are made for a blind person, much of the "unessential" symbology is eliminated in order to reduce the display to a manageable size. Although there have been no major attempts to investigate the effect of display size on readability, it has been suggested by Wiedel and Groves (1969) that tangible displays be kept within a hand span.

To date, only limited information is available to guide the designers of haptic displays on the size and nature of the symbols to be used. It is obvious that there are physical limitations; a given symbol or figure can be reduced only so much and remain discriminable. However, currently there is no way of determining how small a symbol could be made. The recognition threshold for a symbol will vary with its configuration or the elements contained in it. Just as important for the designers of tangible displays is whether beyond a threshold, the size of a tactual figure affects haptic performance.

Lobb and Friend (1967) investigated the effects of absolute size and relative differences in size on the recognition of randomly shaped polygons using sighted adult subjects performing tactually. In this experiment, the absolute size of a polygon had no effect on the accuracy of recognition performance, but relative size differences did. If the subjects were given a polygon that was either larger or smaller than the polygon initially presented, there was a significant increase in errors. Berlá (1972b) also investigated the discriminability of different-size histoforms (2.5, 5.1, and 7.6 cm [1, 2, and 4 in]) that varied over three levels of complexity using blind children in grades one and two as subjects. Neither the absolute size nor the variations in complexity affected the accuracy of discrimination. However, increases in either absolute size or complexity significantly increased the time necessary to examine the figures.

Relative differences in size have also been found to affect the discrimination of textural patterns. Morris and Nolan (1963) had blind students in grades four through twelve inspect a 5.1 by 5.1 cm (2 by 2 in) textural pattern and then gave them seven figures from which to choose the same pattern. In general, as the size of the choice figures decreased from 5.1 to 0.6 cm (2.0 to 0.25 in) through 0.6 cm (0.25 in) steps, discriminability of the patterns decreased. However, small-grain patterns remained more discriminable at smaller sizes than did large-grain patterns, and older children were able to discriminate more patterns at smaller sizes than younger children. All textures were recognized 90 percent of the time when the choice figures were the same size as the standard figure. Although relative differences in size decrease the accuracy of recognition, there has been no research to determine whether training could facilitate performance.

In constructing tangible graphic displays, judgments have to be made concerning the size of elements to be placed on the display. If the elements are too small, they become unrecognizable; if they are to be judged on the basis of differences in size, then differences that are too small result in nondiscriminable symbols. In visual displays, the reader can alter the angular size of the elements by moving the display closer to the eyes. Tactually, no such adjustments are possible, and therefore the absolute size of the elements is critical. Technically, producers of tangible graphic displays need not only sets of empirically derived, highly discriminable symbols but also sets of values that indicate discriminability along different physical dimensions. For example, Berlá and Murr (1975b) empirically derived a set of values for the tactual discrimination of line width using the method of constant stimuli in a psychophysical experiment with blind children. These values could be used to determine mathematically the smallest differences that were discriminable 90 percent of the time by blind children. On the average, a line had to be approximately 25 percent wider than a comparison line for 90 percent of the blind students to be able to recognize the difference between them. For example, suppose a teacher is making a tactile display for the sixth-grade class. One line put on the display is 0.76 cm (0.30) in width. Wanting to add another line that the class can perceive as wider, the teacher is not sure how much wider the second line should be. Multiplying the width of the first line (0.76 cm) by 25 percent yields 0.19 cm, the minimum difference in size for a line to be discriminable from a 0.76 cm (0.30 in) line, 90 percent of the time. Adding the 0.19 cm (0.075 in) to the line gives a value of 0.95 cm (0.375 in). This means that as long as the value is at least 0.19 cm wider than the 0.76 cm line, it will be discriminable. Although a teacher may never need to perform this specific calculation, by having tables of information such as this one on a variety of physical dimensions, he or she can design tactile displays with a great deal of technical specificity.

Another finding in the Berlá and Murr study (1975b) was that when the blind students were given repeated trials (without feedback) in discriminating line width, their ability to discriminate increased significantly. Even without feedback or reward, blind students learn to make increasingly fine discriminations provided they are given the opportunity.

In reading graphic displays, the reader is often required to estimate the distance between two points or the size of a symbol. No studies have investigated the extent to which blind children can estimate the size of areas or the distance between two points on a haptic display. However, Duran and Tufenkjian (1969) did investigate the strategies blind children spontaneously employed in comparing the size of two rods. The most frequent strategy was to place the rods side by side and use the fingertip or palm to determine which end extended farther. When blind children were prevented from using this strategy, they used other methods such as estimating the size of the rods with finger spans, tracing each rod with their fingertips or hands, or using a body part as a measuring instrument. Although all these methods can be used effectively to estimate size or distance on a graphic display, no attempt was made to determine which one was most accurate. However, a few studies have been reported with haptic observations by sighted subjects that may have generality to the blind population.

Studies by Mashhour and Hosman (1968), Stevens and Stone (1959), and Teghtsoonian and Teghtsoonian (1970) have shown that sighted subjects observing haptically overestimate the size of stimuli held between the thumb and forefinger. But other studies by Teghtsoonian and Teghtsoonian (1965) and Stanley (1966) have shown that when subjects estimate the size of stimuli by holding the fingers of separate hands at the end of a line, or by tracing length of a line from beginning to end with the fingertip, they are more accurate in estimating the distance than they are using a finger span technique.

Figure–ground

In designing tangible displays, it is important to determine what relationships provide maximum differentiation between figure and ground. Until very recently, it was common to use both raised and incised lines on graphics for blind children. However, Nolan (1971) found that raised figures could be discriminated much faster and more accurately than incised figures. In his study, blind children in grades four through twelve were presented with identical sets of raised and incised geometric forms in a five-choice recognition task. The students made 7 percent more correct responses with the raised figures and required 38 percent more time to recognize the incised figures.

In a related study, Nolan and Morris (1971) compared the performance of blind students on three map-reading tasks on six pseudomaps that differed on symbol height and symbol separation. Each map contained areal, point, and linear symbols. There were three conditions of symbol height. In one condition, the symbols were all raised to the same height above the ground, 0.46 mm (0.018 in); in a second condition, the point and line symbols were raised higher than the areal symbols, 0.64 and 0.38 mm (0.025 and 0.015 in), respectively; and in the third condition, the point symbols were raised higher than the line symbols, which were higher than the areal symbols 0.89, 0.63, and 0.38 mm (0.035, 0.025, and 0.015 in), respectively. There were two conditions of symbol separation, either 2.28 or 0.38 mm (0.09 or 0.015 in). Combining each condition of relative symbol height with each condition of separation resulted in six maps. Separate groups of blind students were given the task of locating the point and areal symbols and asked to follow a dotted line "path" on the different maps. The students were able to locate the point symbols significantly faster and more accurately under the condition of maximum differences in symbol height and symbol separation. Following the dotted line was significantly faster with increases in line height but not symbol separation. Neither relative height nor separation affected the speed or accuracy of locating areal symbols.

Designers of tactile displays commonly use texture in a way that is analagous to the use of color on ink-print maps. Color is often used to differentiate adjacent areas from one another as well as to enhance the contrast between figure and ground. Berlá and Murr (1975a) compared the performance of blind children reading a tactile pseudomap that contained background textures with that of a group of blind children reading the same pseudomap without textures. Both groups were asked to perform two tasks: locating a series of identical point symbols on the map and tracking a line with their fingertips from a starting point to a goal.

The use of textures on one pseudomap significantly degraded performance. Blind students located 20 percent fewer symbols and took 36 percent more time on the textured map. They also took 41 percent longer to track the line. This study showed that the addition of texture to a map made it more difficult to detect tactual figures. Unlike color, texture did not enhance performance but degraded it.

The problems blind children encounter in reading tangible maps depend to some degree on the nature of the map. In braille textbooks, one of the most frequent tangible maps is a raised-line political map (Arampatta, 1970). In its simplest form, a political map can be conceived as a series of contiguous shapes. From a perceptual standpoint, the blind child's task is to differentiate one shape from another and remember its relative position in the context of the map as a whole. Berlá and Butterfield (1977a) investigated the design of tangible political maps by having blind children locate and trace specific shapes on three differently designed political pseudomaps. Each map contained five U.S. states randomly placed and connected to each other by lines that gave the appearance of a political map. This map was then reproduced in plastic in three different ways by using either a thin raised line, a broad raised line, or a broad incised line. Each child was shown a cue card that contained an identical representation of one of the shapes on the map and was asked to locate and trace each of the five shapes on one map. Of the three types of maps, the one with broad raised lines was easiest to read. Significantly more shapes were located, and significantly faster, on this map than on the other two types. A reason for this is that blind children typically trace a raised line on its top surface and erroneously follow lines that intersect with the shape they are tracing. However, a raised line can be conceived as having three parts, namely, a top surface and two edges. If a relatively broad line is used on a political map, the contiguous shapes are defined by two different edges. If the haptic reader traces the inside edge of the line of the shape that has been located, he or she will avoid making contact with lines that intersect with the shape to be traced. Consequently, the contour of the figure can be traced without distraction from intersecting lines.

Spatial orientation

For visually presented forms, children are quite consistent in identifying the phenomenal orientation of a shape (Ghent, 1961; Ghent & Bernstein, 1961), that is, visually presented stimuli perceptually appear to have a phenomenal top and bottom. Children are quite consistent in recognizing that an unfamiliar figure is upside down or right side up, based on its overall configuration and distinctive features. However, when shapes are presented tactually to blindfolded sighted subjects or blind subjects (Pick, Klein, & Pick, 1966), the subjects are inconsistent in identifying

370

the phenomenal orientation of a series of shapes. For specific types of shapes, it has been found that a change in orientation is more difficult to discriminate than a change in shape presented visually, but haptically a change in the orientation of the same shape is as easy to discriminate as a change in shape (Goodnow, 1969; Pick et al., 1966). This is true for both blind and sighted subjects observing haptically. When a tangible shape is rotated, it is not recognized as a rotated shape but instead is perceived as an entirely different shape. Blind children are also very poor in reorienting tangible shapes that have been presented in one orientation and then rotated. When asked to restore the figure to its original orientation, their performance is very poor, averaging more than 58 degrees of error for children in grade two and more than 30 degrees of error for children in grade eight (Berlá, 1974). It is clear from these studies that the orientation of a figure is *not* a good cue for the tactual modality and that blind children have poorly developed spatial orientation skills. However, there has been little, if any, training of blind children's ability to use orientation cues on graphic displays.

Symmetry

According to the principles of Gestalt psychology, figures that are symmetrical with respect to a common axis are rated as "better figures" by observers and remembered or identified more easily than asymmetrical figures. However, Walk (1965) performed an experiment in which sighted college students associated nonsense syllables with either visual or tangible graphics. The visual learning group learned to associate the nonsense syllables with the symmetrical figures in fewer trials than with the asymmetrical figures, whereas the tactual group learned to associate the nonsense syllables with the asymmetrical figures more quickly. This experiment suggests that symmetry does not provide the haptic reader with the same qualitative sense of balance and uniqueness that it does for the visual reader. Another possibility is that asymmetrical shapes provide more variations in contour than symmetrical ones and therefore permit the haptic reader a larger set of distinctive features that differentiate it from other shapes. However, effects of symmetry will probably depend upon the set of shapes being used. It appears that a single symmetrical shape is haptically more outstanding among a set of asymmetrical shapes than it is among other symmetrical shapes (as is the case in vision). However, no such experiment has been performed with blind children.

Redundancy

If two stimuli differ on two dimensions such as color and shape, the information is said to be redundant because the stimuli could be differentiated on either dimension alone. Discrimination is usually facilitated in difficult tasks by redundancy. Schiff and Isikow (1966) investigated the influence of redundant tactile information on the ability of blind subjects to discriminate differences in the length of bars on a tangible histogram. The basic approach was to correlate varying degrees of roughness and relief with increases in the length of the bars. For example, the longer the bar, the coarser the texture. The use of redundant information was found to facilitate discrimination when there were small differences in length between the bars. When there were large differences, the use of redundant information had no effect on performance. The principle of redundancy has potentially wide application in tangible graphics for the blind. By making symbology on tangible graphs highly redundant, it might be possible to reduce the size of tangible displays substantially and/or to increase the amount of information contained on such displays because smaller differences between stimuli would become more discriminable.

Perceptual training

The fact that blind children have difficulty making discriminations among tactile stimuli along a number of dimensions does not mean they are incapable of doing so. It is frequently noted that blind children have very poor tactile skills. However, the fact that young blind children can learn to read the complex braille code is enough to show how training can facilitate the development of perceptual abilities. One important demonstration of this fact was a study by Maron (1973). He showed that retarded blind children could significantly improve their ability to discriminate shape and texture when given specific types of perceptual training. The training consisted of either a perceptual isolation procedure, in which the relevant cue (texture or shape) was presented first in isolation with additional cues being faded in, or a functional procedure in which students practiced matching materials on the basis of a single cue (texture or shape). Either procedure alone or in combination resulted in a significant increase in discrimination performance on subsequent test tasks compared with that of equivalent untrained groups. This and other studies to be discussed indicate the importance of training as a significant area for further research and application to the interpretation of tangible graphic displays by blind children.

Discriminable symbols

Because there is no extensive body of research on tactual perception with blind children, attempts have been made to identify sets of tactually discriminable symbols.

A few researchers have worked with geometric forms, attempting to determine which ones are most tactually discriminable (Austin & Sleight, 1952; Degowin & Dimmick, 1928). The circle has been reported to be the clear winner. This is because researchers have used the circle in combination with other geometric forms that have corners or angles. Now, the discriminability of any tactual symbol depends upon the other forms in the series, so that a circle becomes far less discriminable when the other members of the series are ellipses. Therefore, the research findings on discriminable symbols are not generalizable beyond the set of stimuli in a given series (Schiff, 1967). As such, a few studies have reported that a square is the least discriminable figure (Degowin & Dimmick, 1928: Rosenbloom, 1929), whereas at least one other study has reported it to be one of the most highly discriminable forms (Austin & Sleight, 1952). Researchers would do well to determine the amount of similarity between various forms and the degree of accuracy that can be obtained with a given level of similarity.

In addition to geometric forms, a few studies have reported on the discriminability and identification of letters (Austin & Sleight, 1952; Dinnerstein & Wolfe, 1962; Schiff, 1967). These studies have used letters that varied in size. Dinnerstein and Wolfe (1962), using four sighted adults with letters ranging in size from 3.18 to 8.90 cm wide (1.25 to 3.5 in) and 8.90 cm (3.5 in) high and 1.5 mm (0.06 in) in depth, found 100 percent accuracy in recognition for letters *A, E, Γ, I, J, L, P, T, W, X, Y*, and *Z*; 90 to 99 percent accuracy for *B, C, G, O*, and *V*; 80 to 89 percent accuracy for *D, H, M, N, Q, R, S*, and *U*; and 70 to 79 percent accuracy for *K*. Schiff (1967) presented two random orders of the alphabet, reported as 1.42 cm (.56 in) high to 12 blind and 12 sighted college students. The blind students were significantly faster, but there was no significant difference in terms of error scores. Seventeen letters (*A, B, C, E, F, H, I, J, L, Q, P, R, S, T, U, Y, Z*) were found to be highly identifiable (three errors or less). Schiff noted that the letters showing the greatest number of errors also produced the greatest number of errors when presented visually via the tachistoscope. In a related study, Schiff and Dytell (1971) compared the performance of deaf and hearing children on the tactile identification of letters. The tactual errors for both groups were very similar to the visual errors made by sighted children and adults. These studies suggest that errors in letter identification are specific to the features of the letters themselves rather than to the modality through which they are perceived or the nature of the subject population (Gibson, 1969).

Another study by Austin and Sleight (1952) investigated the recognition of the entire alphabet under four conditions: (1) solid figures, no movement; (2) solid figures, with movement; (3) point figures, no movement; and (4) point figures, with movement. The letters were all inscribed in a 1.27 cm (0.5 in) circle, that is the figure was drawn with a maximum dimension of 1.27 cm (0.5 in). The solid figures with movement present resulted in the greatest accuracy of identification, with approximately 60 percent of the letters being discriminable at or above the 90 percent level. Those letters were *C, D, E, G, I, J, K, L, O, P, Q, T, U, V, W, X, Y*. The letters *I, X*, and *L*, were identified 100 percent of the time under all conditions, and the letters *C, O, T*, and *U* were recognized 90 percent of the time under all conditions.

Recent research with the Optacon has shown that blind children can very rapidly learn to recognize capital letters of the alphabet in a variety of print styles. This fact, combined with the previously reported research on letter recognition, suggests that with a minimum of training, blind children could learn to identify raised-line representations of most, if not all, capital letters, which could then be used as symbols on tangible graphic displays.

In addition to geometric forms and alphanumeric figures, attempts have been made to identify those ink-print symbols that are also tactually discriminable when made tangible. Three general classes of symbols are needed to construct graphic displays for the blind, namely, areal, point, and linear symbols.

The identification of a set of highly discriminable symbols is complicated by the medium in which the symbols are reproduced. The most frequently used medium for tangible graphic displays is paper. However, paper has one serious disadvantage. It limits the amount of relief that can be obtained, and figures embossed on it often do not have the relatively sharp edges that provide the best tactual stimulation. Plastic, on the other hand, permits greater variations in relief and, when embossed, typically results in symbols with sharp edges for maximum stimulation and legibility. From a perceptual standpoint, plastic is clearly the better medium. However, it poses other problems, particularly in relation to braille books, in which the substitution of plastic for paper would add considerably to the book's bulk. Consequently, it appears that research on symbology in particular and tactile graphic displays in general must use both paper and plastic.

374

An extensive series of studies on tactile symbols was conducted by Nolan and Morris (1971), who used a paired-comparison procedure to investigate the discriminability of areal, point, and linear symbols. Using stringent criteria,[1] they identified sets of point and linear symbols that were highly discriminable in paper and a set of areal, point, and linear symbols that were highly discriminable in plastic.[2] Additional research (Gill & James, 1973; James & Gill, 1975) has enlarged the set of discriminable symbols available.

Inspection of the symbols found to be highly discriminable suggests that certain symbol characteristics contribute to legibility. These characteristics are as follows: areal symbols – continuous versus interrupted, regular versus irregular, size of the elements making up the pattern; linear symbols – continuous versus interrupted, thick versus thin, smooth versus ragged edge, single versus double lines; point symbols – shape, size, solid versus outline, continuous versus dotted (Nolan & Morris, 1971). It should be pointed out, however, that these characteristics were intuitively derived from a limited set of items rather than from empirical comparisons. On the other hand, certain research has identified symbol characteristics not contributing to symbol legibility; these include the shape of the elements that make up the areal symbol (Nolan & Morris, 1971; Schiff, 1967), the directional orientation of the elements comprising the areal symbol (Schiff, 1967), and the complexity or number of sides (Foulke & Warm, 1967). One unique symbol that takes particular advantage of the tactual system is the directional arrow tested by Schiff, Kaufer, and Mosak (1966). This tactual symbol resembles a sawtooth. When stroked in one direction, it feels rough, but when stroked in the opposite direction, it feels smooth. This symbol can be substituted for the conventional visual arrow that is commonly used in visual graphic displays.

Exploring and reading graphic displays

The tactual perceptual process, by its very nature, may be serial and fragmentary (Lashley, 1951; Révész, 1950). Unlike vision, a total perception of a display cannot be obtained in one micro act. The haptic observer must explore the stimulus in successive movements, perhaps analyzing each separate percept and integrating it with previous percepts. Consequently, haptic exploration is an exceedingly slow and fragmentary process compared with vision. Relative to the other sense organs, the hand is the only perceptual system in which the freely roaming members (fingertips) determine the order of critical information (distinctive features) for processing. In the visual system, a single fixation provides a simultaneous (parallel) processing of distinctive features and their spatial relationships. For audition, the serial temporal order of the stimulus events is relatively fixed. By analogy, the critical information in a melody is the temporal relations among the notes (frequency ratios). If the sequence of the notes is altered either by changing the temporal pattern (the time values among the notes) or the arrangement of the notes within the tune, a new melody is created. In essence, the nature of the emergent pattern (the melody) is a function of serial order (Lashley, 1951). However, for the freely roaming hand, the serial order of features is subject to wide variation depending upon the consistency of the system used in inspecting tactile displays. For example, if a shape had six distinctive features, a blind child could feel them in 720 different sequences (Berlá, Butterfield, & Murr, 1976). In reality, there are other factors, such as the position of the stimulus with respect to the observer and the habitual ways of responding, that would substantially reduce the number of possible alternatives. However, if the identical display is presented to the same child on two or more occasions, variations in inspection strategies will alter the sequence of the features so extracted, and thus may determine whether the child perceives the two stimulus events as the same or different.

There has been empirical research on the function of hand and finger movements in tactual perception. Russian researchers' work described by Pick (1963, 1964) and research by Zaporozhets (1965) and Zemtsova (1969) has investigated hand and finger movements, mostly by observing children as they explore tangible figures and analyzing motion pictures of their performance. As a basic premise, they assume that the movements of the hand over a stimulus allow the reader to form a motor-copy image of the tactual figure. Many of their observations are interpreted within this framework. Their research suggests that the motions of the hand can be divided into micro- and macro-motions that are considered necessary for the adequate perception of tangible figures. The finer micro-motions are necessary for the perception of figure texture and play a minor role in the perception of spatial properties. Macro-motions are divided into (1) search and directing and (2) pursuit movements. These movements purportedly locate and measure objects, construct motor copies of them, and check and correct the previous functions. The observations of these researchers suggest that haptic exploration usually begins by locating a reference point, frequently the top part of the figure. Then the fingers trace the contour of the figure, using the thumbs as anchors in a discontinuous motion.

With respect to the development of hand and finger movements, Gin-evskaya (in Zaporozhets, 1965) has observed that young children between the ages of 3 and 4.5 years show rather primitive movements characterized by incomplete exploration and lack of a systematic approach. By ages 6 to 7.5, the hand motions become purposeful and contour tracing becomes the rule rather than the exception. Zaporozhets (1969) reports the research of Russian investigators who have observed that children under 5 years of age characteristically do not trace contours and make significantly more errors than 6-years-olds, who usually do trace the contour. These observations are congruent with those of Piaget and Inhelder (1956), who have characterized the tactual perceptual development of sighted children in three stages. During the first stage, children of 3 to 4 years of age can recognize common objects tactually but do not abstract the concept of shape, primarily because of a lack of exploration. A child at this age tends to discriminate shapes based on the particular part of the shape fortuitously touched by the hand. Thus, very different shapes, such as a triangle and a square, are often perceived as identical because the child happens to touch a corner of each. The child's lack of exploration also prevents integration of separate parts of a tangible figure into a whole to form a percept. In a second stage, which occurs between 4 and 6 years, the child begins to recognize common geometric forms and to explore tangible shapes more purposefully. However, at this stage exploration is not systematic, and the child fails to use a reference point around which to organize the separate parts of the figure. It is only during stage three, between 6 and 7 years, that the child begins to explore tangible shapes systematically and to use a reference point (starting and end point) to integrate the individual parts of the figure.

Thus, for the sighted child performing tactually, the development of hand and finger movements appears to progress from a fragmentary, unsystematic, and incomplete exploration to one that is systematic, detailed, complete, and integrated (Piaget & Inhelder, 1956).*

It might be assumed that observing blind children performing tactually would provide the researcher with a sophisticated model of the development of haptic skills. This assumption might be based on the belief that blind children, out of necessity, depend more heavily on haptic skills to acquire information or because of the emphasis in their education on learning specific haptic skills, most notably braille. However, this assumption would be wrong. Research on blind children in grades one

* Editor's note: Piaget's influential conception of tactual perception and its development is widely accepted but is at odds with many psychologists' research findings and observations. (W. S.)

through twelve has generally indicated that their haptic skills are extremely poor (Nolan & Morris, 1971). For example, on haptic map-reading tasks, blind children characteristically fail to define and explore the extent of the area (map) they have been asked to examine, are very unsystematic when instructed to explore a tangible display, and exhibit poor tracing and shape discrimination skills (Berlá & Butterfield, 1977b; Berlá, Butterfield, & Murr, 1976; Nolan & Morris, 1971). Furthermore, the lack of these skills permeates all grade levels, and the steadily increasing ability with years in school seems to be more the exception than the rule.

However, research with a select and highly educated sample of blind adults (Berlá, 1972a) showed them to be highly systematic and analytic in their scanning of tangible displays. Although no specific scanning strategy was used consistently by this group, their strategies could be categorized generally as a horizontal (left to right or right to left) or a vertical (top to bottom or bottom to top) search of the tangible display. In subsequent studies (Berlá, 1973; Berlá & Murr, 1974), blind children in grades four through twelve were trained to search a tangible display for specific symbols with either a horizontal or vertical search pattern. The vertical pattern group was superior both to the horizontal patterns group and to an untrained group. Observations of children performing the task were more revealing of the factors involved in searching a display than the specific outcome of the study. When the children scanned the display in a horizontal pattern (left to right), they tended to describe arcs in moving their hands from left to right because they would pivot on their elbows. In addition, they would move their hands up, covering a section of the map they had covered before, or move their hands down and skip sections of the map. There was little or no arcing or skipping of map parts by the students trained in the vertical scanning pattern (top to bottom) because of the motion to and from the body. Another difference between the horizontal and vertical scanning patterns had to do with the amount of information that could be obtained in one horizontal or vertical sweep of the display. The tactual field of view can be defined by the number of fingertips used in scanning. It was observed that the primary fingers used for gathering information were the index, middle, and ring fingers of both hands. The thumbs and little fingers were primarily used for support. In many instances, the students were observed to raise their little fingers from the display as they scanned. Consequently, the tactual field of view or so-called perceptual window was equivalent to six fingers, three on each hand. When the vertical scan is compared with the horizontal scan, the vertical scan has a much larger perceptual window and therefore provides more information. As the hands scan down the map, each of the six fingers is in contact with a different part of the map. Thus, the perceptual window is approximately equivalent to the width of six fingers. However, when the tactile display is scanned horizontally (left to right), each finger covers approximately the same area of the map. In essence, the same information is presented to each finger. Therefore, the perceptual window and the amount of information obtained in one horizontal sweep are much smaller compared with a vertical sweep. Consequently, fewer vertical sweeps than horizontal sweeps are needed to cover the same tangible display.

The haptic skills of blind children in examining and discriminating shapes are poor. In an attempt to delineate the problems and the potential skills needed by blind children to discriminate shapes and read tangible political maps, a videomatic behavioral analysis was undertaken to examine the behaviors of good and poor haptic map readers (Berlá, Butterfield, & Murr, 1976). Thirty-six blind students in grades four through twelve were videotaped as they attempted to locate specific shapes (U.S. states) on a pseudopolitical map. On the basis of error and time scores, the videotapes of the nine best and the nine poorest map readers were analyzed in order to identify specific behaviors that differentiated them. Good map readers were much more systematic and complete in their exploration of shapes. Using their index fingers, they faithfully traced the outline of a shape, stopping at various points to inspect carefully a distinctive feature. (Distinctive features were behaviorally defined as the degree of perseveration on specific features as determined by two judges.) The good map readers appeared to be able to locate and identify a particular shape on the map based on two or three distinctive features. Poor map readers were generally unsystematic and incomplete in their exploration of a shape. They had difficulty tracing the outlines of the shapes and paid little attention to the distinctive features of a given shape.

In two subsequent studies (Berlá & Butterfield, 1977a,b), blind students were trained to examine shapes first by locating a reference point on a shape, then by tracing the contour of the shape in a clockwise or counterclockwise motion, and finally by returning to a reference point. They were then asked to retrace the shape in the same way but to pick out the parts of the shape that were different (distinctive features) and remember them. On a subsequent shape recognition task, they were given a shape for examination that was then removed and replaced by four choice figures from which they had to choose the correct shape. The students trained to examine the shapes systematically significantly outperformed a matched untrained group on the same task. On another task, two equivalent groups of blind students were asked to locate shapes on a political map. One group received the training described above with the instruction to locate a target shape on the map by searching for its distinctive features. The trained students again significantly outperformed an equivalent untrained group. It should be noted that training in each of the previously reported studies was less than 1.5 hr per child, yet it resulted in a 20 to 40 percent gain in accuracy and speed of performance.

Map concepts

Educators of blind children have stated that before maps can be used in classroom instruction, blind children must be oriented to their immediate environment such as their classroom, dormitory, home, and school. This orientation should include basic knowledge about objects and their spatial relationships, basic concepts related to time–distance relationships, and geographical concepts. Teachers have indicated that the most important and difficult concept in teaching maps to blind children is having them relate a map to a known environment (Berlá, 1974). From an educational standpoint it is essential that a child's first tangible map be a representation of an environment with which he or she is totally familiar. Theoretically, it should be easier for a child to relate an abstraction such as a map to a known, concrete environment rather than to an unknown area. One suggested procedure was to develop a simplified map of a child's classroom that would represent furniture by simple geometric forms. Teaching would begin by relating these geometric map forms to actual furniture in the room. For instance, small squares might be used to represent desks. The next step would be to have children describe the spatial arrangement of furniture in the classroom and to demonstrate their knowledge by showing those same relationships on the tangible map. Subsequently, students could be given a variety of mobility tasks in the classroom and required to indicate the paths they would or did follow. In this way, they would begin to learn the relationship of the map to the environment and vice versa. Once children have demonstrated their understanding of the relationships between the classroom and the map, the map's complexity can gradually be increased by using additional symbols to represent other significant features of the classroom. The map can then be enlarged to represent an area that includes hallways and other classrooms. As the complexity of the map and the physical space it represents are gradually increased, blind children would come to develop more concrete knowledge about their environment and its abstract representation in map form. Blind children first have to learn that a map can represent their personal environment; then they can use maps to acquire knowledge about environments they have never directly experienced.

Another dimension of the mapping problem is the blind person's cognitive map or memorial representation of the physical environment. Casey (1978) studied the cognitive maps of both congenitally blind and partially sighted (legally blind) students aged 16 to 21 years. Each student was asked to reconstruct a model of his or her campus using wooden blocks for buildings and Velcro cloth strips for pathways. Each map thus constructed was evaluated for organizational accuracy by two independent judges. The partially sighted students, who were blindfolded while performing the task, significantly outperformed the congenitally blind students. However, the most important part of the study concerned the nature of the maps constructed by the two groups. For the most part, the totally blind students organized the maps of their environments into a number of separate sections, whereas the partially sighted students organized theirs as a single unified space. It was as if the blind students had cognitively separated the physical space into separate, independent areas. In addition, the curved walkways placed on the map by the blind students were much straighter than those of the partially sighted students. Casey notes, however, that some blind students constructed maps that were integrated schemas, and these students were the ones who appeared to have more highly developed travel skills.

Other research (Franks & Nolan, 1970, 1971) has shown that young blind children are deficient in basic geographical concepts related to the physical features of the earth such as lakes, islands, mountains, valleys, and peninsulas. These concepts are more difficult to learn because of the practical limitation of providing blind children with concrete experiences with physical features. Blind children's perception of these features is limited due to their inability to perceive them in their entirety. As a consequence, whatever concrete experiences a blind child can obtain need to be combined with verbal descriptions and models.

The preceding discussion has been concerned primarily with tangible maps and the skills and concepts necessary to read and interpret them. The fact is that there has been little research on graphs or diagrams for the haptic reader. There has been no research, for example, on the design of line graphs and whether blind children can extract information presented in them or whether, for that matter, verbal descriptions could substitute for many graphic displays now incorporated into braille books.

381

Summary and conclusions

It is apparent from the preceding review that the state of the art leaves much to be done. Although there is a small body of knowledge on the design of graphics, the skills necessary for reading them, and the knowledge the reader needs to bring to the task, very little of this information has been incorporated into the commercial production of graphics or into the curriculum for blind children in the United States. Although there are many problems to be solved and many steps taken to remedy the situation, it is apparent to this writer that little will be accomplished unless major thrusts are made simultaneously. The first priority must be the use of more sophisticated technology commercially in making tangible displays for the blind. There is sufficient information to enable producers to make graphic displays substantially more legible than those that currently exist. Among other things, guidelines for the design of tangible displays need to be established and standardized so that the decisions regarding symbols and their placement are not left to individuals who have neither a knowledge of tactual perception nor training in education of the blind. Without this initial thrust, all the research and training in perception, reading skills, and concept development will not make illegible, poorly designed graphics comprehensible to the most sophisticated haptic reader.

Another important thrust is more extensive development of curriculum materials that could be incorporated into existing educational programs for the blind. At this time, so little is being done at the classroom level that any modest changes in curriculum would result in substantial gains. Curriculum development could be achieved largely by a group of educators of the blind working in concert with tactual researchers to establish a developmental sequence of skills, concepts, and materials that could be incorporated into existing educational programs. It is important that the curriculum be initially geared to blind children in the primary grades, who could most benefit from training in basic skills and concepts.

With respect to research, one of the most fruitful areas appears to be that of perceptual–motor skills training. The few existing studies have demonstrated substantial improvement in performance with only short periods of instruction. This is not to say that important and meaningful research cannot be conducted on symbology, design, and concept development; these areas are certainly in need of continued efforts.

There has been no systematic research on tangible graphs and diagram reading; this is a relatively new research area. This research could take several approaches. One would be to analyze graphs and diagrams to determine the kinds of information intended to be communicated to the haptic reader, and under what conditions verbal descriptions could be substituted. A second approach could be to analyze and delineate skills and concepts needed to read graphs and diagrams. Although it may not be practical to do this for all types of graphs and diagrams, it may be possible to delineate subsets of displays based on subject areas such as mathematics books in general or geometry in particular, or on the frequency of occurrence of different displays in the most popular series of braille textbooks. For example, line graphs may occur most often in braille books. Once this has been determined, a number of potentially researchable questions can be posed. These include the nature of lines to be used on the display; whether blind children can accurately determine the specific value of the data points represented by the functions depicted on the graph; whether blind children can determine the slope and/or curvature of a line; whether a background grid facilitates or inhibits the reading of graphs; and the physical characteristics of graphs such as overall size, relative symbol size, height, separation and labeling, which optimize reading performance. A third approach could undertake perceptual-training studies to determine to what extent blind children can learn the skills and concepts needed to abstract the information contained in these displays and the systems for facilitating such learning.

Because tangible displays involve independently researchable but interrelated problems, any development or improvement in one area will affect the nature and outcome of research in other areas. For example, innovations in production technology would greatly improve the legibility of graphic displays, which might increase the use of tangible displays in the classroom curriculum, which, in turn, might affect the development of children's skills and concepts. Most important, however, is the implementation of information and techniques in the educational system.

Notes

1. "Criteria for a symbol to be considered discriminable were (1) that average confusion with other acceptable symbols should be 5 percent or less and (2) that confusion with itself or any other single symbol acceptable by criterion (1) should be 10% or less. In addition, for any set of symbols acceptable by criteria (1) and (2), there should be no significant differences in discriminability of acceptable symbols among students in grades ranging from 4 through 12" (Nolan & Morris, 1971, p. 19).
2. The reader should consult Nolan and Morris (1971) for the actual physical dimensions of each symbol.

References

Arampatta, D. Illustrations in social studies textbooks as they affect the visually handicapped. Specialist in education thesis, George Peabody College for Teachers, 1970.

Austin, T., & Sleight, R. Accuracy of tactual discrimination of letters, numerals, and geometric forms. *Journal of Experimental Psychology*, 1952, *43*, 239–247.

Berlá, E. Behavioral strategies and problems in scanning and interpreting tactual displays. *The New Outlook for the Blind*, 1972, *66*, 277–286. (a)

Effects of physical size and complexity on tactual discrimination performance of primary age blind children. *Exceptional Children*, 1972, *39*, 120–124. (b)

Strategies in scanning a tactual pseudomap. *Education of the Visually Handicapped*, 1973, *5*, 8–19.

Tactual orientation performance of blind children in different grade levels. *American Foundation for the Blind Research Bulletin*, 1974, *27*, 1–10.

Berlá, E., & Butterfield, L., Jr. Teachers' views on tactile maps for blind students: problems and needs. *Education of the Visually Handicapped*, 1975, *7*, 116–118.

Tactile political maps: two experimental designs. *Journal of Visual Impairment and Blindness*, 1977, *71*, 262–264. (a)

Tactual distinctive features analysis: training blind students in shape recognition and in locating shapes on a map. *Journal of Special Education*, 1977, *11*, 335–346. (b)

Berlá, E., Butterfield, L., Jr. & Murr, M. Tactile political map reading by blind students. A videomatic behavioral analysis. *Journal of Special Education*, 1976, *10*, 265–276.

Berlá, E., & Murr, M. Searching tactual space. *Education of the Visually Handicapped*, 1974, *6*, 49–58.

The effects of tactual noise on locating point symbols and tracking a line on a tactile pseudomap. *Journal of Special Education*, 1975, *9* 183–190. (a)

Psychophysical functions for active tactual discrimination on line width for blind children. *Perception & Psychophysics*, 1975, *17*, 607–612. (b)

Casey, S. Cognitive mapping by the blind. *Journal of Visual Impairment and Blindness*, 1978, *72*, 297–301.

DeGowin, E., & Dimmick, F. The tactual perception of simple geometric forms. *Journal of General Psychology*, 1928, *1*, 114–122.

Dinnerstein, A., & Wolfe, M. Tactile slit scanning of letters. *Perceptual & Motor Skills*, 1962, *15*, 135–138.

Duran, P., & Tufenkjian, S. Tactile-kinesthetic methods for measuring length used by congenitally blind children. *Perceptual & Motor Skills*, 1969, *28*, 395–400.

Foulke, E., & Warm, J. Effects of complexity and redundancy on the tactual recognition of metric figures. *Perceptual & Motor Skills*, 1967, *25*, 177–187.

Franks, F. Introduction to map study: teaching locational and directional referents to young blind students. Unpublished doctoral thesis, George Peabody College for Teachers, 1974.

Franks, F., & Nolan, C. Development of geographical concepts in blind children. *Education of the Visually Handicapped*, 1970, *2*, 1–8.

Measuring geographical concept attainment in visually handicapped students. *Education of the Visually Handicapped*, 1971, *3*, 11–17.

Ghent, L. Form and its orientation: a child's eye view. *American Journal of Psychology*, 1961, *74*, 177–190.

Ghent, L., & Bernstein, L. Influence of the orientation of geometric forms on their recognition by children. *Perceptual & Motor Skills*, 1961, *12*, 95–101.

Gibson, E. J. *Principles of perceptual learning and development.* New York: Appleton-Century-Crofts, 1969.

Gibson, J. J. Observations on active touch. *Psychological Review,* 1962, *49,* 477–691.

Gill, J., & James, G. A study of the discriminability of tactual point symbols. *American Foundation for the Blind Research Bulletin,* 1973, *26,* 19–34.

Goodnow, J. Eye and hand: differential sampling of form and orientation properties. *Neuropsychologica,* 1969, *7,* 365–373.

James, G., & Gill, J. A pilot study on the discriminability of tactile area and line symbols for the blind. *American Foundation for the Blind Research Bulletin,* 1975, *29,* 23–31.

Lashley, K. The problem of serial order in behavior. In L. A. Jeffress (Ed.), *Cerebral mechanisms in behavior.* New York: Wiley, 1951, pp. 112–136.

Lobb, H., & Friend, R. Tactual form discrimination with varying size and duration of exposure. *Psychonomic Science,* 1967, *7,* 415–416.

Maron, S. The use of dimensional-highlighting procedures to facilitate tactile discrimination learning in visually handicapped and mentally retarded adolescents. Unpublished doctoral thesis. University of Michigan, 1973.

Mashhour, M. & Hosman, J. On the new "psychophysical law": a validation study. *Perception & Psychophysics,* 1968, *3,* 367–375.

Merry, F. A further investigation to determine the value of enclosed pictures for blind children. *Teachers Forum,* 1932, *4,* 96–99.

Merry, R. To what extent can blind children recognize tactually, simple embossed pictures? *Teachers Forum,* 1930, *3,* 2–5.

Merry, R., & Merry, F. Tactual recognition of embossed pictures by blind children. *Journal of Applied Psychology,* 1933, *17,* 148–163.

Morris, J., & Nolan, C. Minimum sizes for areal type tactual symbols. *International Journal for the Education of the Blind,* 1963, *13,* 48–51.

Nolan, C. Relative legibility of raised and incised tactual figures. *Education of the Visually Handicapped,* 1971, *3,* 33–36.

Nolan, C., & Kederis, C. *Perceptual factors in braille word recognition.* New York: American Foundation for the Blind, 1969.

Nolan, C., & Morris, J. *Improvement of tactual symbols for blind children: final report.* Louisville, Ky.: American Printing House for the Blind, 1971.

Piaget, J., & Inhelder, B. *The child's conception of space.* London: Routledge & Kegan Paul, 1956.

Pick, H. Some Soviet research on learning and perception in children. In J. C. Wright & J. Kagan (Eds.), *Basic cognitive processes in children. Monographs of the Society for Research in Child Development,* 1963, *28,* 185–190.

Perception in Soviet psychology. *Psychological Bulletin,* 1964, *62,* 21–35.

Pick, H. L., Jr., Klein, R. E., & Pick, A. D. Visual and tactual identification of form orientation. *Journal of Experimental Child Psychology,* 1966, *4,* 391–397.

Révész, G. *Psychology and art of the blind.* (Translated by H. A. Wolff.) New York: Longmans, Green, 1950.

Rodabaugh, B. *Optacon: Ink print reading for the blind.* Palo Alto, Calif.: American Institutes for Research, 1974.

Rosenbloom, B. Configurational perception of tactual stimuli. *American Journal of Psychology.* 1929, *41,* 87–90.

Schiff, W. *Using raised line drawings as tactual supplements to recorded books for the blind* (Final Report No. RD-1571-S). Washington, D.C.: Vocational Rehabilitation Administration, 1967.

Schiff, W., & Dytell, R. S. Tactile identification of letters: a comparison of deaf and hearing children's performances. *Journal of Experimental Child Psychology,* 1971, *11,* 150–164.

Schiff, W., & Isikow, H. Stimulus redundancy in the tactile perception of histograms. *International Journal for the Education of the Blind*, 1966, *16*, 1–11.

Schiff, W., Kaufer, L., & Mosak, S. Informative tactile stimuli in the perception of direction. *Perceptual & Motor Skills*, 1966, *23*, 1315–1335.

Stanley, G. Haptic and kinesthetic estimates of length. *Psychonomic Science*, 1966, *5*, 377–378.

Stevens, S. S., & Stone, G. Finger span: ratio scale, category scale and jnd scale. *Journal of Experimental Psychology*, 1959, *57*, 91–95.

Teghtsoonian, M., & Teghtsoonian, R. Seen and felt length. *Psychonomic Science*, 1965, *3*, 465–466.

Teghtsoonian, R., & Teghtsoonian, M. Two varieties of perceived length. *Perception & Psychophysics*, 1970, *8*, 389–392.

Walk, R. Tactual and visual learning of forms differing in degree of symmetry. *Psychonomic Science*, 1965, *2*, 93–94.

Wiedel, J., & Groves, P. *Tactual mapping: design, reproduction, reading and interpretation* (Final Report No. RD-2557S). Washington, D.C.: Dept. of Health, Education and Welfare, 1969.

Zaporozhets, A. The development of perception in the preschool child. In P. H. Mussen (Ed.), *European research in child development. Monographs of the Society for Research in Child Development*, 1965, *30*, 82–101.

Some of the psychological problems of sensory training in early childhood and the preschool period. In M. Cole & I. Maltzman (Eds.), *A handbook of contemporary Soviet psychology*. New York: Basic Books, 1969.

Zemtsova, M. Characteristics of perceptual activity in the blind. In M. Cole and I. Maltzman (Eds.), *A handbook of contemporary Soviet psychology*. New York: Basic Books, 1969.

12. Tangible graphic displays in the education of the blind persons

BILLIE L. BENTZEN

In Chapter 12, Billie Bentzen reviews educational aspects of tangible graphic displays, primarily from a teacher's perspective. She briefly examines the history of tangible graphics production, reviewing both commercial or mass-production sources of tangible graphics and small-scale individual techniques that teachers or parents might utilize to produce inexpensive tangible displays. Tools, techniques, and specific suppliers of graphic materials are noted, making this chapter especially valuable to teachers who may use tangible graphic materials only occasionally. Bentzen describes the available materials and briefly notes their relative advantages and disadvantages for various educational purposes. This chapter provides a compact and useful guide for teachers of visually handicapped students. Together with the preceding chapter and those that follow, it provides a complete analysis of the practical considerations of tangible graphics production.

WILLIAM SCHIFF

Introduction

Some of the earliest educators of the blind created tangible graphic displays for their students, yet the value of such displays is not accepted automatically today. The meaning behind the old adage "a picture is worth a thousand words" is questioned now, even by creators of visual graphic displays (Robinson & Petchenik, 1976), so it is not surprising that educators of the blind are far from unanimous in their attitudes toward the use of visual and/or tangible graphic displays as tools for teaching.

Producers of educational materials for the blind have recognized a responsibility to make information presented graphically in texts available to touch readers. This has been done in two ways: (1) the information has been presented verbally and (2) tangible graphic displays have been produced and reproduced by a variety of techniques.

Teachers' responses to available graphics have varied. In many cases, they have not used them because students seemed to find them difficult and sometimes uninformative. Students did not know how to use the displays; they had had no systematic training. Symbols were difficult to discriminate. The displays seemed too complex and perhaps too large. It was often difficult for students to associate drawings or maps with reality. In short, tangible graphic displays did not seem to do for blind students what visual graphics do for sighted students (Berlá & Butterfield, 1975; Best, 1967).

Perhaps tangible counterparts of visual displays were not appropriate for blind students, or perhaps there were important differences in haptic and visual perception, indicating that graphic displays for blind persons should be designed differently.

There is no agreement on whether tangible graphic displays should reproduce exactly what is present in visual form. Some educators believe that it is important for the tangible and visual representations to be as similar as possible so that blind students in integrated settings will not be confused and will learn the principles of visual graphic representation (Krebs, 1964; Pickles, 1967). Although graphic displays that are essentially two-dimensional are informative to many persons, it is seldom possible to give the haptic impressions of three dimensions in a two-dimensional presentation, and drawings of three-dimensional objects are among the most difficult for blind students to interpret (but see Chapter 9).

Teachers have responded to this dilemma in three different ways:

1. Some teachers have persisted in the use of available tangible graphics, evaluating them through experience. This has led to recognition of the need for research on principles of haptic perception as applied to the problem of tangible graphic displays (see Chapter 11), and to the development of new techniques of commercial production and reproduction (see Chapter 13).
2. Some teachers have not used available tangible graphics. Disappointed by their students' lack of success, they have decided that tangible graphics are not useful teaching tools. The apparent inability of blind students to use tangible graphics has led to research on techniques of interpreting these materials – especially geographic maps (Berlá, 1972, 1973; Berlá, Butterfield, & Murr, 1976).
3. Some teachers have created their own tangible graphic displays. This has encouraged research on techniques for teacher or volunteer production and has led to the development of commercially available materials for the production of one or a few displays.

The issues in relation to maps for orientation and mobility are slightly different. Some teachers, tacitly acknowledging that maps are good aids to spatial orientation, have refused to use them on the basis that they would never be commonly available to blind travelers. They did not want their students to become dependent on an unavailable resource. But as mobility maps are becoming more common, this argument is becoming less valid.

Other mobility teachers, recognizing the need for the kind of spatial information normally conveyed through maps, but convinced that a verbal presentation would be more readily perceived and utilized by blind travelers, have developed various recorded and tactile verbal maps (see Chapter 10).

Still other mobility teachers, frustrated with their attempts to teach spatial concepts and configurations verbally and motorically, and with the apparent limitations of the auditory system as a perceiver and decoder of spatial information, have created their own mobility maps. Some use them whenever particular difficulties arise, as in describing unusually complex intersections or facilitating communication with a student who has a verbal communication problem. Others, however, use them as a standard teaching technique, believing that tactual maps are essential to the formation of accurate and flexible cognitive maps. Through the use of tactual maps, their students are taught to organize information arising via any sensory system into a spatial structure (Gilson, Wurzburger, & Johnson, 1965).

The production of tangible graphic displays

The beginning of commercial production

Some educated blind persons and their teachers, friends, or families have made devices to make graphic displays tangible since at least the seventeenth century, when Mirza Rezi of Persia is said to have employed a wax pencil to create a tangible line (Zahl, 1962). In the early 1700s, the blind mathematician Nicholas Saunderson developed a device employing thread that connected pins to make geometric constructions (Zahl, 1962), and the family of blind Melanie de Salignac, in Paris, is known to have made maps for her using wires, threads, wax, and pins in the mid-1700s (Farrell, 1956).

George Weissembourg, who was blinded at age 5, was probably the first person to be concerned with producing multiple copies of tangible graphic displays. In the 1770s he was experimenting with various ways to emboss paper maps. These products were said to have been illegible, but he did have some satisfactory maps made in which boundaries were embroidered and the maps glued to cardboard (Zahl, 1962). Valentin Haüy, who founded the world's first school for blind children in 1784, was inspired by descriptions of Weissembourg's maps. Haüy made maps for his students by laying wires along the borders of a print map, carefully pasting an identical map over the first, marking towns and islands with nails having different heads, and finally shellacking the maps (Zahl, 1962).

Other developments in Europe in the late 1700s and early 1800s included various systems for drawing in wax and pricking lines in soft paper. Special pincushions were created for making geometric designs using pins, wires, string, and rubber bands. Some of these systems were reproduced in quantity, chiefly at the schools where they were developed, and were sold commercially. From 1783 to 1893, experiments were made to produce a fountain pen with ink that would congeal into a raised line (Zahl, 1962).

A technique for using plates to emboss maps, introduced by Kunz of Ilzach, became common in Germany, Switzerland, and Scandinavia in the late nineteenth century (Zahl, 1962).

Concern with commercial production of tangible graphic displays in the United States, as in Europe, dates to the beginning of a school for the blind. Dr. Samuel Gridley Howe, who founded Perkins School for the Blind, simultaneously started a press (now known as the Howe Memorial Press of Perkins School for the Blind) that began producing maps and diagrams as well as books. These were available to blind persons throughout the country. By 1836, Howe had designed and produced an edition of diagrams for illustrating problems in mechanics, an atlas, and a geography book. The latter two are believed to be the first attempts ever made to give the blind maps in the form of a book. Dr. Howe's maps were embossed on paper, using metal plates. They were much less expensive than anything else available at the time and included more information (Lane, 1911).

The Howe Press remains a major supplier of braille maps in the United States today, although most of the maps available were produced as a Works Progress Administration project during the Depression. This project employed 40 men and women, 15 of whom were blind, in the design and embossing of geographical and historical atlases containing 350 maps (Waterhouse, 1975).

By far the largest producer of all types of tangible graphic displays in the United States is the American Printing House for the Blind. Its first book was published in 1866. An early and continuing concern has been the tangible reproduction of graphic displays in textbooks (Nolan, 1976).

Major producers of braille reading materials in Europe and Asia are also engaged in the production of tangible graphics (*International guide to aids and appliances for blind and visually impaired persons*, 1977).

Current commercial production techniques will be described in Chapter 13.

Volunteer production: selected approaches

Braille presses, geared for quantity production of embossed reading material, have never met the total need for reading material or for tangible graphics. Volunteers have frequently been the source for braille transcription or recordings of books desired by one or a few blind persons. For some time, efforts have been made to coordinate the production of tangible graphic displays to accompany these books. Just two of these efforts, representative of two different approaches to the problem, will be mentioned here.

In 1945, the National Braille Association was formed as an informal clearinghouse and advisory body to professionals and volunteers engaged in the production of braille reading materials. Scattered individuals and groups throughout the United States had sometimes produced tangible graphic displays to accompany braille books. These products were often labors of love, painstaking reproductions of the illustrations in print books, whether or not the detail was haptically perceivable or intelligible. The displays were usually produced by embossing with a stylus and/or tracing wheel in paper and glueing on a variety of materials for additional line, point, and areal symbols. Multiple copies were sometimes made by vacuum forming. There is now a coordinated effort through the National Braille Association to teach interested persons to translate their visual perceptions of graphic displays into tangible equivalents and to produce these displays using the techniques mentioned above (Epstein, pers. comm., 1979).

Recording for the Blind began officially exploring the possibility of producing raised-line drawings in 1962. Prior to this time, drawings were translated into verbal descriptions where they logically fall in text. In 1964, the Vocational Rehabilitation Administration awarded a grant to Recording for the Blind, enabling them to develop design criteria and sets of discriminable symbols producible by embossing in aluminum foil with special wheels (Schiff, 1965, 1967). This project produced the first tangible symbol for use in graphic displays designed especially for haptic perception. It was a line that is rough when traced in one direction and smooth when traced in the opposite direction. It conveys directionality to the finger far better than any raised translation of a visual arrow (Schiff, Kaufer, & Mosak, 1966). The design criteria, symbols, and techniques resulting from this project have been implemented in regular production of raised-line drawings by Recording for the Blind.

The Recording for the Blind system is unique in producing drawings by trained volunteers who are specialists in their subjects. Drawings are selected for their meaning and importance for teaching. All drawings are also described verbally. The verbal description can provide additional information not easily included in a complex drawing, and it can guide the reader in exploration and interpretation. Simple drawings may be only verbally described (Amick, pers. comm., 1979; Levi, pers. comm., 1979).

Individual production of tangible graphic displays: materials and techniques

Teachers and volunteers have found many materials and techniques suitable for the production of displays. Some techniques use common household or crafts supplies, whereas others use commercially available systems. Some of the displays can be duplicated by vacuum forming.

One common technique consists of glueing such materials as string, wire, sandpaper, fabric, and buttons on a paper or cardboard backing. Although many of these products are rather crude in appearance, they may be much more perceptible to the haptic system than their vacuum-formed counterparts because they take advantage of minute differences in density, thermal conductivity, and texture that can be provided only through the use of different materials. This technique is useful for presenting all kinds of graphic information.

Another common technique consists of freehand embossing of symbols in paper, aluminum foil, or plastic sheets to create a raised graphic display. Paper is the least expensive material and is well suited for production of simple displays, requiring only one or two types of broken lines and braille labels. Foil is easily embossed into smooth and broken lines varying in width and height. Point symbols of varied sizes, shapes, and heights can be embossed, and varied textures can be created. Labeling can be done in either braille or large type. Suitable tools include ballpoint pens, tracing wheels, leather-working tools, and mimeograph stencil-cutting tools. (Special embossing tooth wheels may be purchased in the United States from the Howe Press.) Aluminum foil of an appropriate weight may be purchased from crafts suppliers or from the American Printing House for the Blind. Scrap offset printing plates are also suitable (Craven, 1972). Plastics such as Brailon (American Thermoform Corporation, 8640 East Slauson Avenue, Pico Rivera, CA. 90660) may also be used. Plastic sheets cannot be vacuum formed, in contrast to paper and foil displays, but single copies may be more durable.

Paper, foil, and plastics can be used in hybrid systems, combining both the glueing and embossing techniques. The paper and foil displays can be vacuum formed, providing no symbols are undercut, or melted at low temperatures.

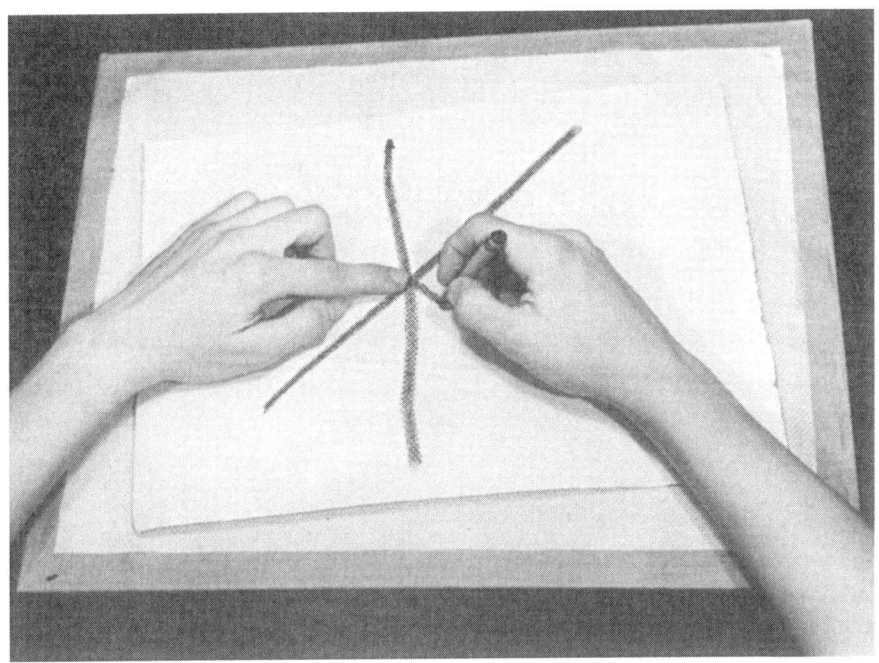

Figure 12.1. Screen board with a student drawing a configuration of a complex intersection. (From Welsh & Blasch, *Foundations of orientation and mobility*, American Foundation for the Blind, New York, 1980)

A variety of systems and materials, some resembling those of the eighteenth and nineteenth centuries, are commercially available especially for making single copies of tangible graphic displays. Some of these also produce displays that can be reproduced by vacuum forming. Some of these systems are easily manipulated by blind persons, enabling them to make their own displays for future use and to communicate graphically with either blind or sighted persons.

The simplest materials commercially sold (American Printing House) consist of a piece of wire screen taped to a masonite backing, a pad of newsprint, and a crayon (Figure 12.1). The chief advantages of such a screen board are that it is inexpensive, relatively easy for students to manipulate, and produces an upright image. The primary disadvantage is lack of definition in symbols. Lines can be varied only in width and length. Point symbols must be very large to be perceived as different in shape, and textures can be varied only in their extent.

Another simple concept, marketed in several countries and with some variations under various names (Raised Line Drawing Kit, American

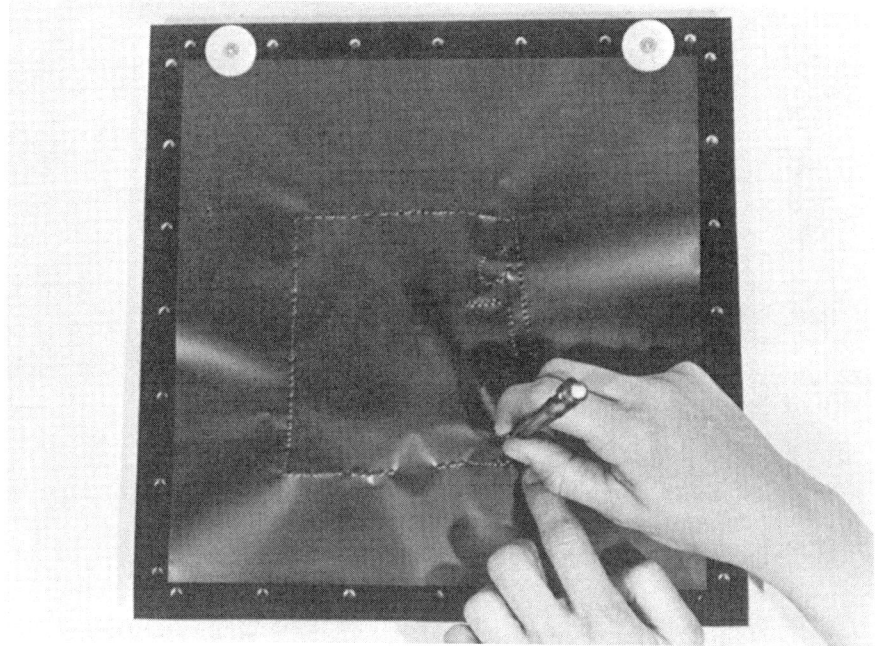

Figure 12.2. Raised Line Drawing Board (Howe Press) with a student drawing a conceptualization of a room shape and positions of furniture in the room. (From Welsh & Blasch, *Foundations of orientation and mobility*, American Foundation for the Blind, New York, 1980)

Foundation for the Blind; Raised Line Drawing Kit, Howe Press [Figure 12.2]; Plastic Sheets for Maps, De Blindas Forenings Forsaljningsaktiebolag, Sweden), consists of a sheet of plastic or cellophane on which a tangible image is produced by drawing with a ball-point pen or stylus (Sewell, 1952). Some include a writing board having a dense rubber surface, whereas others are backed with paper; the plastic or cellophane may be attached by clips, knurled washers, or droplets of water; and some are fashioned into a sleeve that can contain a print display. All of these systems can be used to produce diagrams, graphs, and maps, and several are accompanied by tools for geometric drawing (*International Guide to Aids and Appliances for Blind and Visually Impaired Persons*, 1977). All of the systems are relatively inexpensive and produce upright images having moderate durability. There is, however, limited potential for variation among symbols produced using these materials; some students have difficulty exerting sufficient downward pressure to produce distinct lines, and others have difficulty controlling the thin sheets.

Steel boards and magnetic materials, sometimes created by individual

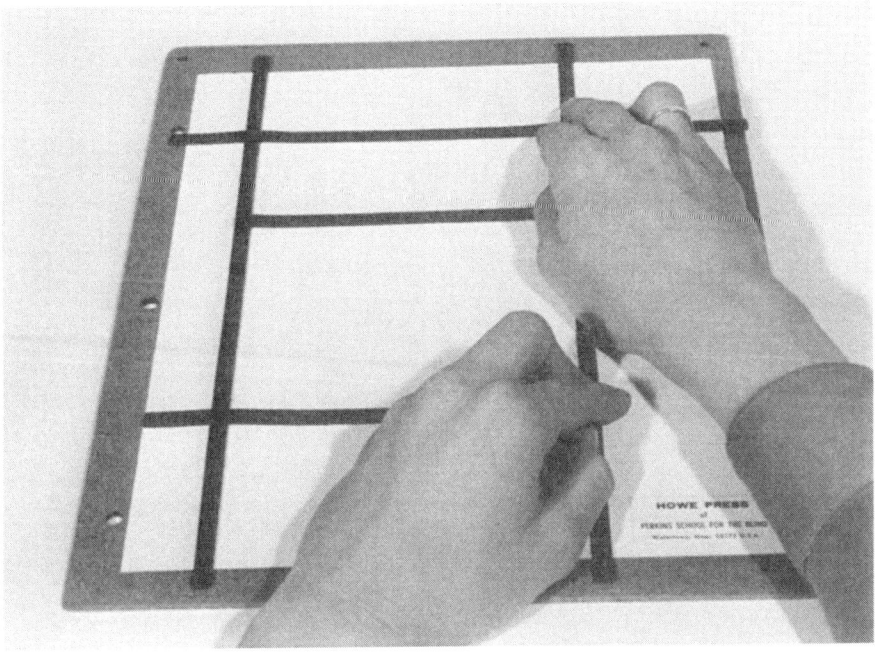

Figure 12.3. Jr. Magstix with a student determining the configuration of small neighborhood intersections. (From Welsh & Blasch, *Foundations of orientation and mobility*, American Foundation for the Blind, New York, 1980)

teachers from available materials, are marked by Howe Press as systems for producing graphic displays for mathematics or for creating simple mobility maps. Magstix consists of a 61 by 46 cm (24 by 18 in) green steel board, with a grid of fine raised black lines, magnetic rubber strips 2.54 cm (1 in) and 0.64 cm (0.25 in) wide, a magnetic rubber cord, and an 18 by 28 cm (7 by 11 in) sheet of magnetic rubber. Jr. Magstix consists of a double sided, 23 by 28 cm (9 by 11 in), white magnetic board accompanied by assorted strips, cord, and a sheet of magnetic rubber (see Figure 12.3). The materials are easily manipulated by both teachers and students and are relatively pleasing to touch. Additional types of magnetic symbols can be purchased from graphics supply houses, and common household materials can be utilized by backing them with bits of magnetic rubber. These materials are most useful for teaching basic spatial concepts or constructing simple shapes and diagrams.

Self-adhesive fabrics (hook-and-pile combinations such as Velcro) are used in two commercially available systems for making diagrams (Chang & Johnson, 1968). An elaborate system called the Chang Tactual Diagram

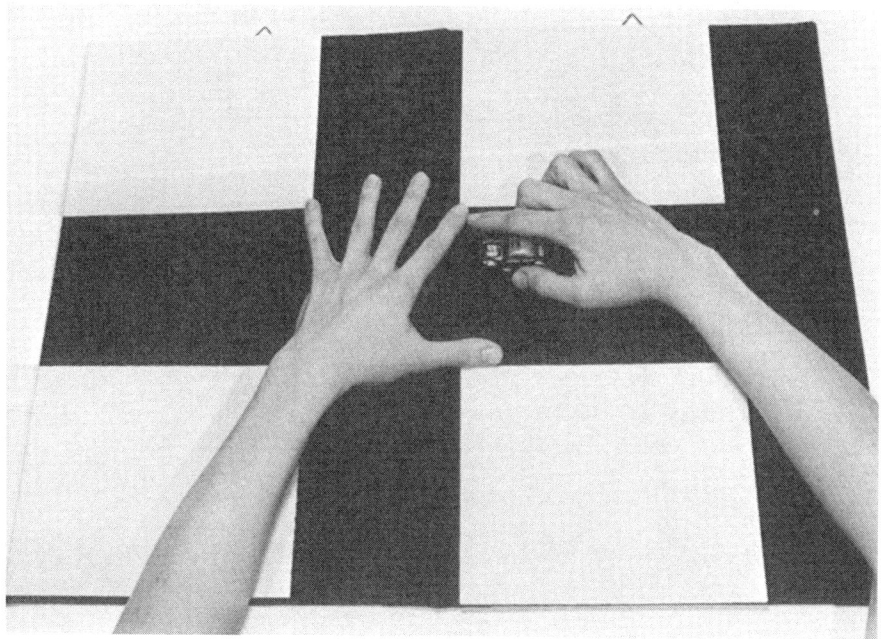

Figure 12.4. Chang Tactual Diagram Kit with a student demonstrating the possible motions of a car at an intersection. (From Welsh & Blasch, *Foundations of orientation and mobility*, American Foundation for the Blind, New York, 1980)

Kit is marketed by the American Printing House and consists of a 61 by 46 cm black pile board, 104 yellow flat geometric forms of 27 different shapes and sizes backed with Velcro (hook), 27 additional Velcro (hook) strips for making other shapes and materials usable with the kit, two molded stick men, an instructional guide, and a carrying case (see Figure 12.4). A 28 by 43 cm (11 by 17 in) pile board (the Hook and Loop Board) is marketed by the De Signs Company in Los Angeles. It comes with a limited supply of cardboard and hook material for teacher construction of needed symbols. Like the magnetic materials previously mentioned, these materials are relatively easy for both teacher and student to manipulate, but their best use is limited to very simple displays.

Special materials are available to enable blind students to construct graphs and geometric figures. Rubber or cork grid boards are used with pins and rubber bands or steel springs. They are marketed by the American Printing House (Louisville, Ky.) and the Royal National Institute for the Blind, London. Tangible grid paper is available from the same sources, to be used in conjunction with cork or rubber backing boards.

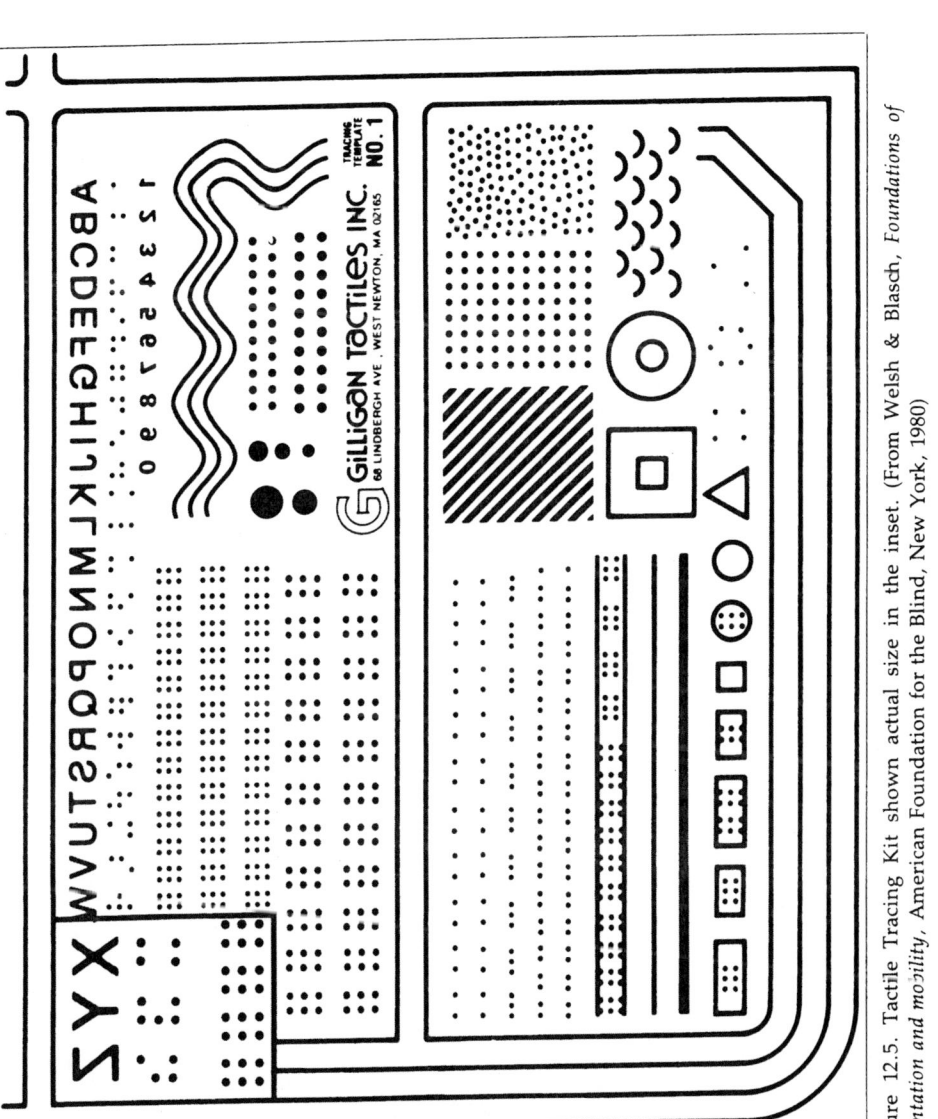

Figure 12.5. Tactile Tracing Kit shown actual size in the inset. (From Welsh & Blasch, *Foundations of orientation and mobility*, American Foundation for the Blind, New York, 1980)

Symbols

Linoleum

Sand paper

Wire mesh

Plastic screen

Symbol	Profile	Symbol	Profile

Symbol	Profile

A Tactile Embossing Kit, manufactured by Gilligan Tactiles, Inc., and distributed by the National Braille Press in Boston, includes a tracing template especially designed for mobility maps but equally useful for other tangible graphic displays (see Figure 12.5). Displays are embossed by drawing in transparent plastic with the round-tipped styli or wheel included in the kit. A large variety of point, line, and areal symbols, braille, and large print can be embossed using the template. Displays can be produced with both high information density and good haptic properties, although little variation in height can be achieved. Embossing must be done in reverse, so the materials are most suitable for teacher or volunteer production of graphic displays. A special technique is said to be available for making master copies for vacuum forming. The system, as supplied, is suitable only for single copies.

A kit of Map Making Parts, designed at and available through the Blind Mobility Research Unit of Nottingham University, Nottingham, England, is especially suitable for the production of individual or vacuum-formed master copies of mobility maps (James, 1975; Figures 12.6 and 12.7). Other types of displays can also be created with the materials. Included in the kit are 27 by 27 cm (10.5 by 10.5 in) cellulose sheets backed with Twinstick, 30 sets of 12 plastic point symbols, 6 rolled solder line symbols, 4 sheets of areal symbols, and glass powder for negating the sticky surface of the cellulose when all desired symbols have been adhered. These materials are relatively time-consuming and difficult to manipulate properly, but they can be used to produce maps that are both small in scale and high in information content. The line and point symbols included have been tested for discriminability (James, 1975).

The Perkins Brailler (a manual machine for rapid embossing of single copies of braille) is frequently used for the production of graphs and charts that are rectilinear, and points along an X–Y axis can be plotted accurately (Kerr, 1974). Simple grid patterns (mobility maps) can also be produced. The image is upright, so students can produce their own displays using this system (see Figure 12.8).

Teaching the use of tangible graphic displays

There has been a paradox in discussions about teaching the use of tangible graphic displays. On the one hand, students have limited success in

Figure 12.6. Kit of Map Making Parts: symbols are the same size as in the kit. (From Welsh & Blasch *Foundation of orientation and mobility*, American Foundation for the Blind, New York, 1980)

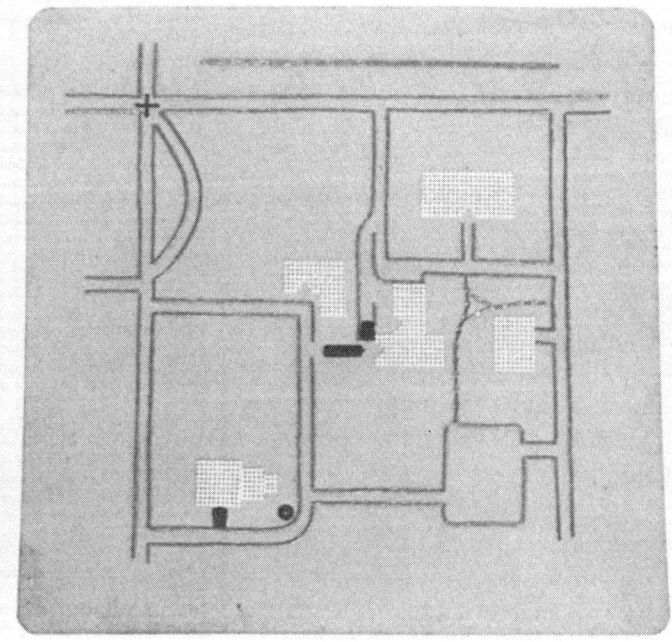

Figure 12.7. Map master made from a kit. (From Welsh & Blasch, *Foundations of orientation and mobility*, American Foundation for the Blind, New York, 1980)

understanding the content of these materials unless they have had extensive experience manipulating objects and moving in the environment (Berlá, 1973; Franks & Nolan, 1970; James, 1967). Therefore some persons have argued that use of tangible graphics should be delayed until concepts of objects and environments are well developed through observation of reality. On the other hand, tangible graphics assist students in developing systematic observation skills. Therefore some persons recommend their introduction as early as practicable or as soon as a child begins to learn to read braille (Pickles, 1967).

Skill in the acquisition of information from tangible graphic displays improves with instruction and practice (Berlá & Butterfield, 1977; Wiedel & Groves, 1969).

Given the lack of both good tangible graphic displays and instructional materials to teach their use, teachers and students are unable to get maximal use from such displays. However, tangible graphic representations of things that are either too small or too large to be readily apprehended through actual manipulation and exploration have been invaluable to many students.

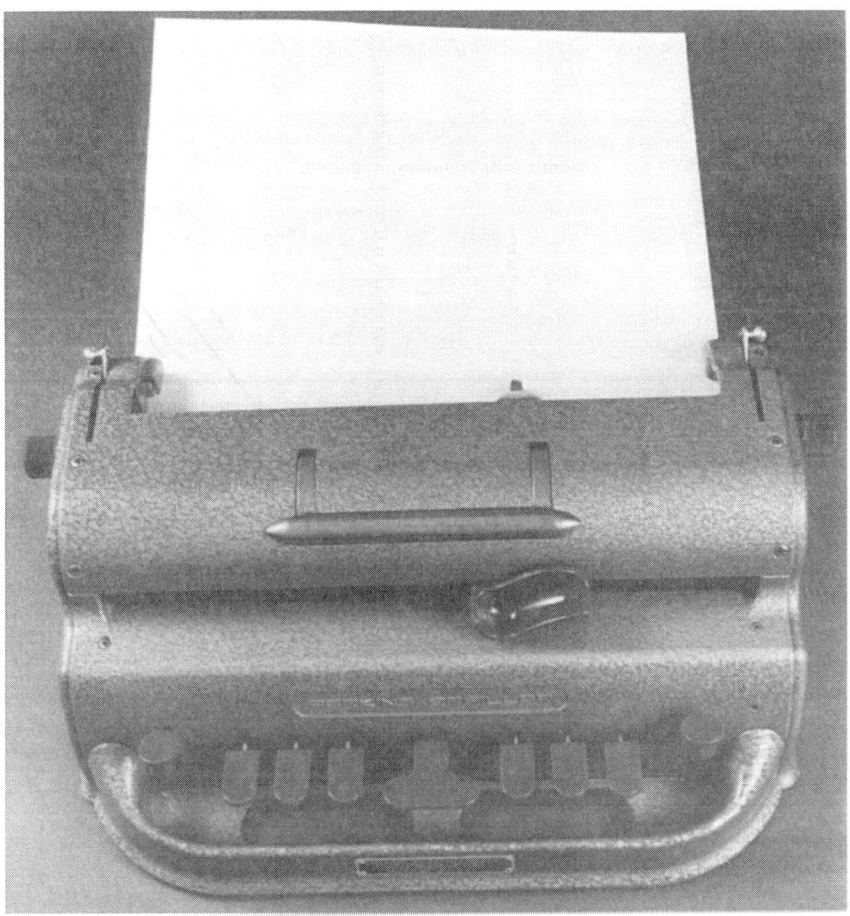

Figure 12.8. The Perkins Brailler being used to emboss a grid. Variations in dot pattern and line width can easily be achieved. (Photograph by Rich Friedman)

Two complementary sets of instructional materials for teaching the use of tangible maps have been developed by Frank Franks at the American Printing House for the Blind (Introduction to Map Study I and II). These materials, designed for kindergarten and younger elementary school blind children, do an excellent job of teaching the systematic exploration and the abstract representation of space using graphic symbols. Such curricula are excellent introductions to geography and spatial orientation as well as to maps as a special form of graphic display. They are developed in sufficient detail for a relatively untrained teacher to utilize successfully. This is important if they are to be readily available to blind

401

children in integrated programs, who may spend very little time with a trained teacher of the visually handicapped.

Recommendations on the use of tangible graphic displays in education

The success of many blind persons in gaining, through tangible graphic displays, information that is not readily apprehended in any other way is reason enough to continue their use in education of the visually handicapped, despite our small knowledge of optimal design and production techniques and the use of such displays. Many teachers also feel that it is important for their students to understand graphic displays simply because of their common use in communication with sighted persons.

However, this author believes that no attempt should be made to present tangibly everything presented in graphic form for the sighted. Those things should be presented that are difficult to describe verbally or to experience directly through nonvisual exploration. Pictures or diagrams of three-dimensional objects can probably best be presented by two-dimensional views, verbal descriptions, or models. Displays should be designed according to principles of haptic perception and not merely be raised visual displays. This will, at times, mean altering both the content and the organization of a display as well as making intelligent choices of symbols. Verbal descriptions or explanations should regularly accompany the graphic displays so that students will need no further assistance to get maximum information from them.

Tangible graphic displays must be both readily available and easy for teachers, volunteers, or blind persons to make. High-quality displays should accompany all commercially produced texts, where appropriate, and production materials that are quick and easy for teachers or volunteers to manipulate should be readily available. Continued attention should be given to development of materials that blind students can utilize to record their own observations. Teachers and volunteers should be trained in the design and production of tangible graphic displays.

Students should be taught to understand graphic displays when they are learning to read tactually. If introduced at this early stage, tangible graphic displays can be utilized to maximum advantage in guiding and organizing students' perceptions of the world.

The skills of display users improve with instruction and practice. Therefore appropriate materials and curricula should be developed for the instruction of blind students in the use of tangible graphic displays. Teachers should be taught to teach their use.

References

Berlá, E. P. Behavioral strategies and problems in scanning and interpreting tactual displays. *New Outlook for the Blind*, 1972, 66, 277–286.

Strategies in scanning a tactual pseudomap. *Education of the Visually Handicapped*, 1973, 5, 8–19.

Berlá, E. P., & Butterfield, L. H. Teachers' views on tactile maps for blind students: problems and needs. *Education of the Visually Handicapped*, 1975, 7, 116–118.

Tactual distinctive features analysis: training blind students in shape recognition and in locating shapes on a map. *Journal of Special Education*, 1977, 11, 335–346.

Berlá, E. P., Butterfield, L. H., & Murr, M. J. Tactual reading of political maps by blind students: a videomatic behavioral analysis. *Journal of Special Education*, 1976, 10, 266–276.

Best, B. D. Geography workshop. *International Conference of Educators of Blind Youth, Proceedings of the Fourth Quinquennial Conference*, Watertown, Mass., September, 1967, p. 238.

Chang, C., & Johnson, D. E. Tactual maps with interchangeable parts. *New Outlook for the Blind*, 1968, 62, 122–124.

Craven, R. W. The use of aluminum sheets in producing tactual maps for blind persons. *New Outlook for the Blind*, 1972, 66, 323–330.

Farrell, G. *Story of blindness*. Cambridge, Mass.: Harvard University Press, 1956.

Foulke, E. Transfer of a complex perceptual skill. *Perceptual & Motor Skills*, 1964, 18, 733–740.

Franks, F. L., & Nolan, C. Y. Development of geographical concepts in blind children. *Education of the Visually Handicapped*, 1970, 3, 2–11.

Gilson, C., Wurzburger, B., & Johnson, D. E. The use of the raised map in teaching mobility to blind children. *New Outlook for the Blind*, 1965, 59, 59–62.

Hill, J. W. Limited field of view in reading letter-shapes with the fingers. In F. Geldard (Ed.), *Cutaneous communication systems and devices*. Austin, Tex.: Psychonomic Society, 1973.

International guide to aids and appliances for blind and visually impaired persons (ed. 2). New York: American Foundation for the Blind, 1977.

James, G. A. The use of maps in schools for blind children. *International Conference of Educators of Blind Youth, Proceedings of the Fourth Quinquennial Conference*, Watertown, Mass., September 1967, pp. 235–236.

Kit for making raised maps. *New Beacon*, 1975, 59, 85–90.

Kerr, J. J. British and American arithmetic devices for the blind – an analytical description. Unpublished doctoral thesis, Temple University, 1974, Ann Arbor, Mich: Xerox University Microfilms.

Krebs, B. M. Illustrations and educational devices for the blind: development of standards for embossed illustrations. *American Association of Instructors of the Blind, Proceedings*, June 1964.

Lane, S. E. History of the Howe Memorial Press and Library of Embossed Books. Unpublished manuscript, Research Library, Perkins School for the Blind, 1911.

Lappin, J. S., & Foulke, E. Expanding the tactual field of view. *Perception & Psychophysics*, 1973, 14, 237–241.

Nolan, C. Y. Educational materials: yesterday, today and tomorrow. *Association of Educators of the Visually Handicapped, 53rd Biennial Conference.* July 1976, pp. 21–28.

Pickles, W. J. Presentation, Teaching of science to the blind. *International Conference of Educators of Blind Youth, Proceedings of the Fourth Quinquennial Conference,* Watertown, Mass., September 1967, pp. 219–222.

Robinson, A. H., & Petchenik, B. B. *The nature of maps: essays toward understanding maps and mapping.* Chicago: University of Chicago Press, 1976.

Schiff, W. Research on raised line drawings. *New Outlook for the Blind,* 1965, *59,* 134–137.

Development of raised line drawings as supplementary tools in the education of the blind (Final Report, Project No. RD-1571-S). Washington, D.C.: Vocational Rehabilitation Administration, 1967.

Schiff, W., Kaufer, L., & Mosak, S. Informative tactile stimuli in the perception of direction. *Perceptual & Motor Skills,* 1966, *23,* 1315–1335.

Sewell, H. P. Patent for "Method & apparatus for forming raised characters & lines" granted Nov. 11, 1952, by the U.S. Patent Office, Washington, D.C.

Waterhouse, E. J. History of the Howe Press of Perkins School for the Blind, Watertown, Mass.: The Howe Press of Perkins School for the Blind, 1975.

Welsh, R. A., & Blasch, B. B. *Foundations of orientation and mobility.* New York: American Foundation for the Blind, 1980.

Wiedel, J. W. & Groves, P. A. Tactual mapping: Design, reproduction, reading and interpretation (Final Report, Project No. RD-2557-S). Washington, D.C: Department of Health, Education and Welfare, 1969.

Zahl, P. A. (Ed.), *Blindness, modern approaches to the unseen environment.* New York: Hafner, 1962.

13. Production of tangible graphic displays

JOHN M. GILL

John Gill, an engineer and human factors psychologist, presents a brief chapter describing methods for producing single-and multicopy haptic maps and diagrams. Gill's computer-guided engraving systems produce tactual diagrams that most blind and sighted perceivers agree are the best-defined materials currently available. However, the technology is not widely available, other methods are often better suited for certain purposes (e.g., single diagrams), and a designer is still needed to program the system to select the way symbols and displays are to be made and which symbols and other display features will be utilized. Chapter 13, in combination with Chapters 12, 14, and 15, yields a valuable picture of methods, materials, and techniques available for the production of effective tactual graphics for visually impaired people. WILLIAM SCHIFF

Introduction

The earliest reported method of producing embossed material was in 1517 by Francesco Lucas, who engraved alphanumerics in wooden blocks. The first single-copy tactual maps were probably made by Jeorg Weissembourg in the early eighteenth century by sewing beads and threads on linen. In 1785 Valentin Haüy successfully embossed raised images in paper, but it was not until the last decade that embossed maps and diagrams became widely available to the blind population.

The main characteristics of systems for producing tactual maps are summarized in Table 13.1. The choice of method will depend on the ultimate use of the map and on financial considerations. Traditionally copies have been made on manila paper, but this material imposes physical limitations on the design; there is a limited range of discriminable symbols, relatively low height of embossing, and the paper is not suitable for outdoor use. Many of the systems developed in recent years have employed vacuum forming of plastic sheets, which are more durable and capable of better symbol definition (Figure 13.1). Wiedel (1971) and Gill (1973) have studied the suitability of various commercially avail-

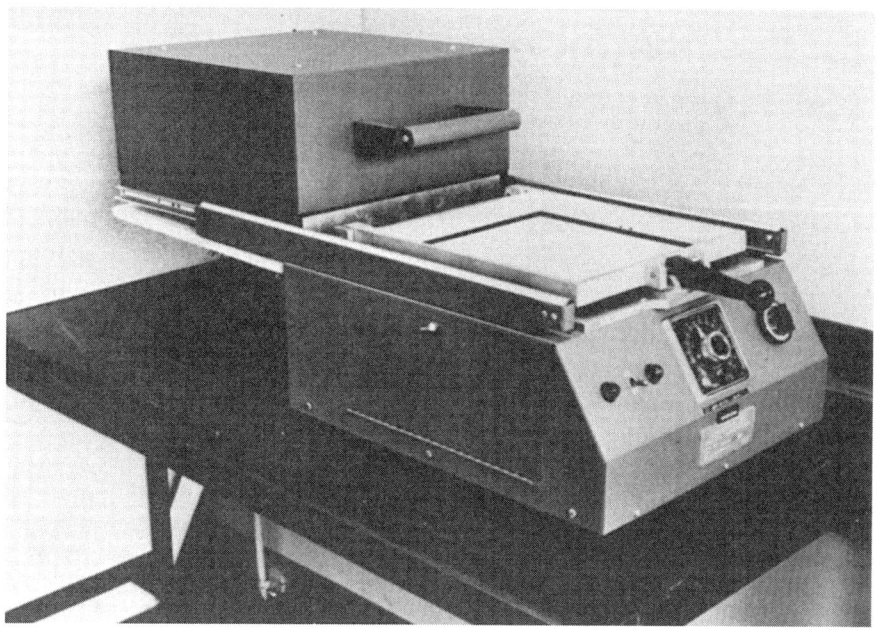

Figure 13.1. Vacuum-forming machine. Heating elements soften a vinyl sheet placed over a master on the horizontal platform when the upper unit is slid closed. A vacuum pump draws the softened vinyl down over the raised materials on the master, creating copies such as those shown in Figures 15.2 to 15.10.

able thermoplastics and found that calendered polyvinyl chloride gives the best results.

It has been found desirable to use more than one height of embossing, but many production systems are limited to a single elevation. The optimum elevation of symbols will depend on whether the copies are monolithic, whether the map is for outdoor use, and how tactually sensitive the user is. If the production system requires an accurate visual master for each elevation of embossing, then the maps will be very expensive when only a few copies are required.

Raised-line drawing kit

These kits have been designed for drawing by the blind or by teachers who need to produce a map or diagram quickly. The most usual method is to use a ballpoint pen on Mylar or Melinex, which puckers under the pressure of the pen. This system can produce only one type of line and braille cannot be added easily.

Table 13.1. *Characteristics of 19 systems for producing tactual maps*

System	Base material	Method of duplicating	Capable of operation by a blind person	Needs accurate visual master	Cost[a]				Quality[a]			
					Time to make master	Capital cost of equipment	Cost materials for master	Cost materials for copies	Maximum elevation	No. different elevations	Accuracy	Durability
Raised-line drawing kit	Thin plastic		Yes		C	D	D		D	D	D	D
Metal foil	Plastic	Vacuum forming			C	B	D		C	C	C	B
String master	Plastic	Vacuum forming			B	B	D	C	B	B	C	B
Wire master	Plastic	Vacuum forming			B	B	D	C	B	B	B	B
Solid dot	Paper	Screen printing		Yes	B	D	D	C	D	D	B	D
Sewing machine	Plastic	Vacuum forming	Yes	Yes	C	B	C	D	C	C	C	B
Embossed zinc plates	Paper	Press			C	B	C	D	C	D	C	D
Sintered bronze	Plastic	Vacuum forming		Yes	A	B	A	D	B	A	C	B
Metal and epoxy	Plastic	Vacuum forming			B	C	C	C	A	A	B	B
Virkotype	Paper	Deposition		Yes	C	B	B	C	D	D	B	D
Polyvinyl	PVC	Deposition		Yes	C	B	B	C	C	C	C	B
Photoetching	Paper	Press		Yes	C	B	B	A	B	B	B	B
Photolathe	Paper	Press		Yes	C	B	C	C	C	B	A	B
Drum embosser	Paper			Yes	C	C	D	C	C	D	B	C
Relief printer	Paper		Yes		D	B	D		C	D	D	D
Sensory quill	Plastic or metal foil	Vacuum forming	Yes		D	B	D	C	C	D	D	B
Line embosser	Paper	Paper	Yes		C	A	D	C	D	D	D	D
Numerically controlled machine tool	Plastic	Vacuum forming			D	A	C	C	B	A	A	B

[a] A = very high; B = high; C = medium; D = low.

Metal foil

A master for vacuum forming is made by embossing a sheet of aluminum foil (Craven 1972, Schiff, 1966). The map has to be drawn in mirror image on the back of the foil, which is then placed on a rubber mat; the lines are then embossed with a spur wheel. Textured areas can be produced by glueing sandpaper to the front surface of the foil.

String master

This method involves building up a master on transparent cellulose. Various thicknesses of string are used for line symbols; sandpapers, linoleum and fabrics are used for textures.

Wire master

The wire master method is very similar to the previous method except that solder wire is used in place of string (Armstrong & James, 1978; Fletcher, 1970). Solder can be rolled to give solid, dotted, or dashed lines with a triangular cross section. This system is superior to the string method because the solder is easier to manipulate and the lines have sharper crests.

Solid dot

Nippon Lighthouse in Japan has developed this technique for screen-printing embossed maps. The system requires no special equipment and can produce multicolored maps. The disadvantages include low-elevation embossing and poor control over dot profile. Because the visual quality is good but the tactual quality is relatively poor, the main application is for people with some useful vision who use both visual and tactual senses to read a map.

Sewing machine

A master for vacuum forming is made by machine-sewing a fibrous material with thick thread. Areal and point symbols can be glued to the top surface of the master.

Embossed zinc plates

A system based on the traditional method for printing braille books involves embossing a pair of zinc plates on a special machine (Figure

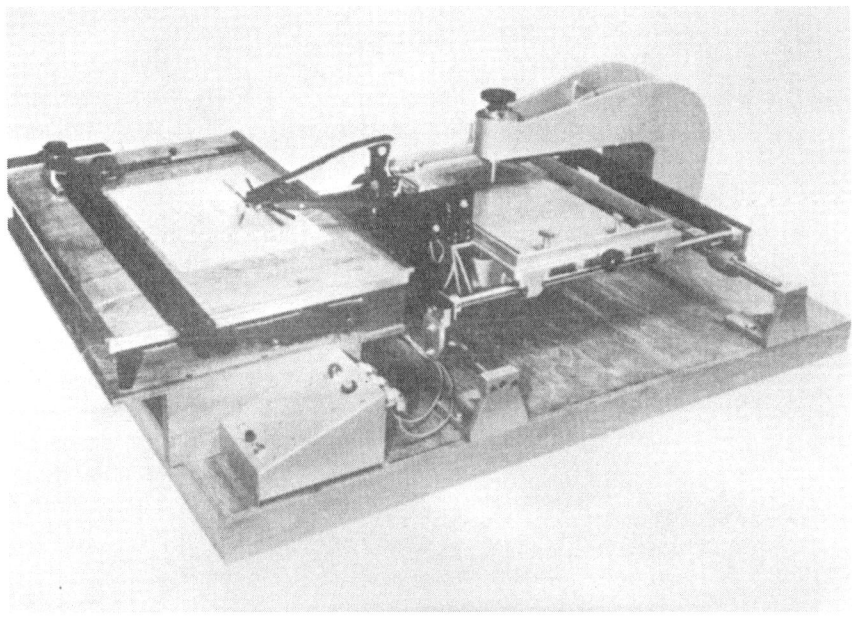

Figure 13.2. A machine for embossing dots on a pair of zinc plates. (Courtesy of Royal National Institute for the Blind, London)

13.2). The plates are used in a press for making copies on manila paper. This system is usually limited to producing maps in a punctate form with only one elevation of embossing.

Sintered bronze master

A sheet of sintered bronze is manually engraved to make a female master for vacuum-forming plastic sheets (Figure 13.3). This system can produce high-quality maps, but the bronze is very expensive and engraving can take several months. The use of a female master gives poor control over the shape of the line crest or point symbol crest, which strongly affects the discriminability of the symbol.

Metal and epoxy resin master

The male master is made from metal and epoxy resin. Blocks of resin are used for regular shapes, and epoxy resin is molded for the remainder. Because the master is not porous, one must drill air holes in it before vacuum forming plastic copies. Manufacturing the master is so time-consuming that the method is viable only for enthusiastic amateurs.

409

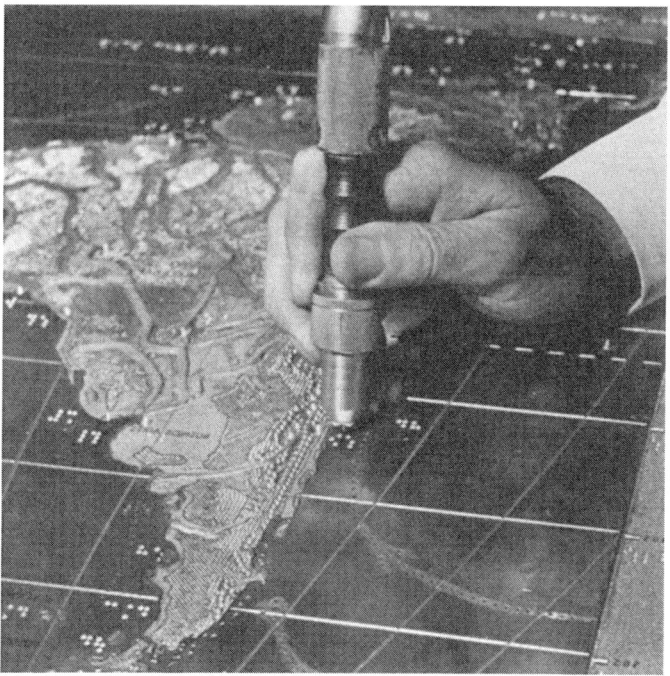

Figure 13.3. Manual engraving of a sheet of sintered bronze. (Courtesy of National Institute for the Blind, London)

Virkotype

Wet ink print is dusted with a fine resinous powder that adheres to the wet ink as a raised plastic symbol when heated (Wiedel, 1964). The maximum elevation is relatively low, and the system is reliable only under laboratory conditions.

Polyvinyl chloride base (PVC)

This process involves heating resinous powders to form a core about 0.38 mm (0.015 in) thick. During the heating process, a master surface mold prepared from a photo-engraved plate applies a raised layer of pigmented vinyl that permanently affixes to the base. The map can be embossed on both sides, providing an alternative to overlays (Kidwell & Greer, 1973).

Photoetching

A photographic copy of a map is placed on top of a sheet of photosensitive plastic that is exposed to ultraviolet light, and the master is chemically etched to the required depth. It is necessary to repeat the whole process for each different elevation on the map. Because both male and female masters can be produced, copies can be made by vacuum forming plastic sheets or by embossing paper, plastic, or metal in a conventional press. This latter facility can be very important when a large number of copies are required.

Photolathe

A machine developed by Jens Scheel (1969) in Germany, in which a lathe is controlled by a photoelectric scanner, is limited to a single elevation. Because both male and female masters can be produced, copies can be made of paper in a conventional press.

Drum embosser

In principle, this machine is very similar to the photolathe, but the cutting tool is replaced by a solenoid. The system is limited to producing diagrams in punctate form.

Relief printer

Saab-Scania (1972) in Sweden has developed a flatbed embosser for use in the classroom. The equipment consists of a drawing table and one or more reading desks. The reading desk contains a punch for embossing manila paper. The output is in punctate form with either three or five dots per centimeter. The picture can be either enlarged or reduced and the data stored on a conventional stereo tape. Thus diagrams could be stored on the same tape as a talking book.

Sensory quill

Traylor (1972) developed a system for embossing either plastic or aluminum foil. The system uses a motor-driven hammer to emboss the plastic or metal foil. The system is limited to a single elevation of embossing, but the operator can produce dotted or dashed lines by making them from short sections of continuous lines.

Line embosser

A computer line printer can be modified to produce tactual diagrams by removing the ribbon, increasing the pressure on the hammers, and put-

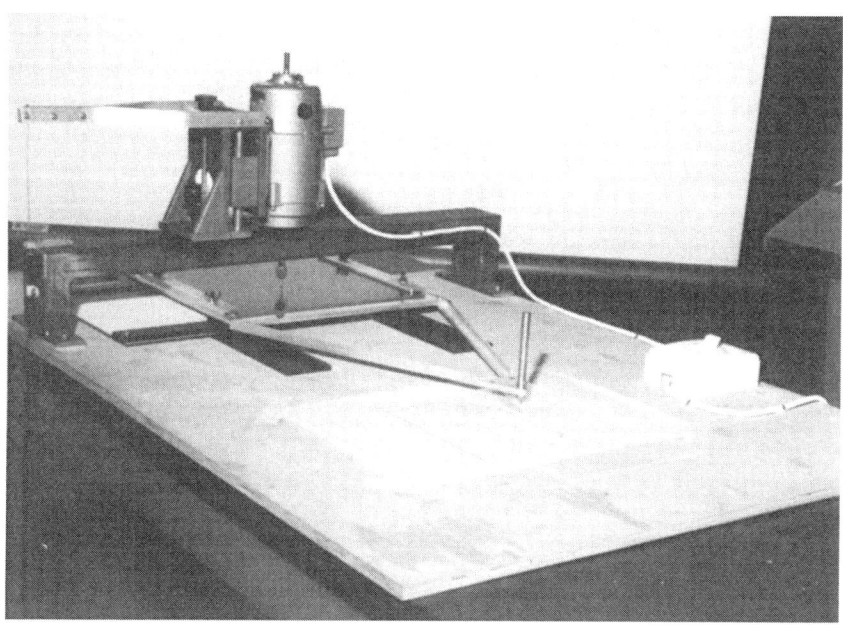

Figure 13.4. Manual engraver for producing a female master on a sheet of laminated plastic.

ting some rubber behind the paper. Different textures can be produced by using different characters. The physical quality of the output is poor, but the significance of the system is that it can be operated by blind users. Hallenbeck (1969) has written software for the graphic output from computer programs as well as diagrams produced by direct instructions on a teletype.

Manual engraver

Gill (1973) developed a machine for manually engraving a sheet of laminated plastic; a Perspex stencil provides precise dimensions for standard symbols (Figure 13.4). An epoxy resin male copy is then used as a master for the vacuum forming of plastic sheets. The system has the advantage of low capital expenditure, but it is labor intensive because there is no interactive design capability.

Numerically controlled machine tool

Gill (1973) developed a system using computer-aided design for a map layout and a numerically controlled machine tool for engraving a lami-

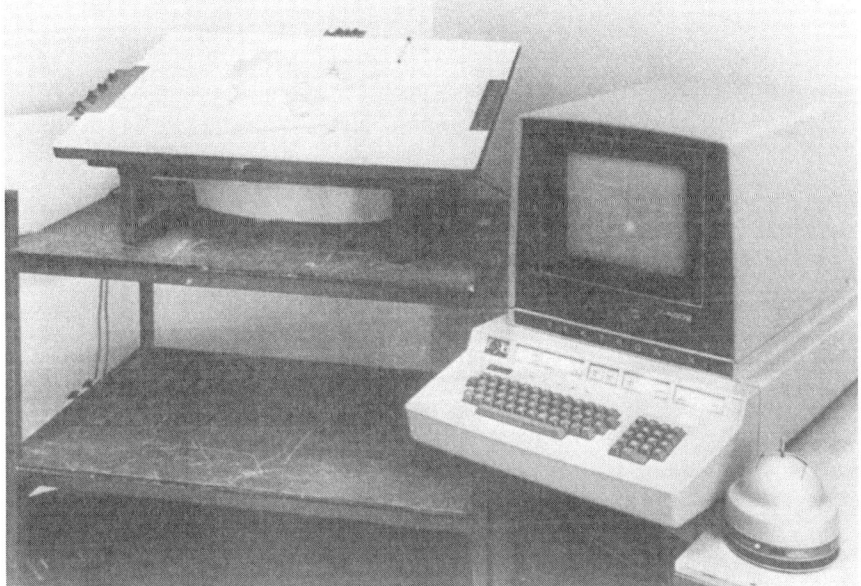

Figure 13.5. Coordinate table and visual display for automatic production of consistent, high-quality tangible displays.

nated plastic sheet. The topographical information is entered into a computer from a coordinate table. Editing on the visual display unit permits the insertion or deletion of individual lines, movement of endpoints of lines, and change of scale. A wide variety of line types (solid, dotted, and dashed) can be specified from the keyboard, and the operator controls the height of the symbols on final copies. A joystick can be used to position standard symbols. Alphanumeric text can be entered from the keyboard; the text is automatically converted to grade I braille, with a choice of four different cell sizes.

When a satisfactory display is obtained, output is requested. This can include output on a digital plotter, magnetic tape, or punched paper tape. A map can be stored on tape and then quickly modified at a later date. The engraving machine can be controlled either directly from the computer used in the design stage or from a smaller computer with the data transferred on punched paper tape. The engraving machine is used for making a mirror-image female copy of the map on a sheet of laminated plastic. Thermoplastic copies are produced from a male epoxy resin master on a vacuum-forming machine.

413

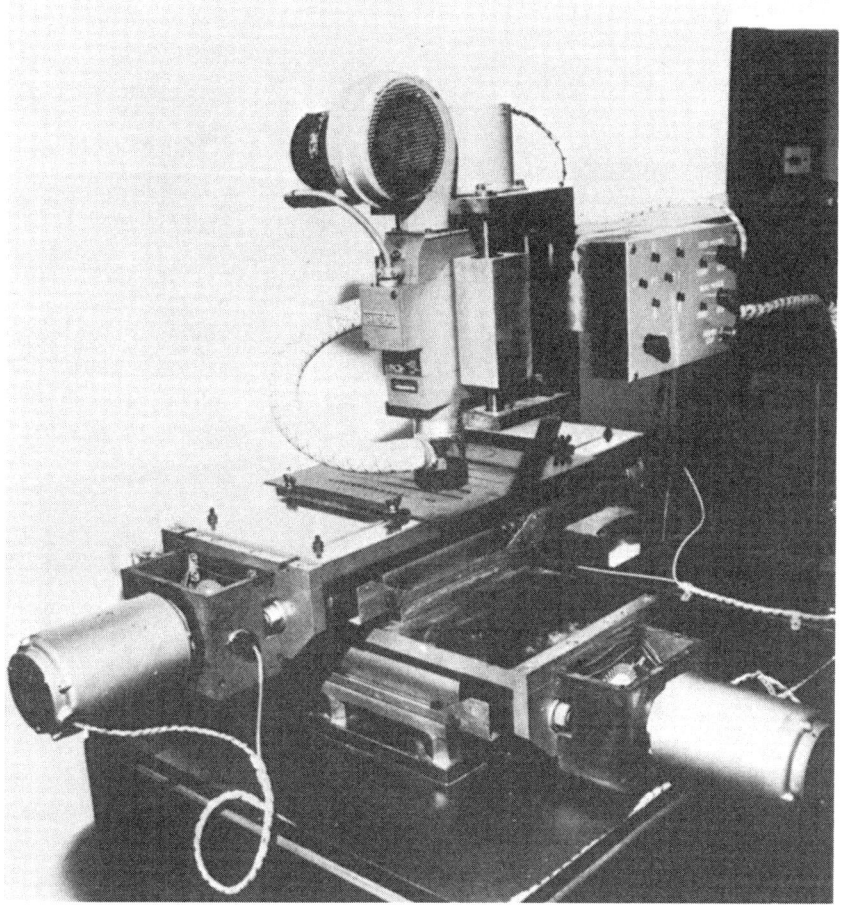

Figure 13.6. Engraving machine for automatic production of consistent, high-quality tangible displays.

Embossed maps with visual markings

It is often desirable to include visual markings on a tactual map for the partially sighted and the sighted. The PVC base production system, used by Kidwell and Greer (1973), can produce the embossing with a different color than the background.

Transparent plastics have the advantage that visual markings can be put on the underside of the map after vacuum forming. This avoids problems of alignment and deterioration of markings by abrasion during

414

use. Ink can be rolled across the back of the plastic sheet so that the embossed lines are left clear, resulting in light colored lines on a black background, as recommended by Greenberg (1968).

Other methods generally involve adding the markings to the plastic before vacuum forming. Generation of the artwork can be labor intensive unless the system is computer based.

Ogrosky (1973) tried using mimeography with some success, but the contrast was inferior to that produced by offset printing. However, offset printing is economically viable only for large production runs. Photocopying, although unsuccessful to date, would keep markings from being rubbed off because the visual image is fused to the top surface of the plastic. Screen printing appears to be the best system currently available, although it is labor intensive.

References

Armstrong, J. D., & James, G. A. *Handbook on mobility maps*. Nottingham: University of Nottingham, 1978.

Craven, R. W. The use of aluminum sheets in producing tactual maps for blind persons. *New Outlook for the Blind*, 1972, 66, 323–330.

Fletcher, R. C. (Ed.), *The teaching of science and mathematics to the blind (with section on raised diagrams)*. London: Royal National Institute for the Blind, 1970.

Gill, J. M. Design, production and evaluation of tactual maps for the blind. Unpublished doctoral thesis, University of Warwick, England, 1973.

   Tactual mapping. *Research Bulletin of the American Foundation for the Blind*, 1974, no. 28, 57–80.

Greenberg, G. L. Map design for partially seeing students: an investigation of white versus black line symbology. Unpublished doctoral thesis, University of Washington, 1968.

Hallenbeck, C. E. Computer displays as occupational aids for the blind: preliminary report on research in progress. *Research Bulletin of the American Foundation for the Blind*, 1969, no. 19, 248–251.

Kidwell, A. M., & Greer, P. S. *Sites, perception, and the nonvisual experience: designing and manufacturing mobility maps*. New York: American Foundation for the Blind, 1973.

Ogrosky, C. E. New approaches to the preparation and reproduction of tactual and enhanced image graphics for the visually handicapped. Unpublished master's thesis, University of Washington, 1973.

Saab-Scania. *Handicap equipment: relief printer Saab EPP 370*. Saab, 1972.

Scheel, J. *Electronic tracer*. J. Scheel, 1969.

Schiff, W. Manual for the construction of raised line diagrams. New York: Recording for the Blind, 1966.

Traylor, D. R. The Huegel quill: A new tactile development for the blind. *Proceedings of the 1972 Conference on Electronic Prosthetics*. Lexington, Ky.: University of Kentucky, 1972, 147–149.

Wiedel, J. W. Virkotype process of raised printing (Circular 64-10). Washington, D.C.: Library of Congress, Division for the Blind, 1964.

Pre-printed thermoformed mobility maps. Unpublished manuscript, University of Maryland, 1971.

Wiedel, J. W., & Groves, P. A. *Tactual mapping: design, reproduction, reading and interpretation* (Final Report No. RD-2557-S). Washington, D.C.: Dept. of Health, Education and Welfare, 1969.

14. Tangible graphics: producers' views

JASHA M. LEVI & NANCY S. AMICK

In Chapter 14, Jasha Levi and Nancy Amick provide a view of tactual diagrams too seldom considered by psychologists and rehabilitation specialists – that of producers of tangible graphics. Part of this chapter emerged from the Louisville Workshop and Symposium, the foundation for this volume. Both authors of this chapter have had lengthy experience with tangible diagram construction.

Jasha Levi was a pioneer in the production and distribution of tangible supplements for textbooks and has made a substantial contribution to this field. His efforts to apply tactual perception to reading and understanding illustrated texts in scientific and technical areas were seminal. He first reviews the historical development of raised-line drawing supplements for recorded books for the blind student and professional. He then discusses such practical issues as the need for and role of verbal descriptions (on tape or in braille) in assisting the haptic perceiver to obtain maximum information from tangible graphics associated with books.

Nancy Amick has probably designed, produced, and supervised the production of more tangible graphics for blind readers than anyone in the United States. Her pioneering work and considerable experience are brought to bear on practical aspects of producing effective diagrams for blind perceivers. She provides a step-by-step guide for anyone considering the construction of such materials. Diagrams having minimum clutter and maximum discriminability may be designed by following the relatively small set of guidelines provided in this chapter. Psychophysical discriminability data are here translated into concrete guidelines for constructing maps and diagrams in a multitude of technical areas. The issue of which visual diagrams to transform into tangible representations is discussed, as is the related issue of whether to copy or alter a diagram designed to be seen to one to be felt. Anyone involved with the production or construction of tangible materials to be used by visually impaired persons must read this informative chapter. WILLIAM SCHIFF

Part 1. Raised-line drawings as supplements to verbal descriptions in recorded textbooks

Jasha M. Levi

In the late 1950s, and early 1960s, blind students in American schools and universities began entering progressively more complex fields of

417

study. The textbooks they were ordering from various sources reflected that trend.

A large number of these students had been blind since birth or had lost their sight early in life. They showed a generally well-developed tactual ability: The percentage of braille readers among them was much higher than in the visually handicapped population as a whole. This difference in proficiency was expected since the degree of tactual dexterity is inversely related to age.

Some standard textbooks needed by these students were available in braille. However, it was obvious that a great deal of time is required for braille transcribers to produce a new braille volume, and if one was not already available, as was (and is) generally the case with all new textbooks, recording them on magnetic tape was (and is) the only practical way to get them to the student on time.

Recorded textbooks had an advantage over their braille counterparts. They could be produced faster, and volunteer reader-specialists could describe the drawings the way an instructor does in a class.

Most of the required textbooks were recorded for these students by a number of individuals, including family members and colleagues, and by thousands of volunteers in local and national organizations.

Of the latter, Recording for the Blind (RFB) was by far the largest supplier. RFB was providing copies of textbooks already recorded in its extensive library and recording new textbooks on request. As a matter of course, drawings, diagrams, and other textbook illustrations were described verbally.

Soon it became apparent that the main difficulty here was in preparing appropriate verbal descriptions of complex illustrations. The more complicated the printed drawings, the more challenging was the task of explaining them by words alone. The problem was addressed by the introduction of raised-line drawings as supplements to verbal descriptions.

The demographics of the blind student population served by RFB indicated that only 34 percent could read braille; a small additional number showed some tactual ability. The raised drawings were primarily intended for the use of this group, and even if their number had been much smaller, serving them with tactual supplements would have made the effort worthwhile.

However, a print-handicapped student does not necessarily have to be a proficient braille reader to make use of raised drawings, but tactual ability does make a difference. This is why raised-line drawings have become such a useful tool, not only for students who are braille readers but for many more young nonreaders of braille among the visually handicapped population in schools and universities.

The idea of producing raised-line drawings was not new. Some of the braille books, in particular those produced by the late Cecily Bryant of the Thayer Chapter of Telephone Pioneers, not only faithfully reproduced the text but also gave a tactile version of the drawings that accompanied it. The skill of this transcriber and the beautiful execution of her drawings deserve special recognition and a permanent place in the annals of services to the blind.

The first experimental drawing to accompany a recorded textbook was made at RFB by this writer. It was a representation of a fission reaction; several materials of differing textures were used in a pasteup.

With volunteer consultant Clyde Keith, we next conducted an informal, pragmatic project to determine the most practical method of making master drawings that could be reproduced on plastic Brailon sheets in small as well as large quantities. Metal foil (copper at first and aluminum later) and various toothed and solid wheels were introduced. Metal masters proved particularly useful because of the ease with which corrections could be made on them, and because they lent themselves to the use of a large variety of tools for many different discriminable raised-line configurations. Furthermore, mistakes cannot be corrected as simply on braille paper masters. The first complete booklet of raised drawings to accompany an RFB text was made in 1960.

Several RFB recording studios joined in producing raised drawings, led at first by the Louisville, Ky., and Princeton, N.J., units. Among the first RFB volunteer participants in this effort were Ruth Drennan Carmichael and Marion Harcourt (and somewhat later, Billy Marx) in Kentucky, and Nancy S. Amick in the Princeton Unit. Nancy Amick has stayed on to become the chairman of the Raised Line Drawings Committee of Recording for the Blind. Through her participation, in both the administrative organizational work and the actual development of techniques, manuals, and practical execution of drawings, Mrs. Amick has made a contribution of major importance to this new field. She has rightfully come to be recognized as the leading practitioner of the art of producing raised-line drawings as supplements to recorded textbooks in all fields of study.

Eventually, thousands of drawings were made to accompany hundreds of recorded textbooks. Close to 900 titles with raised-line supplements are circulated yearly in up to 3,000 copies. There are indications, however, that questions are being raised at RFB on whether that agency should continue with this task or pass it on to some other organization.

419

It is hoped that the final decision will be made in favor of not only continuing production but also increasing the number of raised-line additions to their recorded textbook service.

The next step was a structured research project conducted by Schiff and Levi to determine discriminable lines and textures and to set up guidelines for the production of drawings. One of the major results of this project was the development and introduction of a conceptually unique tactual counterpart of the arrow symbol – the *tactual arrow*. Recognizable immediately by touch, the line flows smoothly in the intended direction and is rough when scanned the other way.

The need for verbal descriptions of drawings for those with little tactual ability was obvious. It soon became apparent that verbal guides to the illustrations also added a dimension of better comprehension of the tactile drawings to those who could read them.

A sighted person takes in the whole of a drawing or illustration and then examines the details with some background knowledge of its complete meaning. For those who cannot see, the verbal description takes the place of that overview. The raised-line drawing can then be observed in its particulars with much more understanding than without the oral description.

Based on this consideration, work was continued on coordinating the verbal and tactual presentations of drawings during the introductory phases of the project and beyond. The need for this mix of the two media in no way detracts from the vital importance of each in its own right. On the contrary, those who describe drawings verbally should be trained further to do so precisely and in specific terms. It does no good to say: "And this point up here . . . "; one must give the location of the point.

Parallel efforts must continue to train those who draft raised-line drawings to make them tactually meaningful. Also, of the utmost importance, training of blind students in the use of tactile drawings must start as early as possible in life. Timely training is imperative for the development of better skills in scanning raised lines and thus achieving speed and efficiency to comprehend them under the pressure of today's overwhelming informational workload.

Part 2. Designing useful drawings for the blind

Nancy S. Amick

Although a great deal of work has been done on the discriminability of individual lines and textures, little has been done on the problem of

420

combining these lines and textures into useful tactual drawings for the blind. Since 1962, RFB has been experimenting in the field of tactual drawings; currently it produces supplements of drawings to accompany recorded texts in such fields as biology, mathematics, physics, electronics, and economics. The usefulness of drawings in any of these fields depends on proper planning of the size, choice of textures and line heights, and labeling so that the important features are emphasized and the material is presented in an accurate, clear, and uncluttered manner. Consequently, good drawings, whether made by hand or by computer, require intelligent planning by a drawing designer–someone who is familiar with both the subject matter and the needs of the blind and who can translate the visual representation into a useful tactual form. The ideas offered here on drawing design are based on 18 years of experience and experimentation, along with feedback from students and evaluation by participants in the Louisville Workshop and Symposium.

Planning the drawing: translation from visual to tactual format

When a sighted person is presented with a drawing, the eye scans the page, picking out the most important features with the help of boldface lines, varying type sizes, and perhaps some colored lines. When presented with a good tactile drawing, the blind person should also be able to locate the important information by quickly scanning the page with the hand. The important lines must attract attention immediately by being rough or highly embossed. The size must be adequate for individual lines to be traced, and the labels must be placed so that they do not detract from the figure itself. Important parts of the drawing must stand out, and the page must not blend into an undefined, overall texture of lines and braille. In short, it must not seem cluttered or undifferentiated.

To the blind person, variations in height and texture are the counterpart of boldface type or colored ink. The rougher the line texture or the more elevated the line, the quicker it is noticed and the more important the line will seem. Given two lines of the same height, the rough-textured line will always seem more important than the smooth one. Consequently, height and texture can be combined in a variety of ways to produce discriminable lines of differing importance. In a successful raised drawing, line heights and textures are selected so that the tactual effect is compatible with the importance of the lines. This means that lines of primary importance, such as the main curves in a graph, should be shown by either rough lines or high-rise smooth lines; secondary lines such as guidelines or grid lines in graphs should either be light and smooth or finely serrated. By playing rough textures against smooth ones, the designer can further enhance the contrast between lines and improve their discriminability. For instance, two closely spaced lines are far more discriminable when one is drawn in a rough texture and the other in a higher-rise, smooth texture. Clearly, not every combination of height and texture produces lines that can be distinguished from one another, and even individual lines that have been tested for discriminability may not seem clear in the context of a complicated drawing. The tendency is to overestimate the ability of the blind to make fine distinctions between lines that visually may seem different but feel identical. The best advice is to choose textures and heights that maximize the *contrast* between adjacent lines and that are *compatible* with their overall importance. Then, *feel* the finished drawing yourself to see if the desired effect has been achieved.

The drawing designer can make a fairly accurate judgment of the usefulness of a drawing by feeling it. Although one need not be able to understand or interpret the drawing, one must be able to feel and follow the individual lines without losing track of them. The braille labels should feel close enough to the lines that one barely notices the braille as the finger traces the line. There should be no question about what the labels identify, but they must not interfere with the ability to feel the lines or complicate the overall page so that the lines are hard to find. One should learn to watch out for places where the lines and braille degenerate into textured areas. Such areas occur when the overall size of the drawing is too small, when there is too much braille or it is too close to the lines, or when there is not enough texture variation in the lines to make them discriminable. One must think about problems from a tactual point of view. For instance, if a dashed line is to seem continuous, the finger must be able to feel the second dash before leaving the first one. The drawing designer should develop this sense of feel and learn to anticipate problems in order to minimize them by proper choice of size, spacing, and texture.

Selecting the drawing

The first problem for the drawing designer, and one that is often overlooked, is to assess the figure as a teaching tool and decide whether it is worthwhile to convert it into a raised drawing. In addition to knowledge of the subject, this requires consideration of the text itself and the grade level of the student. The most important questions are: What is the purpose of the figure? Does the figure show something about shape, position, or relative size that can be shown only by a drawing? If not, substitute a verbal description, either brailled or recorded, that will be more useful and less time-consuming to the student. Graphs, geometric figures, and line drawings in physics and biology are examples of figures that make useful raised drawings. Drawings of simple geometric shapes may be very important for the grade school student but may not need to be shown more than once, if at all, in a high school text. Sketches or any drawings in which the information is not entirely clear should not be made into raised drawings without clarification. Drawings showing a car moving along a road or students performing experiments, or others showing that bugs hide from the sun under logs and stones, should not be reproduced. However, an enlarged view of the equipment that students are using, or a detailed view of the bug itself, might be a useful accompaniment to the verbal description. Be sure to ask yourself what the drawing shows that makes it worth your time and that of the student.

If a drawing is deemed worthwhile, the next question should be, where and what are the important parts of the figure, or what is it trying to teach? The final question should always be, can this figure be made into a successful, useful drawing as it stands, or does it need to be modified or presented in a different manner? Answers to these questions influence the three main decisions that the designer must make – the *size*, the choice of *textures and line heights*, and the final *layout* of the drawing.

Size

The most popular word at the Louisville Workshop was *clutter*. *Clutter* is a hard word to define. In many cases, it comes down to choosing the wrong size for the drawing so that the lines are too close together or the labeling is too crowded. Although texture plays a role, the size of the drawing is probably the most important factor in avoiding clutter. The proper size depends in large part on the answer to the question, where and what are the important parts of the figure, or what is it trying to teach? Examine all important areas and check them for potential trouble spots such as multiple lines crossing one another or in close proximity, small angles or small areas that are significant, and braille labels that must fit into tight spots. As a first estimate of the minimum useful size for the raised drawing, apply these two rules of thumb to the enlarged image or sketch: First, any lines that are separated by less than 6 mm (0.25 in) tend to feel like a single wide line instead of two separate lines, although different textures for the two lines will improve their discriminability. Second, areas less than 13 mm (0.5 in) across are too hard to feel, and small shapes such as triangles and squares are hard to recognize if they are less than 13 mm (0.5 in) on a side. Do not overlook the fact that small triangles or multisided regions appear one way or another in most figures and frequently go unrecognized. If the size or shape of these regions is important, the above rule of thumb should be applied.

Next, consider the labeling, as the size of the drawing must often be increased to accommodate the braille. Braille should be spaced about 3 mm (0.125 in) from lines or points. As a rule of thumb, the braille should be positioned so that the finger is just barely aware of its presence as it traces the line or rests on the point. Extra spacing is needed for large fingers to feel braille next to high-rise lines or down in small, recessed areas. In places where the line texture is rough or consists of small dots, the spacing between the line and the braille may need to be increased to avoid any possibility that the two elements will blend into a textured area. When the best possible location for the braille might still lead to ambiguity, dots may be added to call attention to the point being labeled. When an item appears several times, label it more than once; do not count on its being recognized. Direct labeling on the diagram is preferred to keys, but keys are preferred to lead lines. If possible, single letters or numbers should be placed consistently to one side or the other of points. Make any final adjustments in the size of the drawing to accommodate the labels and trace the figure onto the master plate. As a rough estimate, allow 6 mm (0.25 in) for each braille cell that will be needed and sketch out the space that will be required by the braille on the master drawing. If a drawing does not appear in context, allow space to braille a title at the top of the page. The value of a drawing is greatly increased when the blind person knows what he or she is examining. An opaque projector is a boon in selecting the correct drawing size. The magnified image of the figure is projected onto a master plate, and the image size can be studied and adjusted before the figure is traced. In addition to variable magnification, simple projectors can be made to provide the *reversed image* needed by many drawing techniques.

If the size of the drawing cannot be adjusted to accommodate braille, or if the amount of braille overshadows the importance of the lines, plan to use a key. Either letters or numbers can be used. They should be assigned in some logical sequence and placed on the item, if possible, or next to a point. Key letters need not be related to the word they represent, and they can be the single letters *k* through *z* written without a letter sign. The key information should be brailled in a consistent location, preferably below but spaced well away from the figure. Some participants in the Louisville Workshop suggested that a rough-textured outline around the key would help users locate the information quickly. Large keys must be placed on a separate page; the preferred method of binding is as a page facing the drawing.

If the figure is a straightforward line drawing with little labeling, the main problem is to avoid making it too large. It is possible to make a drawing so large that the relationship of the parts is hard to determine. For example, a circle more than a few centimeters in diameter is hard to identify. For simple figures, the concept of a hand span is useful. Keep the figure to a size such that, with the thumb anchored in one spot, the fingers can feel the entire figure without moving the hand.

Simplification

Some figures are too large or complex to fit on a standard-size page. Because the single-page format is by far the most popular, the first thought should be whether the figure can be simplified or modified to fit on one page. A schematic line drawing can be substituted to advantage for a more elaborate picture, or unnecessary detail can be removed. For instance, a rope and sometimes a tube is better shown by a single line than by two parallel lines; a box labeled *house* can be substituted for a detailed view of a house; or the braille word *hand, eye,* or *man* can be substituted for pictures of hands, eyes, or people taking part in scientific experiments. Sometimes the figure contains details that are not necessary, such as realistic pictures of hinges or nuts and bolts when only the pivot point or the point of attachment needs to be indicated by a dot; the label *hinge* or a note of description can be added if desired.

Sometimes information in the original figure can be eliminated. For instance, it may be sufficient to show every other curve in graphs illustrating large families of curves such as the magnetic field around a bar magnet, the shift in position of parabolas for changes in the equation, or characteristic curves for transistors.

Seek ways to reduce the figure to its basic information. For instance, in a simple bar graph where bars are separated by spaces, the length but not the width of the bars is important. Consequently, the bars can be reduced to single lines with a short bar across the end to define the exact length; in figures where the ability to read the bar graph is not an issue, the value associated with the length of each bar can be brailled at the end of the line.

The proportions of some figures, such as electronic circuits, are unimportant and often simply need to be rearranged to fit the shape of the standard-size page.

Complex drawings involving three or more curves on top of one another, such as sine–cosine curves in mathematics or current–voltage–power curves in physics, are difficult to sort out even in a fairly large size. A better solution is to split the figure into several drawings, either by showing each curve individually, followed by a composite view, or by showing a series of views in which the curves are built up to the total number. A biology figure showing the superimposition of the circulatory, nervous, and digestive systems of a small animal might be split into three separate drawings showing each system independently, all drawn to the same scale, with a common outline for reference. If size permits, views that require comparison should be combined on the same page in preference to being shown on successive pages. It is better to produce a drawing that is useful, even though simplified, than to make drawings that are too small or complex.

If it is not practical to fit the drawing on a single page, it can be extended across the binding and onto the left-hand facing page. Facing pages should be avoided if possible, however. One problem is that they require both sides of the book to lie flat on the table; for the standard-size braille book, this requires almost 60 cm (2 ft) of desk space. Although no fold-outs were provided at the workshop, many students thought them preferable to facing pages. For some figures, clarity is not achieved by making the drawing larger. As pointed out earlier, the over-all relationship of the parts will eventually be lost. Some figures have only one small area of importance that needs extra magnification. The combination of a skeleton or overall drawing, plus detailed views of specific areas, is a very useful approach and one that is widely approved, provided a note of explanation is included on the drawings telling how they have been modified. This technique can be applied in several ways. When only one important area needs additional magnification, the skeleton or overall drawing should be complete in all areas other than the one that is to receive additional magnification. Within the complex area, only as many major lines and labels should be included as are clear. The skeleton drawing should not show the entire figure; it must be simplified. Some of the kinds of information that might be omitted are secondary lines or lines showing fine detail, construction lines, horizontal and vertical guidelines; lines marking the extent of angles; arrows showing specific dimensions; textured areas; and complex labels or labels of secondary importance. This information should be included only in the detailed view. The textures, line heights, and general layout of the detailed view must be exactly the same as those used in the skeleton drawing so that there is no problem in correlating the two.

A slightly different version of this technique can be used when all parts of a large drawing need magnification. In this case, the skeleton drawing becomes a schematic diagram showing how the various detailed views are related. A large electronic circuit or a systems analysis could be handled in this manner. The skeleton drawing would then become a kind of block diagram indicating the order and interrelationship of the individual detailed drawings; as many detailed views could be made as are necessary.

Verbal descriptions

There are times when the fine detail of an ink-print figure seems to defy translation into a tactile form. In this case, a verbal description, either brailled or recorded, can be used to explain details that have been omitted from the drawing. Notice the word *omitted;* do not attempt to include anything in the raised drawing that does not feel clear. A short verbal description might also be used to explain and tie together several enlarged, detailed views. The importance of the student's knowing what has been done to modify a figure and what he or she is feeling cannot be overstressed. A short verbal description of any figure makes a world of difference in the value of the drawing. The powerful combination of drawing and verbal description has been underutilized and overlooked. Tape-recorded texts offer the ideal opportunity for combining a general description and a raised drawing, as first recognized by Jasha Levi.

Graphs

Graphs deserve special consideration. A graph is a mathematical picture in which every point on a curve is defined in terms of the horizontal and vertical distance along the axes. Consequently, raised drawings of graphs must be accurate. Some graphs are drawn to show the shape or overall appearance of the curves, in which case the grid is not required and tick marks are sufficient. Some graphs are drawn to show the exact location of points or to illustrate graphing techniques. In these cases, the student must be able to read off values from the graphs, and a grid is both useful and necessary. The purpose of the grid is to act as a guideline. The grid lines must be lower in height and lighter in texture than either the axes or the main curves. The grid lines must be clear, easy to follow, straight, evenly spaced, and separated by at least 13 mm (0.5 in). No preference was found between grids made of light solid or finely serrated lines, but there must be considerable contrast in texture and height between the grid and the main curves. If the spacing between grid lines is less than 13 mm (0.5 in) at the desired magnification for the graph, draw every other line, adding numbers and tick marks along the axes if they are not already present, to indicate the intervals along the axes. On a 16-mm (0.62-in)-square grid, students were able to identify the position of dots at one-half-square locations with no difficulty.

Optacon use

The ever-increasing number of students who have Optacons introduces a new factor in raised-drawing design. Students are using Optacons to scan ink-print figures. When possible, they would like the raised drawing to be similar to the figure in the book so that they can correlate the drawing with the information from the Optacon. All students agree, however, that clarity is the most important consideration and that drawings should be rearranged or expanded as required for utility. The increasing use of the Optacon also brings familiarity with sighted conventions and symbols and adds weight to the idea that the methods of presentation and the symbols used in raised drawings should be essentially the same as those used by the sighted people with whom they will be working and exchanging information.

Materials

One conclusion of the Louisville Workshop was that the participants preferred plastic drawings to those made in paper. There is nothing inherent in the Brailon that produces either a good or a bad drawing; it is simply a copying material. Strictly on the basis of feel, paper is preferred. What was preferred in the plastic may have been the increased height and texture variation that was possible in techniques using a plastic copy as an end product. Although some of these drawings were produced by other methods, the bulk of them were made by the aluminum foil techniques pioneered by RFB. The great advantage of the metal master approach is that both the height and texture of the line can be varied. Smooth as well as rough lines can be made directly in the metal and, unlike paper, both types of lines can be raised to considerable height. Variation of both texture and height allows greater tactile contrast among the lines in the drawing, and roughly two to three times more height is possible in drawings made in metal than in those that are tooled or pressed directly into paper.

Summary

In making drawings, there are two major variables— height and texture. Rough textures attract more attention than smooth ones. For general purposes, use a tool that produces a rough line. Assign a pecking order of importance to your tools, remembering that the texture of a line is more important than the height, and height is more salient than width. In planning a drawing, achieve maximum contrast between adjacent lines or areas by changing both texture and height, but keep the relative importance of the lines compatible with their meaning in the figure. Be accurate, and be consistent in your choice of texture in related drawings. Because variations in height and width have meaning, be sure that all unwanted lumps and bumps are eliminated from your lines. Be sure to *feel* your finished drawing and to *think* about its usefulness.

In conclusion, figures cannot simply be magnified and copied verbatim as raised-line drawings. The process of translating a visual picture into a tactual representation, no matter how it is produced, requires interpretation. What are the factors that make a raised drawing a successful functional translation of the visual picture? A production technique that produces bold lines of varying height and texture; a blind user who has been trained in the use of drawings from an early age; and a verbal description accompanying the drawing that tells what is shown. But most of all, a successful haptic diagram needs proper planning by someone who understands the value of the figure as a teaching tool and who can use variations in height and texture to translate the visual figure into a tactual representation. The skilled drawing designer knows that more is not better. Simplicity is beautiful, and a good raised drawing is certainly worth a lot of words.

15. A user's view of tangible graphics: the Louisville Workshop

WILLIAM SCHIFF

William Schiff provides a last chapter based on the findings of the Louisville Workshop and Symposium on tangible graphics. The views expressed primarily reflect the experiences of blind haptic examiners who inspected materials representing the state of the art in tangible graphics. Some graphics are good; others can be readily improved; still others are not good. Most important, blind students and professionals want more and better diagrams, and want them earlier in their studies than they have been finding them. They want better information dissemination and delivery systems regarding tangible graphics.

The bulk of the chapter reviews the findings and recommendations of the workshop participants. Many of these findings confirm earlier research and speculation regarding tangible graphics. Their summary should provide a useful set of guidelines in producing tangible graphics for the blind. Finally, it is concluded that the field of tactual perception and tangible graphics production is ripe not only for increased knowledge gleaned from more research but also for expanded utilization of what is already known. There is more to be learned, and more to be done with what has already been learned.

WILLIAM SCHIFF

Introduction

For years there have been attempts to improve tangible graphics for blind and visually impaired people. Such materials have been considered supplements to recorded or braille books for blind students and professionals (Schiff, 1967). The primary target audience for supplementary graphics to be felt is students and professionals in science and technology and in fields that traditionally present pictorial and graphic information for instructional purposes.

Conclusions emerging from the workshop are based on certain practical constraints, such as production method or format. These constraints limit the generality of any principles extracted from research or from personal experience with tangible graphics. The conclusions presented in this chapter, then, must always be considered within the context of state-of-the-art materials and methods. As these materials and methods change, so may guidelines for production.

The purpose of the Louisville Workshop was to have a select group of blind examiners encounter sets of tactual graphics representing the state of the art and to evaluate the present and potential usefulness of the formats, materials, and methods presented. Their evaluations were elicited by a set of questions prepared for that purpose, as well as by discussions during inspection of the materials.

The Louisville Workshop

In March 1979, a 2-day workshop was held in Louisville, Kentucky. It was sponsored by a grant from the National Science Foundation to Recording for the Blind (RFB). The workshop was an attempt to evaluate the effectiveness of state-of-the-art materials and techniques used in making tangible graphics. The materials examined represented a variety of systems used for providing tangible graphics both individually and in mass production.

Various disciplines were represented to make broad generalizations possible. These generalizations concerned the effectiveness of current tangible graphics in conveying diagrammatic or pictorial information to blind students and professionals at the high school level and beyond. The workshop further attempted to provide guidelines to improve tangible graphics for the target populations, providing the materials were useful.

Prior to the workshop, samples of tangible graphics were obtained from individuals and organizations involved in their production. Producers were contacted with sufficient advance notice to permit them to provide their best work for evaluation. They were encouraged to produce an entire set of diagrams, but only one organization (RFB) did so, with Nancy Amick supervising the work.

The evaluation was performed by a cross section of paid volunteers solicited from lists of recipients of recorded books for the blind. The volunteers represented several disciplines and educational levels. But because the workshop emphasized *scientific* materials, there was no attempt to include primary or junior high school students as evaluators. This limitation precluded gathering hard data on the training of children to use tangible graphics or the use of tangible graphics by totally naive scientists.

The blind high school and college students and professionals selected all had minimal experience with tangible graphic materials, such as

431

braille, maps, or raised-line supplements to recorded books for the blind. Their level of achievement was very high. Although such selectivity rules out generalizations to the majority of visually impaired persons, it was congruent with the limited aim of the workshop – to examine the value of tangible graphics in scientific and technical fields. Although the technical specialties of the examiners varied, most were conversant with one or more topic areas, such as biology, physics, mathematics, psychology, or electronics. The supposition was that if these highly capable students and professionals did not find tangible graphics of value, they were likely to be of very limited usefulness. It was therefore assumed that only with appropriate scientific or technical backgrounds could observers comprehend technical diagrams – whatever their quality. The assumption thus included a basic premise that some conceptual familiarity was a prerequisite for comprehension. However, not all the information presented was technical; tangible maps whose primary functions were conceptualization, orientation, and mobility were also presented. Although the examiners no doubt had well-developed concepts of space, they might not have had technical expertise in cartography. The maps, then, would presumably be of value to most visually impaired people, regardless of their technical backgrounds.

The workshop was attended by 17 student or professional haptic examiners and by approximately 20 perceptual psychologists, engineers, special educators, and persons involved in the production of tangible graphics or the rehabilitation of blind people. A list of participants and observers may be found in the appendix to this chapter.

Procedures of the workshop

The 17 blind haptic examiners first met as one group. They were then divided into four groups of four to five each. For each group of examiners, there was at least one sighted coordinator. One group contained all functionally blind examiners (totally blind or with light perception only). The other groups each contained one examiner with minor residual vision.

The displays to be examined were primarily raised-line diagrams and maps prepared by several producers. Over a period of 2 days, examiners inspected materials from the following fields: physics, chemistry, biology, botany, physiology, zoology, psychology, sociology, economics, political science, history, mathematics, computer science, electronics, engineering, and mobility, orientation, or geopolitical maps. Some examples of these materials may be found in Figures 15.1 to 15.10. The materials

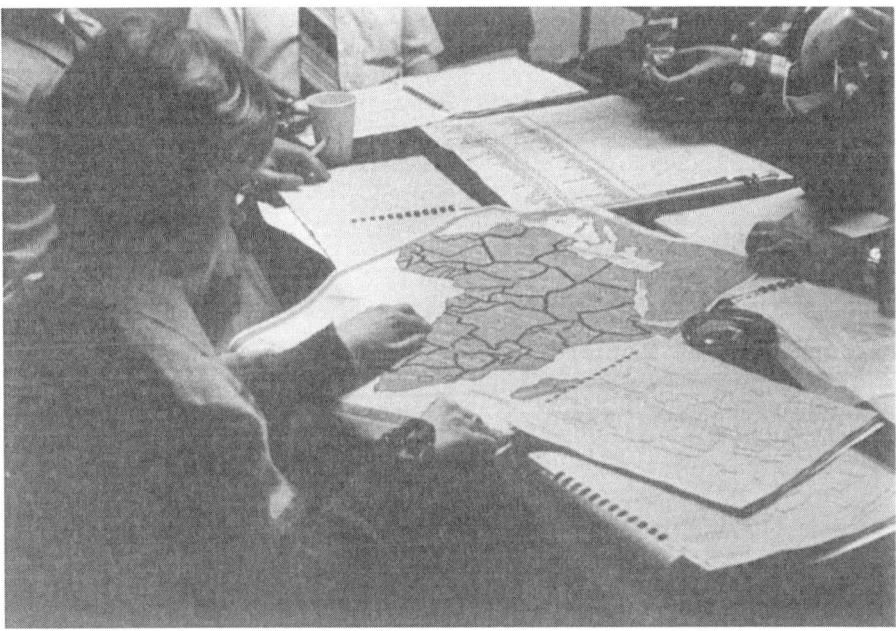

Figure 15.1. Foldable fabric map of Africa. (Courtesy of Howe Press)

were provided by the following persons and organizations: Nancy Amick, RFB; Betty Epstein, National Braille Association; Harry Friedman, Howe Press; John Barth, American Printing House for the Blind; Kathleen Webber, Methstat (Sensory Quill); John Gill, University of Warwick, England; Grahame James, National Mobility Centre, England; and Gilligan Tactiles, Inc. Examiners evaluated each display by responding to and elaborating on the following questions, administered by group leaders:

1. What information did you get from this display?
2. Is this an effective display? If not, what is wrong with it?
3. If the display includes two or more different symbols for marking locations, are they hard to tell apart? How about symbols for lines? For textures?
4. Are any elements in the display so close together that they are hard to distinguish? Which ones?
5. Is the display surface too crowded or cluttered?
6. Is the display the right size? If not, what size should it be?
7. If symbols of different heights have been used, are the heights difficult to distinguish? (Same question for points and lines.)
8. Is the labeling on the display adequate? If not, what is wrong with it?
9. Do braille characters give the display a cluttered appearance? Are braille characters confused with other display elements?
10. Does the display include irrelevant detail?
11. Are the observers examining displays in their own or in other disciplines?

433

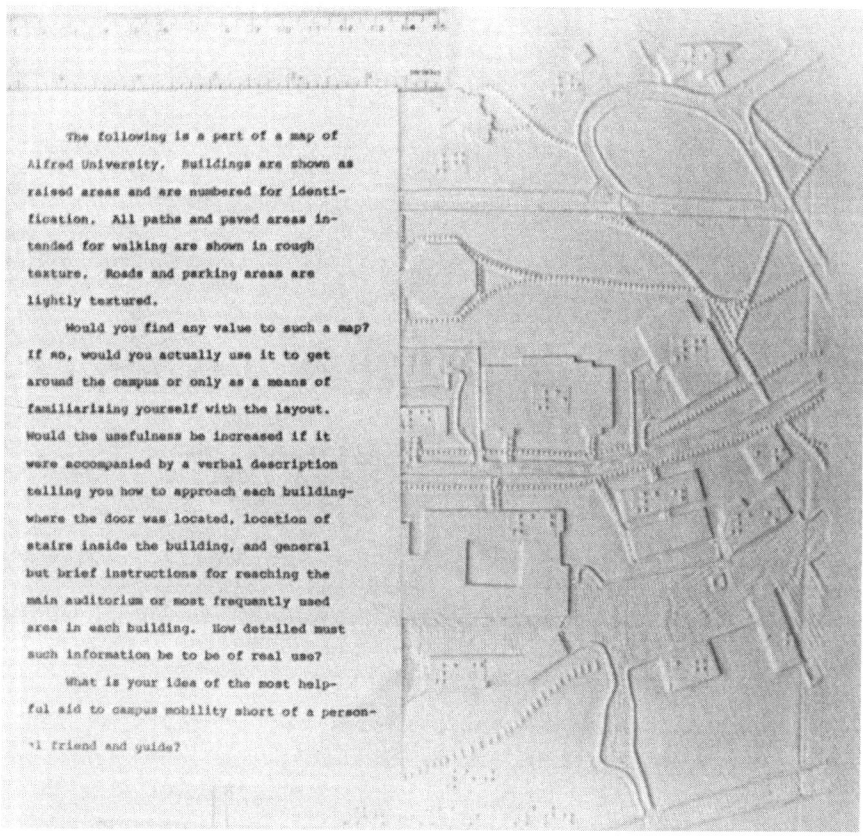

The following is a part of a map of Alfred University. Buildings are shown as raised areas and are numbered for identification. All paths and paved areas intended for walking are shown in rough texture. Roads and parking areas are lightly textured.

Would you find any value to such a map? If so, would you actually use it to get around the campus or only as a means of familiarizing yourself with the layout. Would the usefulness be increased if it were accompanied by a verbal description telling you how to approach each building—where the door was located, location of stairs inside the building, and general but brief instructions for reaching the main auditorium or most frequently used area in each building. How detailed must such information be to be of real use?

What is your idea of the most helpful aid to campus mobility short of a personal friend and guide?

Figure 15.2. Brailon map of Alfred University campus (segment). (Courtesy of RFB)

12. On many displays, some features are more important than others and should be more prominent. Evaluate this display in that regard.
13. Rank displays, and explain the ranking when the same display has been prepared by different methods.
14. What are the characteristics of a good point symbol? A good line symbol? A good texture?
15. Does the unfilled display surface present any problem? Is it too "noisy"?
16. Is the material used to make this display satisfactory? Would a different material have been better? If so, why?
17. Is this display necessary? Could the same information have been conveyed more easily with words or with a table?

The above questions were prepared by the project directors (one of whom is blind) and the project coordinator. The coordinator (Jasha Levi) has had several years of practical experience with student comments on raised-line drawings accompanying recorded books. The questions were

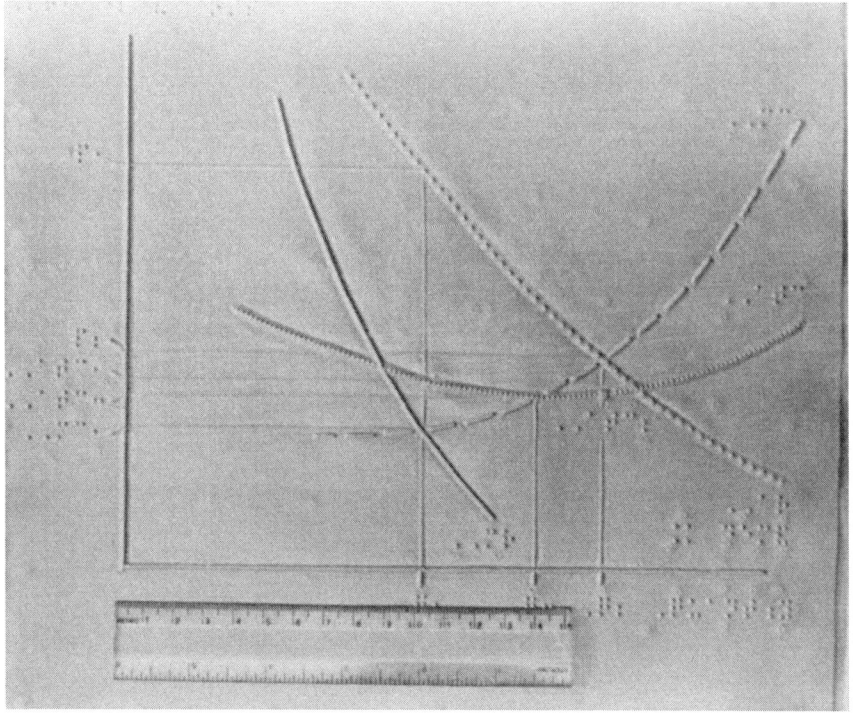

Figure 15.3. Brailon figure, mathematics. (Courtesy of RFB)

thus based on histories of personal, practical, and research experience with raised-line diagrams. They represent the current knowledge of what *goes wrong* in attempts to communicate information with tangible graphics. As such, the bias introduced by asking these questions likely errs on the side of being *too* critical regarding the materials rather than too lax. The list of questions is undoubtedly selective. It is recognized that in developing such a list, biases may be introduced into the outcome. Queries may in some cases create problems that examiners might not otherwise consider. But given the acknowledgment of such potential biases, these questions represent at least 2 decades of experience in researching, producing, and inspecting tangible graphics.

At the close of the meetings, each group developed a set of conclusions and recommendations to be presented by its leaders to the entire group of examiners, perceptual scientists, educators, and producers. These views represented both general and specific findings and recommendations regarding the materials examined and the use of tangible graphics in general.

435

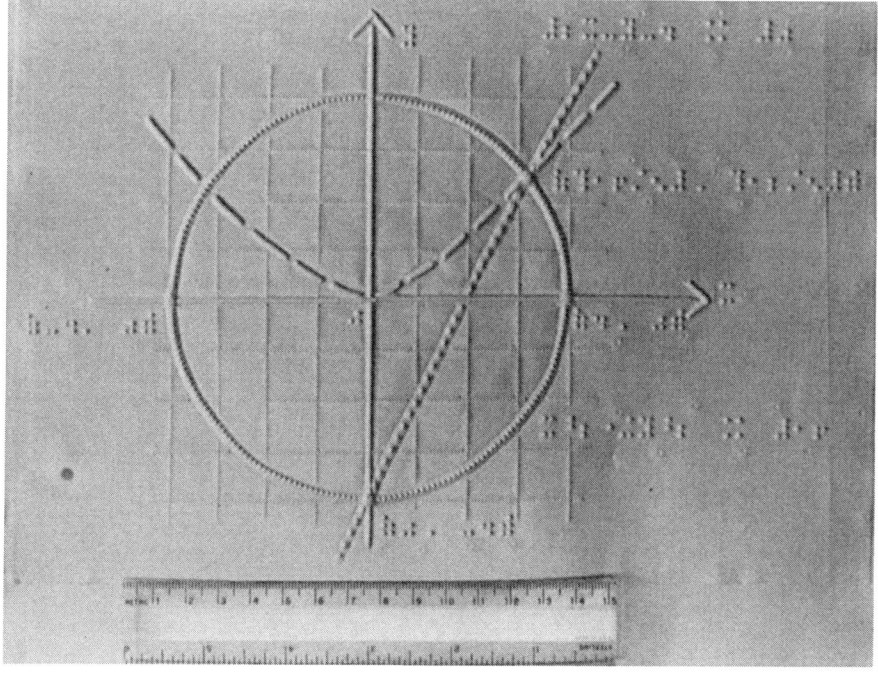

Figure 15.4. Brailon figure, geometry. (Courtesy of RFB)

General findings of the workshop

A consensus was reached on a number of issues. The conclusions are presented below.

1. More raised-line drawings (than are currently available) should be provided with recorded/braille books for the blind.
2. More books now distributed should have raised-line drawings.
3. Tactile/tactual drawings should be provided at the earliest educational level so that blind people do not come upon them suddenly in higher grades.
4. Comprehension of raised graphic displays is usually enhanced by braille or recorded explanations.
5. Brailon (vinyl) copies of displays are ordinarily more intelligible than those presented on paper. Paper, on the other hand, produces less fatigue.[1]
6. Tactual graphic presentations should follow the shape of printed graphic designs (such as circuit symbols in electronics), but display methods geared specifically to tactual recognition are desirable. The tactual arrow symbol (Schiff, Kaufer, & Mosak, 1966) was cited by examiners as an example of direction that further work might take.
7. The following resolution, submitted by one group of examiners, was unanimously passed on voice vote by all participants: that funds be sought from appropriate agencies for the training of additional personnel to prepare raised drawings, charts, diagrams, maps, and similar kinds of materials. Participants

436

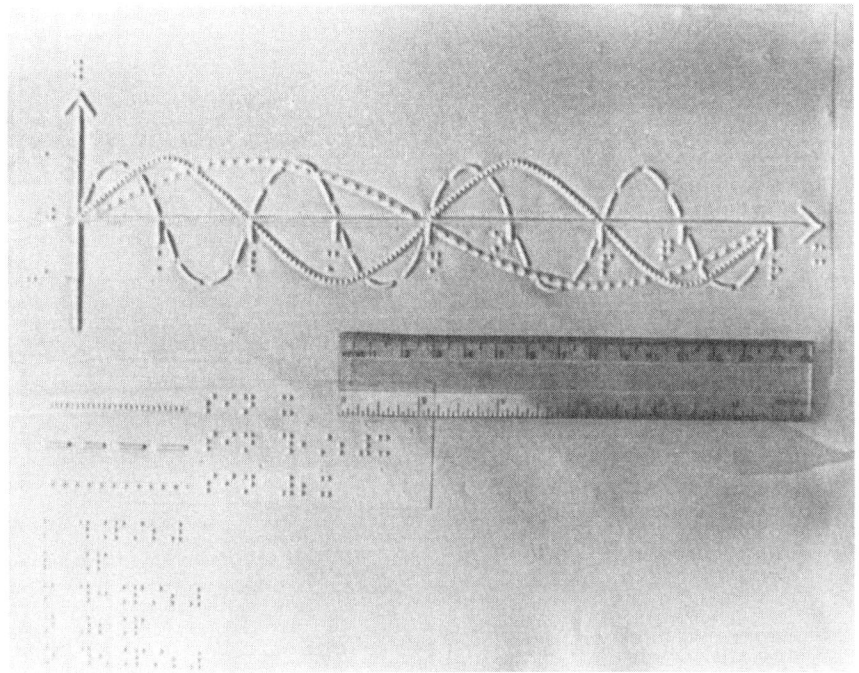

Figure 15.5. Brailon figure, physical sciences. (Courtesy of RFB)

hoped that the importance of tangible graphic displays would be recognized by all agencies involved with education and rehabilitation of the visually handicapped child and adult, and that the process of obtaining graphic information via touch would be given a definite status in the education of blind students.

Specific findings and recommendations of the workshop

In addition to the general conclusions and recommendations of examiner groups, a number of specific findings and recommendations emerged. These points should be of special interest to producers, users, educators, and researchers concerned with tangible graphics. The findings have been organized under several subheadings for convenience.

Format: sizes and materials for tangible graphic displays
Materials. Plastic (or vinyl) is generally superior to paper. (Author's note: There is no evidence of whether this preference is merely a conseqence of the more varied production techniques used with plastics.) Plastics are more durable and permit more varied symbol height, more varied com-

437

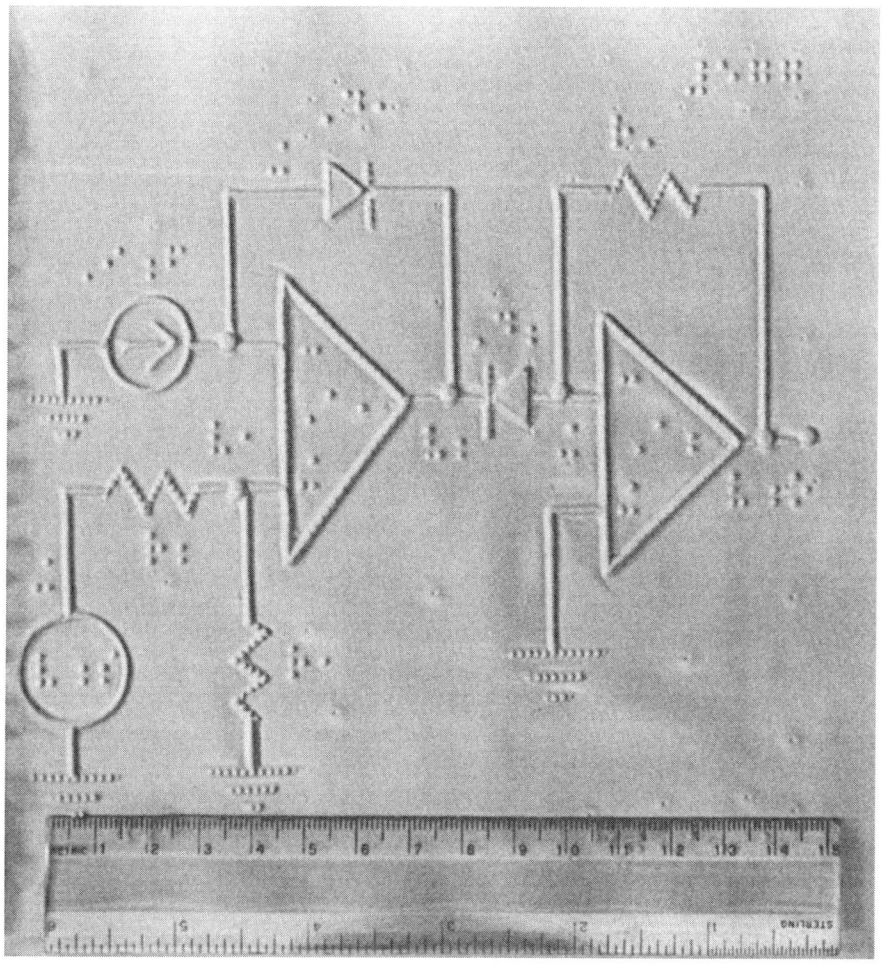

Figure 15.6. Brailon figure, electronics. (Courtesy of RFB)

position and texture. But, plastics are uncomfortable after prolonged inspection, with perspiration of hands and fingers becoming a problem. Perhaps talcum powder might help. Groups agreed that in spite of plastic's slipperiness, it is preferable to paper for graphic presentations. Also, comparisons of mat (matte)-surfaced Brailon with smooth (shiny) Brailon showed mat-surfaced Brailon was preferred for graphic displays.

Size. The larger-format size presented at the workshop (27.9 by 29.2 cm or 11 by 11.5 in) was generally preferred over the traditional (RFB) size (17.8 by 17.8 cm or 7 by 7 in.)[2] Exceptions occurred when very small or simple diagrams or maps were involved. The consensus was that most

438

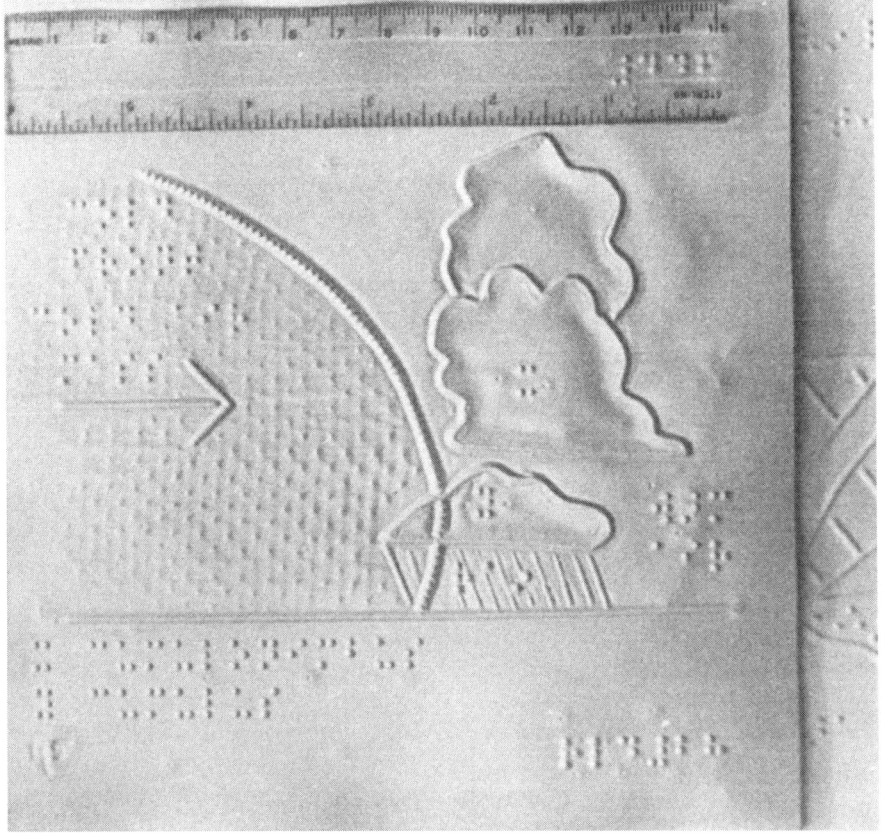

Figure 15.7. Brailon figure, meteorology. (Courtesy of RFB)

diagrams and maps benefit from decreased clutter, a problem with many small-format diagrams. Most examiners agreed that there were tradeoffs between clutter and size. The less cluttered presentation of larger formats was sometimes offset by difficulties in grasping relationships between parts of the diagrams involving more than a single hand span. (Author's note: It is possible that special training to use the hands in *paired* fashion when inspecting tactual diagrams would provide a partial solution.) Most examiners agreed that very large format sizes were cumbersome and of limited value for most purposes. An exception was the large foldable map shown in Figure 15.1. It was believed that fold-outs were likely to be preferred to diagrams much larger than 28 by 29 cm (11 by 11.5 in). The conclusion was that the larger format was better than the smaller, but that format size should be a function of the complexity and nature of the information to be presented.

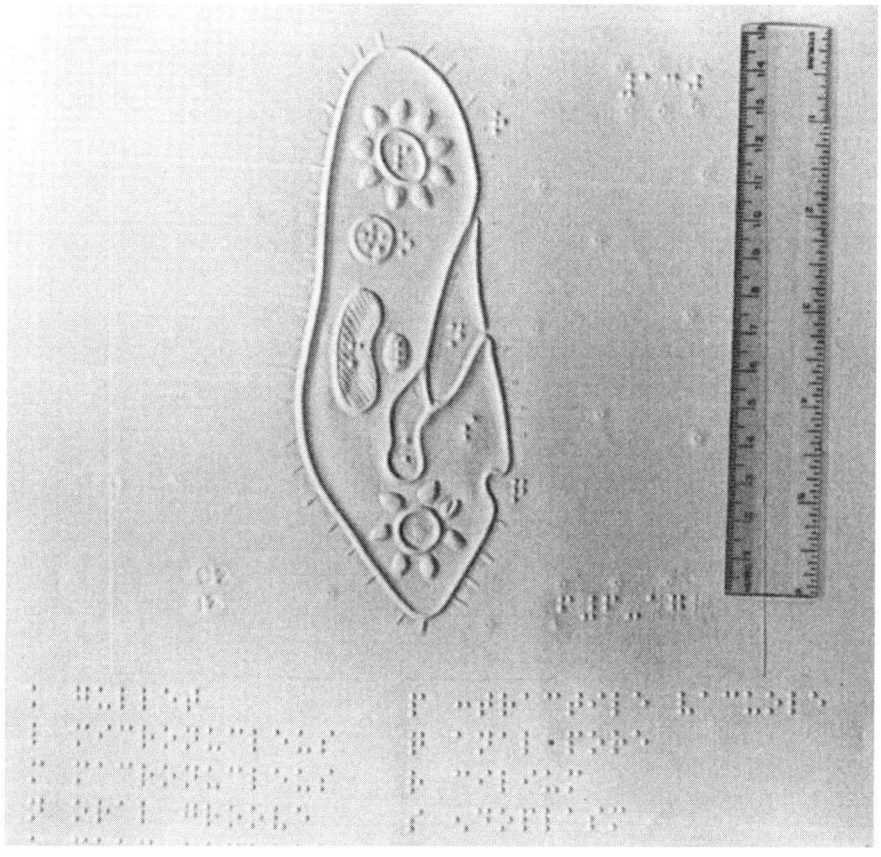

Figure 15.8. Brailon figure, biology. (Courtesy of RFB)

Fold-outs, facing pages, and build-ups. The need to present a great deal of information (graphic and/or braille) in one diagram leads to several other solutions – fold-outs, facing pages, and build-ups. These styles were presented in several diagrams. Examiners found fold-outs a valuable way of extending the effective size of tactual diagrams while avoiding cumbersome sizes. In some instances, facing pages were found to be confusing. An exception was the consistent presentation of braille explanatory material and/or keys on facing pages. These were deemed satisfactory facing-page material. Keys were preferred on facing rather than on preceding or following pages.

Built-up (composite) diagrams were evaluated favorably. There was general agreement that complicated displays should be built up from simpler components, showing the simple components first and then combining them into single complex displays on fold-out or following pages. The consensus was that the most effective strategy was to *build up* from simple components rather than to analyze down from more complex displays. In certain cases (e.g., enlarged or detailed views) analysis is appropriate, however.

Scale. The recommendation was that diagrams should be drawn to scale wherever possible. Exceptions would include representations in which true scale interferes with discriminability or produces clutter, or in which blow-ups of detail are instructive and clarifying. In cases of scale change, these changes should be clearly labeled.

Bindings. The location of bindings was an issue noted by examiners, whereas sighted persons might think the question superficial. For the 18- by 18-cm (7- by 7-in) format (smaller size), interest was expressed for binding at the *top* of the booklet. For the larger 28- by 29-cm (11- by 11.5-in) format, the conventional book-binding location was preferred. Ample blank space should be provided near the binding to prevent it from interfering with scanning fingertips, which proved a problem in a few diagrams inspected.

Titles. Examiners agreed on the need for braille titles at the top of virtually every diagram page. Keys containing symbol, line, or other references should be placed either under the diagram or on the facing page. Placement should be consistent within each set of diagrams and to a degree consistent over all diagrams. Such conventions would eliminate the need for time-wasting searches for relevant title and key information. The same sort of consistency should also be applied to braille labeling. Wherever possible, and especially within a set of diagrams, braille labels should be consistently placed to the right or left of the parts labeled.

Display selection. Examiners were almost evenly divided on the issue of how many diagrams in a book should be made. Some examiners thought *all* diagrams should be produced in a tangible form – given any possibility for comprehension. This strategy would leave selectivity up to readers, who might vary considerably in needs or skill levels. Some might need more or fewer diagrams if reading for different purposes.

The other view was that producing all the diagrams in a book was not only expensive and time-consuming for the producer but could also be time-consuming and confusing for a reader who had to sift through a large number of diagrams to find those that communicated something unique or provided adequate tactual comprehension. This becomes an issue only when books are profusely illustrated. The examiners also pointed out that many printed diagrams in books are really superfluous, and reproducing them in tangible form simply compounds the error. It takes far longer to obtain enough information from a tangible diagram to judge it unnecessary than to do so with a visible diagram. There is no clear resolution of the issue, which might become a serious one only with heavily illustrated science texts and reference books. It is likely that more specific evaluation is required to make each decision.

Descriptions and instructions. Examiners agreed that verbal descriptions without tactual diagrams are typically insufficient for comprehension, as are diagrams without verbal descriptions. Both are typically needed, and it should be general practice to provide braille and/or taped instructions and descriptions with all tangible graphics for the blind. Because all instructions and descriptions at the workshop were in braille rather than on tape, no comparison could be made. It was suggested that for younger students, printed instructions and descriptions might be valuable; the trend toward mainstreaming blind students in sighted classes produces the likelihood that teachers will be unable to read braille, and in classrooms taped instructions might be suboptimal. There was unanimous agreement that aural and/or braille instructions should accompany each booklet of tangible graphics. It is necessary to explain how to use the diagrams, to introduce any special features (e.g., blow-ups, fold-outs, facing-page keys, built-up diagrams), and to describe any special symbols to the reader before he or she begins to use the materials. Special symbols include modified electronic symbols, directional arrow symbols, and the like.

Grids. Most graphs should have grids – especially those used in mathematics. These grids are necessary for the discovery of values associated with lines, curves, points, and so on. Such grids should be made "lighter" (less relief from the page) than the major components of the diagram. Grids do not appear to be necessary for curves when the intent is merely to show the general shape of the curve. If the grid is superfluous, it should not be reproduced. (Author's note: this recommendation violates the more general principle, favored by examiners, that figures should be produced more or less as printed, unless discriminability is sacrificed.)

Content areas. Whether or not a display communicates effectively may be a function of the user's background. Apart from discriminability (mechanical display factors), the major design issue is whether the diagram facilitates understanding. Whenever possible, tangible displays should be designed with a particular audience with a given level of expertise in mind.

In physical and biological sciences, mathematics, electronics, and engineering, the displays were most helpful. One group concluded that "a raised-line drawing is worth a thousand words." The usefulness of diagrams is related to conceptual sophistication in a complicated fashion, however. For the expert, there is likely a point at which diagrams become superfluous–as when a concept is so well understood that words (e.g., *Pacific Coast chain* or *double helix*) have greater communicative economy than a graphic presentation (Schiff, 1980, pp. 355–356).

Biological cross-sectional diagrams *as prepared* were not very satisfactory. Whether this was due to the nature of the material or the methods of presentation was unclear.

Regarding *maps*, particular need was expressed for standardization of symbols and methods of presentation.

Regarding standard *reference texts*, it was recommended that RFB or some agency should prepare them in each field; they could then be used along with other texts assigned for course work. Such reference texts could provide archetypal diagrams. One recommendation suggested that a complete set of Schramm's *College Outline Series* be prepared as an introductory-level set of reference texts.

Symbols

Braille symbols. There should be a braille title at the top of each diagram or map. When there is no room for single braille letters on the diagram, braille labels should be well spaced and connected by low-relief guidelines. (A few examiners objected to such lead lines.) Braille keys should be provided on facing pages or below diagrams. The locus should be uniform for a set of diagrams. Braille symbols or labels should not be very close to lines. English *microbraille* is quite acceptable at this age and educational level. Braille should not be placed in small textured areas; this procedure was totally unacceptable due to confusion between textures and braille codes.

Other symbols. There was complete agreement on the need to standardize symbols. Examiners, educators, and producers noted that there has already been some standardization of symbology in other countries, and that this should occur in the United States as well. Standardization should not preclude change but should be geared to current research findings and technology. Many discriminable lines, point symbols and, to a lesser extent, textures have been identified by research (e.g., Gill & James, 1973; James & Gill, 1974; Jansson, 1973; Nolan & Morris, 1971; Schiff, 1966; Wiedel & Groves, 1969). But standard tools, production methods, and materials have not always been incorporated into the art of making tangible graphics. The result has been confusion among users. The situation is analogous to mathematical notation; a lack of standard notation simply wastes the time of readers. Were notation dependent on the whim of individuals, chaos would reign. The situation with tangible graphic symbols is even worse, however, because the tactual system is inferior to the visual system in distinguishing symbol shapes, and recognition suffers.

Discriminable and unique (memorable) symbols are critical for effective tactual graphics. The linear and point symbols inspected at the workshop were better received than textured areal symbols, which require more work to develop and standardize. A promising possibility is to develop techniques to apply different *substances* (which feel different) to diagrams in order to delineate areas where more than three or four must be coded (see Chapter 4). The following points were noted by examiners as aids to discrimination of focal information in diagrams:

1. Keys are preferred to lead lines.
2. Tick marks on graphs or curves should be prominent, extending beyond the abscissa and ordinate, as opposed to the usual visual conventions.
3. Directional arrow symbols are generally preferred to conventional arrow symbols (see Schiff et al., 1966) because this special symbol is discriminable, unique, and memorable. But its use should be pointed out in braille or aural instructions. Where conventional arrowheads *are* used, they should be small and consist of acute-angle arrowheads with small "wings." All arrows should be placed *outside* textured areas.
4. Nemeth shapes should not be used as symbols in the body of a tactual display.
5. Circles around symbols for vacuum tubes and transistors should be omitted; they confuse the reader.
6. Jump-overs on crossing-wire representations are a preferred convention, and dots should be used to indicate connecting wires in wiring diagrams. Symbolic conventions to be used in wiring diagrams should be keyed at the beginning of every set of electronic or engineering diagrams. Conventions of visual diagrams should be used wherever tactual discriminability permits in order to capitalize on existing knowledge of symbols and to permit access to the information via Optacons used by many technical and scientific persons.
7. Angles should be labeled from within if possible.
8. Differences in symbol height (relief from surface) are a preferred coding procedure. Such coding makes both line and point symbols readily discriminable and more noticeable to tactual perception. Although this point was noted some 15 years ago (Schiff, 1966; 1967; Schiff & Isikow, 1966), it has not found its way into many production techniques. Height–texture redundancy is also a useful coding technique aiding discrimination where it is difficult or where quantities are similar (Schiff & Isikow, 1966).

9. Care should be taken to ensure adequate separation of symbols (see recommendations in Chapter 11 and 14).
10. Sharp dotted lines should generally be avoided. They can cause discomfort as well as tactile adaptation. But one examiner pointed out that such lines might be preferred by blind persons having a concomitant loss of tactile acuity, as found in certain diabetic conditions. A sheet of onion skin paper placed over diagrams can also reduce this problem. (Author's note: the workshop involved hours of continuous diagram inspection, which may have exaggerated this problem.)
11. Identical symbols should be produced as identical. In some cases, the discriminative capacity of tactual perceivers exceeds the production accuracy of diagram producers, and nonidentical symbols meant to be identical confuse readers. This problem bears on production methods and standardization needs, mentioned earlier. If standard tools and methods were used, there would be less variability in symbols within and across diagram sets. The computer-generated lines and areal and point symbols produced by John Gill's production system (see Chapter 13) were rated most favorably by examiners.
12. When precise tracking of lines is required, line symbols should be highly embossed (about 1 mm) and should have steep sides; steepness (sharpness) was considered even more important than elevation.
13. Areal symbols should have low relief when line and point symbols appear on the same page.
14. Large dots should be added to help locate positions labeled by letters or other point symbols.
15. Important information should be indicated by roughness. Rough areas or lines attract more attention or attract it more readily, so that there is a natural focus on rougher coded elements in a display. This focusing should correlate with importance (see Schiff, 1966; Schiff & Isikow, 1966; Chapter 4).

Maps for orientation and mobility

Points relevant to map production have also been listed under other headings, as they concern all diagrams, not just maps. The following issues were thought specific to maps.

1. The Nottingham System for producing maps was very favorably received by examiners. They thought the product was close to optimal (see Chapter 10).
2. For local maps, orientation maps were judged more useful than mobility maps.
3. Small maps are useful only if the area displayed is simple.
4. Use of a compass rose is not effective. Instead, a continuous north edge should consistently mark one side of maps.
5. Textures used on maps were not particularly effective. They were not vivid enough. New technologies should address this problem.
6. Guidelines for mobility maps are covered in James and Armstrong's *Handbook on mobility maps*. These guidelines, and those used by Howe Press in making maps, were evaluated favorably. Again, a pressing need for standardization was expressed by examiners and by Harry Friedman of Howe Press, Perkins School for the Blind. All stressed the need for international standardization.
7. Maps are now available in large-format fabrics (see Figure 15.1). These can be

445

folded and put in pockets. The particular map noted above was highly praised by examiners. Other maps examined have braille information embossed on the *underside* of a large rigid surface. Both the above types of maps are fairly costly to produce, but the examiners thought the effort and cost worthwhile in view of the utility of such maps. The present technology is good and should be more widely utilized.

In contrast to the push for standardization was a counterview endorsed by an entire group of examiners: There is also a need to design displays such as maps according to individual needs. Were this view followed, however, it would be difficult to standardize design criteria for the majority of blind people. On the other hand, symbol standardization could be accomplished while still leaving a number of alternatives to fit individual needs or situational variations.

Three-dimensional diagrams

One lively discussion concerned the utility of diagrams representing the third dimension of space as indicated by the Z coordinate. Forms of three-dimensional diagrams inspected at the workshop included some geometric solids (see Figure 15.10) and biological or earth science cross-sections (see Figure 15.9). Examiners found all these diagrams either completely useless or of minimal value, except for Figure 15.9, which was judged useful. They reported coming to understand the concepts with little help from the diagrams. Their major explanation was that information on the third dimension was based on visual conventions having no clear counterpart for those who had never been able to see.

John Kennedy (Chapter 9) pointed out several qualifications of this argument. First, the diagrams inspected at the workshop were not true three-dimensional diagrams, even though they involved representation of Z-coordinate information. They were either cross-sectional diagrams, involving other unusual representations as well as tridimensionality or transparent geometry solids represented by and consisting only of edge lines. These are not representative of pictorial communication in general; they are a special form of limited information pictures (Schiff, 1980). Such minimal pictures may be the *least* informative (without training) for congenitally blind or early-onset blind people. For example, lines representing the convex intersect of two planar surfaces were constructed precisely like those representing the concave intersect of two planar surfaces. For vision, other information (e.g., shading, linear perspective) may help to make the distinction between convex and concave edges. But current diagrams for blind perceivers do not provide such contextual

446

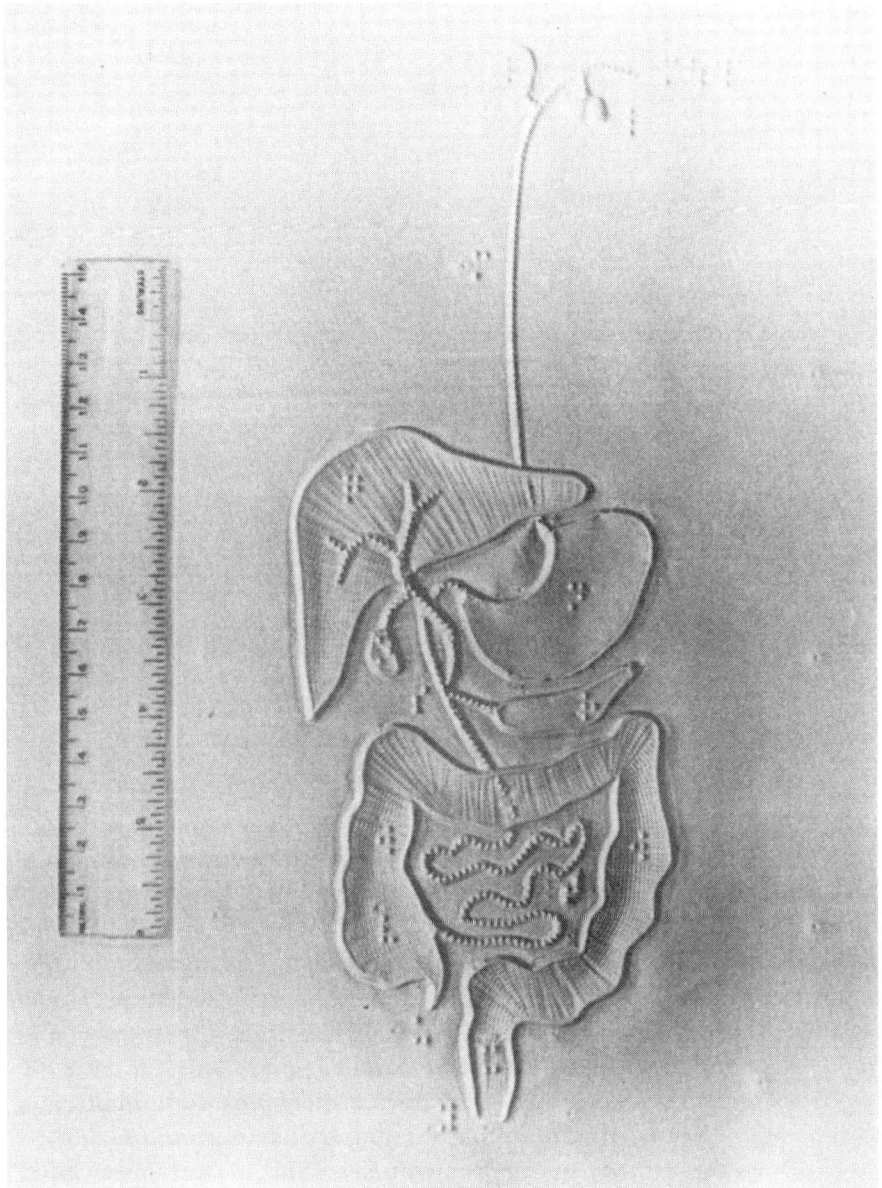

Figure 15.9. *Brailon* figure, "three-dimensional," biological sciences. (Courtesy RFB)

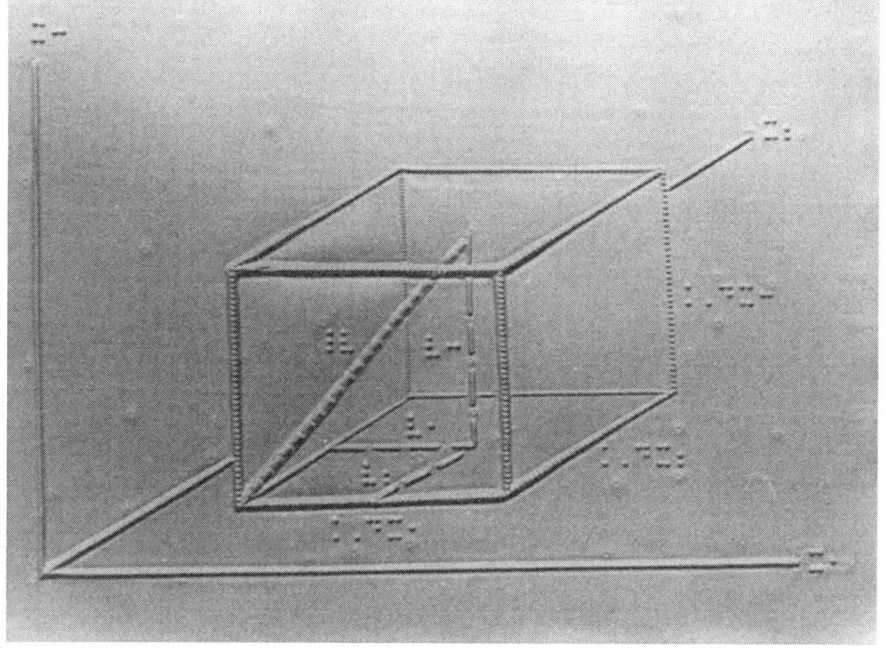

Figure 15.10. *Brailon* figure, "three-dimensional," geometry. (Courtesy RFB)

or redundant information. With more thoughtful techniques of presentation and with more appropriate pictorial information to be represented, it might be possible to make more useful three-dimensional diagrams for blind observers and to convey Z-coordinate information economically and clearly. What is clear is that diagrams involving Z-coordinate information for visual perception cannot simply be copied in tactual forms and presented to people with little or no experience in inspecting three-dimensional worlds at a distance or their pictorial representations. Given examiners' negative evaluations of most of the three-dimensional diagrams inspected, and given the above counterpoints, one can conclude only that these particular three-dimensional diagrams were ineffective. This does not necessarily mean that it is impossible to produce effective three-dimensional diagrams for congenitally blind or early-onset blind people. Chapter 9 further discusses these issues.

Examiners commented on two related points. First, blind students typically receive little or no training in the use of tactual graphics – whether they represent two- or three-dimensional space. Perhaps three-dimensional diagrams require special training or more training than two-dimensional ones. Second, there is a good possibility that three-dimensional diagrams might be used as study tools after training, especially were the training with three-dimensional models. There have been a few reports of the use of models in the education of blind students (e.g., Neumann, 1972), but little research has been done on moving from models to three- or even two-dimensional diagrams for review. Examiners thought this function of three-dimensional diagrams was likely to produce favorable results.

Training for graphics users

The first point made above is clearly a component of a more general issue discussed at length by consumers, educators, and psychologists at the workshop: There should be formal training of visually impaired children and adults in the use of tangible graphics. Most participants thought early training (from grade school) was desirable but admitted that their suggestions were based purely on personal experience and conjecture. They were seriously concerned that little or no instruction is given in such a useful skill. The result is that in the United States, few blind people have used tangible graphics, know about their availability, or realize how useful they can be. The greatest enthusiasm for raised-line diagrams came from students and professionals in scientific or technical fields. But they pointed out that map use extends tangible graphics to areas of value to almost all blind people. Further, early schooling in such fields as geography, mathematics, science, and art might be enriched if there were a serious large-scale effort to train blind children in the uses of tangible graphics. There was a definite mandate favoring the development and implementation of training programs for blind students and their teachers.

Availability and dissemination of tangible graphics

There was virtually unanimous agreement among examiners that there had been very poor dissemination of information regarding the existence and availability of tangible graphics – especially as supplements for recorded books for visually impaired students. Most examiners believed that most blind persons, in the United States at any rate, did not know that raised-line diagrams existed for hundreds of books available on tape distributed by RFB. Nor did they believe many students know that one could request drawings for titles that did not yet have such illustrations. They based these opinions on their own experiences and their contacts with other students. The examiners strongly recommended that RFB use its own resources or seek other support to inform students about this valuable service.

449

There was also concern about the seeming shrinkage in production of tangible graphics. Examiners found this condition serious because the materials were valuable. Examiners acting as representatives for other blind students and professionals proposed recommendations regarding increased publicizing of the availability of tangible graphics and their increased production and dissemination. They stated that not only should blind people themselves be informed about the availability of such materials, but so should professionals, teachers, and others working with blind people. It was further suggested that tangible graphics might be produced by agencies employing experts specifically for this purpose.

General discussion and conclusions

The most general conclusion emerging from the Louisville Workshop is that tangible graphics are a useful and desirable learning aid for blind people. Their main value may be for scientific and technical users, but it also extends to more general utility, such as orientation and mobility maps. In spite of the usefulness of tangible graphics, they appear to be significantly underutilized. Limited resources (e.g., almost all producers of tangible graphics are volunteers) and failures to follow through with user training and dissemination of information about tangible graphics have apparently undercut a valuable service for blind people. A few determined producers (e.g., Nancy Amick) have continued to manufacture high-quality tangible graphic materials over the past 15 years. But available research information has been somewhat neglected by certain producers. Specific design principles recommended by the present group of examiners reflect many of those made by researchers for the past 15 years (see especially the work of James & Gill, 1974, 1975; Jansson, 1973; Nolan & Morris, 1971; Schiff, 1966, 1967). The fact that many of these recommendations have not found their way into most graphics production in the United States is unfortunate.

Tangible graphics for blind people are currently underutilized. Suboptimal diagrams still exist for a variety of reasons, but probably mainly because some producers prefer intuitive guidelines over research findings, because distribution of diagrams and feedback from users is limited, and because standardization has been elusive.

A single agency (in each country) concerned solely with production and dissemination of such tangible graphics supplements is desirable. Although volunteer work is admirable and often of exceptional quality, the volunteer system often lacks systematic control over production

450

techniques, schedules, and quality. There is no doubt that a volunteer agency could be formed, but such delivery systems have achieved only limited success. The need for a large number of raised-line drawings as text and reference supplements makes it difficult to house a tangible graphics production system together with a text-recording or braille book center. Although such an agency might be a subsidiary of one producing braille or recorded books, such systems have not worked well in recent years. This suggests that there are hidden practical problems with this arrangement.

There is now a substantial body of research and practical knowledge of how to make effective tangible graphics. There are persons with administrative, practical, and technical know-how concerning their production at reasonable cost. Further, the Louisville Workshop has shown that tangible graphics are welcomed and encouraged by consumers. Apparently what is now needed is a central agency committed to the production and dissemination of tangible graphics. Such an agency might also oversee attempts to develop training techniques for young and adult students and their teachers. Because the state of the art is changing rapidly, and because our knowledge of tangible graphics is incomplete, basic research in tactual perception and ongoing evaluation of tangible graphics for product improvement should continue.

Acknowledgments

This chapter includes selected excerpts from: Tangible graphics for visually impaired persons: The Louisville Workshop and Symposium. National Science Foundation. Final Report No. SP178-03756, 1980.

Notes

1 Author's suggestion: The generality of the paper–plastic conclusion may be limited by the fact that examiners were feeling diagrams for hours at a time, which may be unusual outside workshop-type settings. Also, one should consider that the alleged superiority of plastic over paper may have been confounded with the fact that symbol relief with plastic is typically far more variable and greater than with paper, and involves steeper edges.
2 The original reason for the 18-cm (7-in) size was to fit the diagram booklet into the package with an 18-cm (7-in) record, and later, a reel of recording tape. This reason no longer exists since Jasha Levi's introduction of smaller long-playing cassette format for recordings for the blind.

References

Gill, J. M., & James, G. A. A study on the discriminability of tactual point symbols. *Research Bulletin of the American Foundation for the Blind*, 1973, 26, 19–34.

451

James, G. A., & Gill, J. M. Mobility maps for the visually handicapped: a study of learning and retention of raised symbols. *Research Bulletin of the American Foundation for the Blind*, 1974, *29*, 87–98.

A pilot study on the discriminability of tactile areal and line symbols for the blind. *Research Bulletin of the American Foundation for the Blind*, 1975, *29*, 23–31.

Jansson, G. *Projektet PUSS: XVI: Linje-och ytsmboler för taktile kartor. (Linear and areal symbols for tactile maps.)* Report No. 44. Uppsala: University of Uppsala, Dept. of Psychology, 1973.

Neumann, F. T. Demonstrating the relationship between three-dimensional figures and their two-dimensional representations. *New Outlook for the Blind*, 1972, *65*, 126–128.

Nolan, C. Y., & Morris, J. E. *Improvement of tactual symbols for blind children* (Final Report No. 5-0421). Washington, D.C.: U.S. Dept. of Health, Education and Welfare, 1971.

Schiff, W. *Manual for the construction of raised line diagrams.* New York: Recording for the Blind, 1966.

Using raised line drawings as tactual supplements to recorded books for the blind (Final Report No. RD-1571-S). Washington, D.C., Vocational Rehabilitation Administration, 1967.

Perception: an applied approach. Boston: Houghton Mifflin, 1980.

Schiff, W., & Isikow, H. Stimulus redundancy in the tactile perception of histograms. *International Journal for the Education of the Blind*, 1966, *15*, 1–11.

Schiff, W., Kaufer, L., & Mosak, S. Informative tactile stimuli in the perception of direction. *Perceptual & Motor Skills*, 1966, *23*, 1315–1335.

Wiedel, J. W., & Groves, P. A. *Tactual mapping: design, reading, and interpretation* (Final Report No. RD-2557-S). Washington D.C.: U.S. Dept. of Health, Education, and Welfare, 1969.

Appendix: participants and observers in the Louisville Workshop

Nancy S. Amick, Recording for the Blind, Princeton, N.J.

John Barth, American Printing House for the Blind, Louisville, Ky.

Billie Bentzen, Department of Special Education and Rehabilitation, Boston College, Boston, Mass.

Edward P. Berlá, Department of Special Education, University of Louisville, Louisville, Ky.

Ruth Bogia, Hopewell, N.J.

James Craig, Department of Psychology, Indiana University, Bloomington, Ind.

Margaret Craig, Canadian Institute for the Blind, Toronto, Ontario, Canada

Tim Cranmer, Bureau for the Blind, Frankfort, Ky.

Kenneth Cross, Tonowanda, N.Y.

Larry Crowe, Health Data Network, Louisville, Ky.

Rony Deaton, Louisville, Ky.

Maxine Dorf, Library of Congress, Washington, D.C.

Walter N. Dotson, Tallahassee, Fla.

Alice P. Eaddy, Utica, N.Y.

Betty Epstein, National Braille Association, Miami, Fla.

Will Evans, Kentucky School for the Blind, Louisville, Ky.

Emerson Foulke, Department of Psychology, University of Louisville, Louisville, Ky.

Tangible graphics: a user's view

Harry Friedman, Howe Press, Perkins School for the Blind, Watertown, Mass.
Sharon E. Garrison, University of North Carolina, Greensboro N.C.
John M. Gill, Warwick Research Unit for the Blind, University of Warwick, Coventry, England.
Betty Gissoni, Kentucky Rehabilitation Center, Louisville, Ky.
Fred Gissoni, Kentucky Rehabilitation Center, Louisville, Ky.
Gerard Guarniero, New York, N.Y.
Abigail Howes, Brockton, Mass.
Gunnar Jansson, Department of Psychology, University of Uppsala, Sweden.
Tim Jones, Kentucky School for the Blind, Louisville, Ky.
John M. Kennedy, Department of Psychology, University of Toronto, Canada.
Lester E. Krueger, Human Performance Center, Ohio State University, Columbus, Ohio.
Susan J. Lederman, Department of Psychology, Queen's University, Kingston, Ontario, Canada.
Jasha M. Levi, In Touch Networks, Inc., New York, N.Y.
Weldon Nail, Monterey Park, Calif.
Anthony Perese, Philadelphia, Pa.
Kenneth Reed, Washington, D.C.
Gerald Richer, Tupper Lake, N.Y.
Larry Scadden, Smith-Kettlewell Institute of Visual Science, University of the Pacific, San Francisco, Calif.
William Schiff, Department of Educational Psychology, New York University, New York, N.Y.
Carl E. Sherrick, Department of Psychology, Princeton University, Princeton, N.J.
Clark Shingledecker, Aerospace Medical Research Laboratory, Wright-Patterson AFB, Ohio.
Stephen Thayer, Department of Psychology, City College of New York, N.Y.
David H. Warren, College of Humanities and Social Sciences, University of California at Riverside, Calif.
Kathleen Webber, Methstat (Sensory Quill), Washington, D.C.
Dorrie Wright, Recording for the Blind, Inc., New York, N.Y.

Name index

Name index

458

Subject index

absolute threshold, 63–6

active touch, xi–xii, 1, 19, 71–3, 108–10, 134

acuity: discrimination, 63, 65–9; tactile/tactual, 63, 168–9; vibrotactile, 63–6, 220–2

adaptation: general, 9, 70; to pressure, 60, 70; to vibration, 70

aesthesiometer, 67–9

aftereffects, 131

amodal perception, 107

amplitude, 242, 246

areal symbols: discrimination of, 369–70, 375, 444; production of, 390, 392, 397, 411–14

atomism, 2, 15, 25

attention, 4, 32–4, 87, 90, 92

audition: tactile substitutes for, 234–58; in texture/roughness judgments, 7, 134, 150–1

basilar membrane, 234, 243, 248

blindness: aids, xii, 73–7, 209–30, 420–9, 448–9; and diagrams, xii, 156, 364–81, 387–402, 420–9, 430–49; and locomotion, 308–9; and maps, 156, 445–6; and mobility, 335, 445; and picture perception, 305–31; and social perception, 275–8; and tactual perception xii, 17, 22, 41, 73–7, 154, 156, 168–9, 209–30, 387–402, 420–9

braille: codes, 40–1, 168–207, 443; displays of, 193, 202–6; history of in U.S., 169–70; kinds of, 443; production of, 390–2, 397, 399, 408–9, 424; reading, 155–8, 168–207, 353–4; research on, 21, 171–205

Brailon, 157, 405–6, 428, 437

clutter, 421–6, 439–40

codes: braille, 39–40, 155, 168–9, 189, 254, 256; development of, 157–61, 373–5; map, 157–61; perception of, 39–41, 168–9; shape, 365, 373–5; size, 366–71; special nature of, 39, 255; speech, 235–58; texture, 157–61; vibrotactile, 74, 210–24

communication: nonverbal, 264–98; pictorial, 216–17; tactile, 57, 266

compass rose, 445

computers: in making maps, 341, 411–13, 445; in making symbols, 341, 411–13, 445; in speech communication devices, 234, 243–5, 252–3, 411–13; in making tangible diagrams, 411–13, 421

contrast, 422, 428–9

cross-modal perception, 103–7, 110–13

cutaneous sensitivities: nature of, 10, 63–71; and perception, xi, 71–4; and skin structures, 10

deafness: and speech perception, 235; and speechreading (lipreading), 236, 253

depth, in haptic diagrams/pictures, 310–11, 322–5

development: of cross-modal perception, 88–9, 152–3; of haptic perception, 84–103, 152, 372–5

difference threshold, 65–6

discrimination: of lines, 444; of surface characteristics, 444; of symbols, 168–9, 186–90, 373–5; of textures, 142–7, 444

distance: optimal spacing in diagrams, 365–8, 445; representation of, 322–5, 388, 446

distinctive features, 77, 370–1, 375–6

drawings: by blind persons, 320–9, 352–3; communication via, 387–8, 420–9, 430–50; copying, 388, 422–3, 429; cross-cultural studies of, 318–31; making, 387–402, 420–9; nature of, 306–13; optimal, 420–9, 436; principles used in raised line, 420–9, 430–50

dynamic tactual displays: of letters, 210–21; of patterns, 209–30; of pictures, 214–17; of speech, 234, 236, 238–9, 257

elasticity, 9, 45–6, 137

environmental design, 229–30